ICU Manual

ICU Manual

Editors

Rahul Anil Pandit
DA MD (Anesthesia) FJFICM FCICM (Australia) FCCP EDIC IFCCM
Chairperson
Department of Critical Care and Emergency Medicine
Sir HN Reliance Foundation Hospital and Research Centre
Mumbai, Maharashtra, India

Charudatt Vaity
MD (Medicine) DNB (Medicine) MRCP (UK) FFICM (UK) EDIC IFCCM
Director
Department of Critical Care
Wockhardt Hospital
Mumbai, Maharashtra, India

Bindu Mulakavalupil
DA DNB (Anesthesia) EDIC IDCCM IFCCM
Chief Intensivist
Department of Liver and Transplant ICU
Sir HN Reliance Foundation Hospital and Research Centre
Mumbai, Maharashtra, India

Darshana Rathod
MBBS MD (Medicine)
Additional Director
Department of Critical Care Medicine
Sir HN Reliance Foundation Hospital and Research Centre
Mumbai, Maharashtra, India

Foreword
Ashit Hegde

JAYPEE

JAYPEE BROTHERS MEDICAL PUBLISHERS
The Health Sciences Publisher
New Delhi | London

Jaypee Brothers Medical Publishers (P) Ltd

Headquarters
Jaypee Brothers Medical Publishers (P) Ltd
EMCA House, 23/23-B
Ansari Road, Daryaganj
New Delhi 110 002, India
Landline: +91-11-23272143, +91-11-23272703
+91-11-23282021, +91-11-23245672
Email: jaypee@jaypeebrothers.com

Corporate Office
Jaypee Brothers Medical Publishers (P) Ltd
4838/24, Ansari Road, Daryaganj
New Delhi 110 002, India
Phone: +91-11-43574357
Fax: +91-11-43574314
Email: jaypee@jaypeebrothers.com

Overseas Office
JP Medical Ltd.
83, Victoria Street, London
SW1H 0HW (UK)
Phone: +44 20 3170 8910
Fax: +44 (0)20 3008 6180
Email: info@jpmedpub.com

Website: www.jaypeebrothers.com
Website: www.jaypeedigital.com

Inquiries for bulk sales may be solicited at: jaypee@jaypeebrothers.com

ICU Manual

First Edition: **2025**

ISBN: 978-93-5696-542-3

Printed in India by Rajkamal Electric Press, Kundli, Haryana-131 028.

Dedication

This *ICU Manual* is dedicated to the tireless healthcare professionals who devote their lives to caring for patients in critical conditions. To the physicians, nurses, respiratory therapists, and support staff who work around the clock, often in the face of immense challenges, your unwavering commitment to saving lives inspires us all. Your resilience, compassion, and expertise are the foundation of modern critical care, and this book is a tribute to your efforts.

We also dedicate this work to the patients and families who entrust their lives and loved ones to the ICU team. Your strength and courage in the most trying moments are a constant reminder of why we do what we do. May this book serve as a tool that helps to improve patient's outcomes, providing the knowledge and "Manuals" necessary to ensure the best possible care in even the most difficult circumstances.

Contributors

Apurva Kakatkar
MBBS TDD IDCCM IFCCM
Consultant
Department of Intensive Care
Sir HN Reliance Foundation Hospital
and Research Centre
Mumbai, Maharashtra, India

Bindu Mulakavalupil
DA DNB (Anesthesia) EDIC IDCCM IFCCM
Chief Intensivist
Department of Liver and Transplant ICU
Sir HN Reliance Foundation Hospital
and Research Centre
Mumbai, Maharashtra, India

Charudatt Vaity
MD (Medicine) DNB (Medicine) MRCP (UK)
FFICM (UK) EDIC IFCCM
Director
Department of Critical Care
Wockhardt Hospital
Mumbai, Maharashtra, India

Darshana Rathod
MBBS MD (Medicine)
Additional Director
Department of Critical Care Medicine
Sir HN Reliance Foundation Hospital
and Research Centre
Mumbai, Maharashtra, India

Eileen Canday PhD
Head Dietician
Department of Nutrition and Dietetics
Sir HN Reliance Foundation Hospital
and Research Centre
Mumbai, Maharashtra, India

Harsh Parikh
DNB (Anesthesiology)
FNB (Critical Care Medicine)
Consultant Intensivist
Department of Intensive Care Unit
DAOH & FWC, Reliance Foundation
Hospital
Jamnagar, Gujarat, India

Jitendra Choudhary
MBBS MD (Anesthesiology)
FNB (CCM) IDCCM EDIC
Senior Consultant
Department of Critical Care Medicine
Sir HN Reliance Foundation Hospital
and Research Centre
Mumbai, Maharashtra, India

Kesari Masaipeta
MBBS MD (AIIMS) PDCC DrNB DNB
Fellow DrNB Critical Care
Department of Critical Care Medicine
Sir HN Reliance Foundation Hospital
and Research Centre
Mumbai, Maharashtra, India

Mehul Shah
FNB IFCCM DNB MNAMS DA MBBS
Chief Intensivist and Head of Surgical ICU
Department of Critical Care Medicine
Sir HN Reliance Foundation Hospital
and Research Centre
Mumbai, Maharashtra, India

Neha Patel
MBBS DNB (Pediatrics) MUHS
Fellowship in Infectious Diseases
Physician
Department of Infectious Diseases
The Children Hospital
Vadodara, Gujarat, India

Poorva Dilip Magarkar
MD (Anesthesia) DNB (Anesthesia)
DrNB (Critical Care Medicine)
Consultant
Department of Critical Care Medicine
HCG Manavata Cancer Centre
Nashik, Maharashtra, India

Pragnasree Ravulapalli
DNB (Anesthesia) IDCCM
Associate Consultant
Department of Critical Care
Sir HN Reliance Foundation Hospital
and Research Centre
Mumbai, Maharashtra, India

Rahul Anil Pandit
DA MD (Anesthesia) FJFICM
FCICM (Australia) FCCP EDIC IFCCM
Chairperson
Department of Critical Care and
Emergency Medicine
Sir HN Reliance Foundation Hospital
and Research Centre
Mumbai, Maharashtra, India

Vedika Premani
MSc (Nutrition) PGD (Nutrition) CDE
Clinical Dietician
Department of Nutrition and Dietetics
Sir HN Reliance Foundation Hospital
and Research Centre
Mumbai, Maharashtra, India

Vikas Gupta
DrNB (Critical Care Med)
DNB EDIC-I FCRS MBBS
Associate Consultant
Department of Critical Care Medicine
Sir HN Reliance Foundation Hospital
and Research Centre
Mumbai, Maharashtra, India

Vivek Jain
MBBS MD FNBCCM EDIC
Consultant
Department of Intensive Care Unit
Sir HN Reliance Foundation Hospital
and Research Centre
Mumbai, Maharashtra, India

Foreword

I am fond of telling people that "Intensive Care" is "Medicine on Steroids." A patient admitted to the ICU often has complex problems, usually encompassing not just one but several of the branches of Medicine, Surgery, Gynecology, and Anesthesia. The severely ill patient in the ICU also does not allow much margin for error.

It is not surprising, therefore, that a resident faced with a critically ill patient feels daunted. This book will go a long way in restoring the confidence of ICU residents in their ability to deal with these sick patients.

This is a concise but comprehensive manual that covers almost all aspects of intensive care. Each chapter is very readable, the recommendations made are based on recent evidence and most important of all, the authors have managed to explain even complex topics in a very simple and easily understandable manner.

Albert Einstein said, *"Everything should be made as simple as possible but not simpler."*

Leonardo Da Vinci said, *"Simplicity is the ultimate sophistication."*

Both Albert Einstein and Leonardo Da Vinci would have been proud of Rahul Anil Pandit and his Co-authors.

Ashit Hegde
MD MRCP
Consultant in Medicine and Critical Care
Head, Section of General Medicine
PD Hinduja Hospital and Medical Research Centre
Mumbai, Maharashtra, India

P.S.: This manual is not just for the resident, I who have been practicing Intensive Care for 36 years and thought that I had seen it all and knew it all and learnt quite a bit from this manual.

Preface

This *ICU Manual* is designed to serve as a practical guide for healthcare professionals working in the intensive care unit (ICU). The complexities of critical care demand a systematic and evidence-based approach to patient's management, and this book aims to provide clear, concise, and up-to-date algorithm to aid in clinical decision-making. It covers a wide range of topics from common medical emergencies to advanced therapeutic interventions, ensuring that healthcare teams can deliver safe and effective care under pressure.

The algorithm outlined here are intended to standardize practices, minimize errors, and promote a collaborative approach to patient's care. Special attention has been given to current guidelines, best practices, and the nuances of critical care in diverse clinical settings. We hope that this book will be an indispensable resource for clinicians, helping them to navigate the challenges of critical care with confidence and competence.

Rahul Anil Pandit
Charudatt Vaity
Bindu Mulakavalupil
Darshana Rathod

Acknowledgments

Writing the *ICU Manual* has been a challenging yet deeply rewarding journey, and we are immensely grateful to all those who have supported and encouraged us throughout the process. We extend our heartfelt thanks to everyone involved in this endeavor. Most importantly, we express our sincere gratitude to the dedicated critical care specialists who tirelessly work on the frontlines, saving lives everyday. We also want to thank our mentors and colleagues for critical care and allied specialties for their invaluable contributions. Additionally, we are deeply appreciative of the patients and their families who have generously allowed us to learn from their experiences. A special thanks goes to Shri Jitendar P Vij (Group Chairman), Mr Ankit Vij (Managing Director), Mr MS Mani (Group President), Ms Chetna Malhotra (Senior Director—Professional Publishing, Marketing, and Business Development), Ms Pooja Bhandari [Director—Production (Books and Journals)], Asmi Bharati (Development Editor), and the team at M/s Jaypee Brothers Medical Publishers (P) Ltd, New Delhi, India, for their support.

Contents

SECTION 5: ABDOMINAL DISORDERS

SECTION 6: NEUROLOGICAL DISORDERS

SECTION

1 Introduction

CHAPTER 1

Approach to a Critically Ill Patient

Bindu Mulakavalupil

DEFINITION

"Critical illness" is any disease process which causes physiological instability leading to disability or death within minutes or hours.

Critically ill patient: A critically ill is one who is at imminent risk of death unless the severity of illness is recognized early and appropriate measures are taken to promptly to assess diagnose and manage the illness.

The sickest of the sick are taken care of by critical care specialists. The ideal place to treat these patients is an intensive care unit (ICU) with well-trained staff. In order to offer the required high intensity of care, including therapy and physiologic parameter monitoring, ICUs maintain a high nurse to patient ratio.

Intensive care units account for 15–25% of patient deaths so doctors should be skilled at end-of-life care (EOLC) too.

Resuscitation: The ABCs—airway, breathing, and circulation (perfusion)—are crucial for the successful resuscitation of a critically ill patient.

After stabilizing the patient's condition, the clinician must choose the best location for additional patient's treatment.

Three key categories can be used to simplify the management of the critically ill patient:

1. Treating the particular critical illness
2. Preventing additional insults
3. Providing supportive care—ventilatory and/or hemodynamic

Restoring vital signs in patients who are at the very end of their physiologic decline is the primary focus of critical care, which necessitates a deep comprehension of pathophysiology. This resuscitation frequently happens quickly and without a thorough understanding of the patient's ongoing medical issues. During the process of physiologic stabilization, intensivists try to get pertinent medical history in order to support the real-time evaluation of the patient's current physiologic status. Intensivists have a wealth of techniques at their disposal to help them accurately to identify the pathophysiology and manage patients with incipient organ failure.

These tools also provide a window of opportunity for the diagnosis and treatment of underlying disease(s) in stabilized patients. Advanced techniques like renal replacement therapy and extracorporeal mechanical support are provided by high-ended ICUs. However, intensivists have a responsibility to counsel and soothe dying patients and their loved ones, as well as to identify when a patient's chances of recovery are slim to nonexistent. If the underlying illness cannot be resolved, critical care physicians frequently have to refocus the aim of care from resuscitation and cure to comfort.

EVALUATION OF THE SEVERITY OF ILLNESS

Illnesses in the ICU are often graded according to severity. Over the past 30 years, many severity-of-illness (SOI) grading systems have been created and proven. Systems for evaluating SOI are crucial for classifying patient groups. SOI scores are helpful in directing the allocation of resources, including nursing and ancillary care, and supporting ongoing evaluations of the quality of ICU treatment.

It is not possible to forecast a patient's survival using SOI rating methods. There are no well-established scoring systems available that claim to guide clinicians in deciding which criteria to use when admitting patients to an ICU **(Flowchart 1)**. Therefore, it is not recommended to utilize SOI scoring systems

Flowchart 1: Approach to a patient in critically ill.

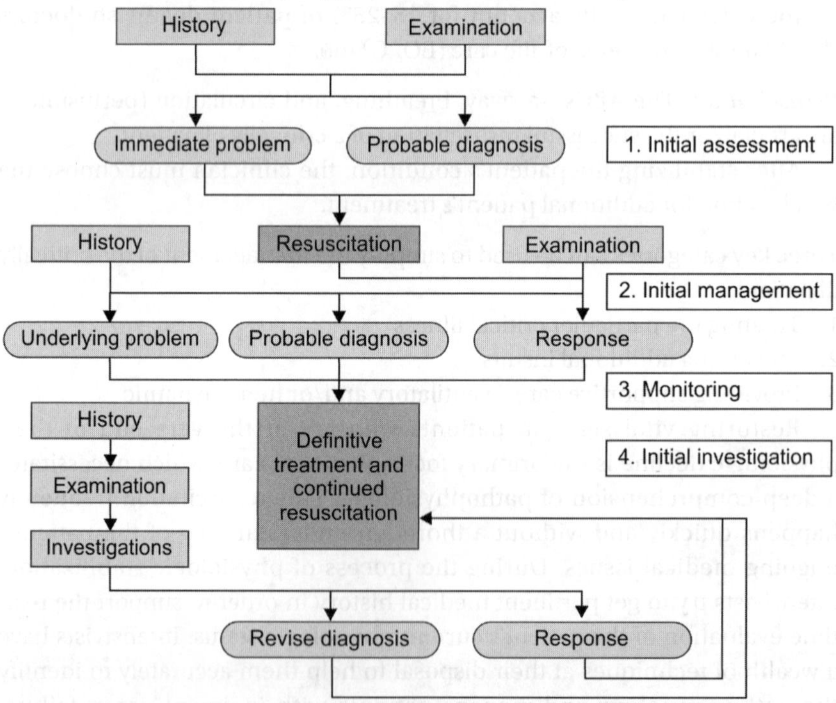

TABLE 1: Categorization of patients based on clinical observations.

Patient category	Clinical observations			
	Appearance	Neurological	Respiratory	Cardiovascular
Not critically ill	Normal	• Alert • Cooperative	• Normal pattern • RR >8 <20 b/min	• HR 60–100 b/min • SBP >90 mm Hg • UO >0.5 mL/kg/h
Potential critical illness	• Sweaty • Pale • Anxious	• Agitation • Confusion • Eyes open to voice only	• Accessory muscle use • RR <8 b/min • RR 20–30 b/min	• HR >100 b/min • SBP <90 mm Hg • UO <0.5 mL/kg/h
Critically ill	• Gray • Blue • Mottled skin	• Unresponsive or eyes open to pain only • Fitting	• Silent chest • RR <8 >30 b/min • Agonal respirations	• HR <50 b/min • HR >150 b/min • SBP <60 mm Hg • Anuric
→	Cardiac arrest or death			

(b/min: breaths/minute; HR: heart rate; RR: respiratory rate; SBP: systolic blood pressure; UO: urine output)

to guide therapy or clinical decision-making. Rather, these instruments ought to be employed as a vital data source in support of clinical bedside decision-making. The sequential organ failure assessment (SOFA), acute physiology and chronic health evaluation (APACHE), and simplified acute physiology scoring (SAPS) systems are the most often used ones.

Admission criteria for ICUs is possible or confirmed organ failure.

The following factors need to be taken into account:

- Diagnosis, sickness severity, age and functional level, coexisting disease, and physiological reserve
- Response to current treatment; availability of appropriate treatment; and prognosis
- Recent cardiopulmonary resuscitation (CPR) episode, expected life expectancy, and the patient's desires

Depending on clinical observations patients can be categorized into not critically ill, potential critical illness, and critically ill **(Table 1)**.

Once you determine the criticality of the patient then a definitive plan can be made according to the **Flowchart 2**.

INITIAL MANAGEMENT OF A CRITICALLY ILL PATIENT IN THE WARD OR EMERGENCY ROOM

When a patient is in the ward/emergency room (ER) and a medical issue arises, communicating with the rapid response team using situation-background-assessment-recommendation (SBAR) will enable all relevant information to be provided, resulting in quicker assistance **(Fig. 1)**.

Flowchart 2: Triaging of a supposedly critically ill patient.

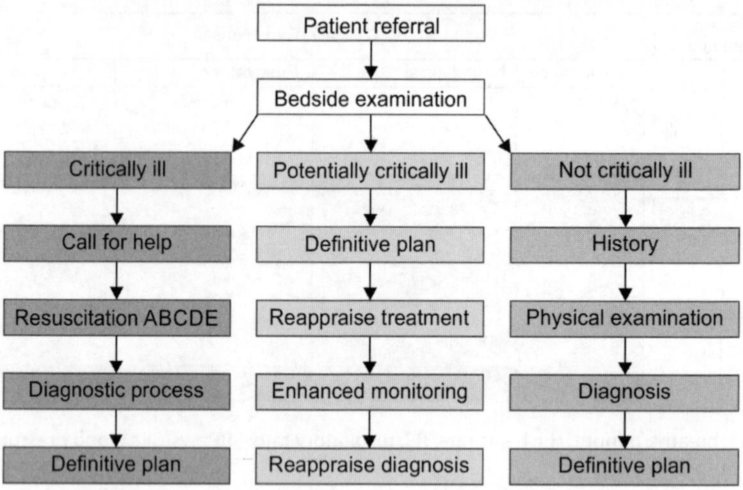

(ABCDE: airway, breathing, circulation, disability, and exposure)

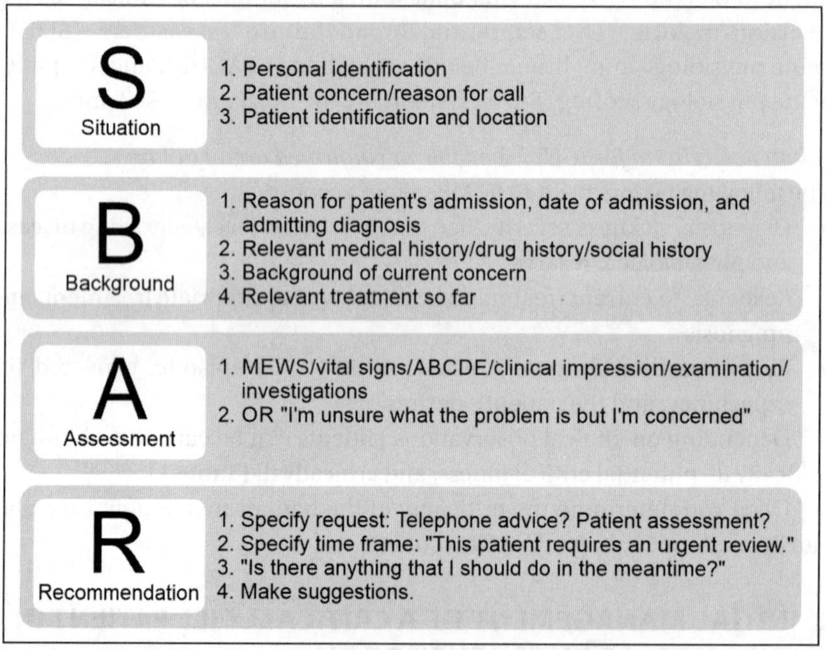

Fig. 1: Situation-background-assessment-recommendation (SBAR) to enable all relevant information for quicker assistance to a patient. (ABCDE: airway, breathing, circulation, disability, and exposure; MEWS: modified early warning score)

Worrying Signs

- Respiratory rate (RR) >30 breaths/min or breaths than 8/min
- Unable to speak in full sentence without pausing
- Agitated/confused/comatose
- Cyanosis/SpO_2 = 90%
- Deteriorating despite therapy

ABCDE approach is most useful approach.

A: Administer high-flow oxygen with 15 L O_2 on nonrebreathing mask (NRBM)—Ensure reservoir bag does not collapse.

B: Measure respiratory rate/SpO_2

C: Monitor the electroencephalogram (EEG) continuously.

- Noninvasive blood pressure (NIBP) every 5 minutes
- Intravenous (IV) cannula large bore
- Take blood samples.

D: Record Glasgow Coma Scale

- Pupil size/reactivity
- Blood glucose

E: Temperature—rectal/tympanic membrane

Others

- Arterial blood gas with lactate
- 12-lead ECG
- Chest X-ray
- Urinary catheter and measure urine output hourly
- Urine analysis—ketones/glucose/pus cells
- Urine pregnancy test (UPT) in young females
- Nasogastric tube, if indicated.

SUMMARY

Critical illness is any disease process which causes physiological instability leading to disability within minutes or hours.

The severity of illness must be recognized as early as possible and appropriate measures are taken promptly to assess diagnoses and management of the illness.

Severity of illness scoring system is useful in guiding hospital administrative policies directing the allocation of resources such as nursing and ancillary care and assisting in assessment of quality of ICU care over time.

SUGGESTED READING

1. Cox D, Donohue P, Costa V. A swallowed toothbrush causing perforation 2 years after ingestion. Br J Hosp Med. 2007;68(10):27330.
2. Jameson JL, Fauci AS, Kasper DL, Hauser SL, Longo DL, Loscalzo J. Harrison's Principles of Internal Medicine, 20th edition. United States: McGraw Hill Education; 2018.
3. Kayambankadzanja RK, Schell CO, Gerdin Wärnberg M, Tamras T, Mollazadegan H, Holmberg M, et al. Towards definitions of critical illness and critical care using concept analysis. BMJ Open. 2022;12(9):e060972.
4. National Institute for Health and Clinical Cases. Acutely ill patients in hospital: NICE pathways. London: National Institute for Health and Clinical Excellence; 2018.
5. Resuscitation Council UK. (2021). The ABCDE approach. [online] Available from: www.resus.org.uk/resuscitation-guidelines/abcde-approach [Last accessed May, 2024].

SECTION 2

Airway and Ventilatory Support

CHAPTER

2 Oxygen Therapy

Bindu Mulakavalupil

INTRODUCTION

Since oxygen (O_2) is a medication, only qualified personnel should prescribe, administer, and oversee its use. High-flow oxygen via a reservoir (nonrebreathe) bag should be administered without a prescription as soon as possible in life-threatening circumstances.

Pathophysiology and types of hypoxia.

Types of hypoxia	*Pathophysiology*
Hypoxic hypoxia	Reduced supply of oxygen to the body leading to a low arterial oxygen tension
Anemic hypoxia	The arterial oxygen tension is normal, but the circulating hemoglobin is reduced or functionally impaired
Stagnant hypoxia	Failure of transport of sufficient oxygen due to inadequate circulation
Histotoxic hypoxia	Impairment of cellular metabolism of oxygen despite adequate delivery

EQUIPMENT

O_2 Administration (Flowchart 1)

- *Nasal cannula:* This is the most popular oxygen delivery method for home usage. It offers comfortable flow rates of 2–6 L/min (LPM), enabling oxygen delivery without compromising the patient's ability to speak, eat, and other oral activities.
- *Face masks:* There are three main categories of face masks—(1) Non-rebreathers, (2) air-entrainment masks (venturi), and (3) basic facemasks. A basic facemask is a mask that distributes oxygen at a rate of 5–8 LPM without a bag attached. By employing jet mixing, an air-entrainment mask (also called a venturi mask) can give the patient preset oxygen levels. The air-to-oxygen ratio falls as the percentage of inspired oxygen rises when wearing one of these masks, resulting in an oxygen concentration of no >40% when using an air-entrainment mask. The inability of the patient to eat, drink, or converse comfortably while wearing this or other full-face masks is a drawback.

Flowchart 1: O_2 administration.

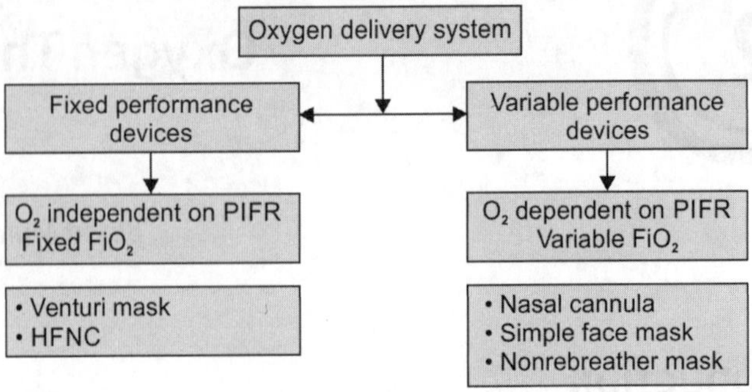

(FiO_2: fraction of inspired oxygen; HFNC: high-flow nasal cannula; PIFR: peak inspiratory flow rate)

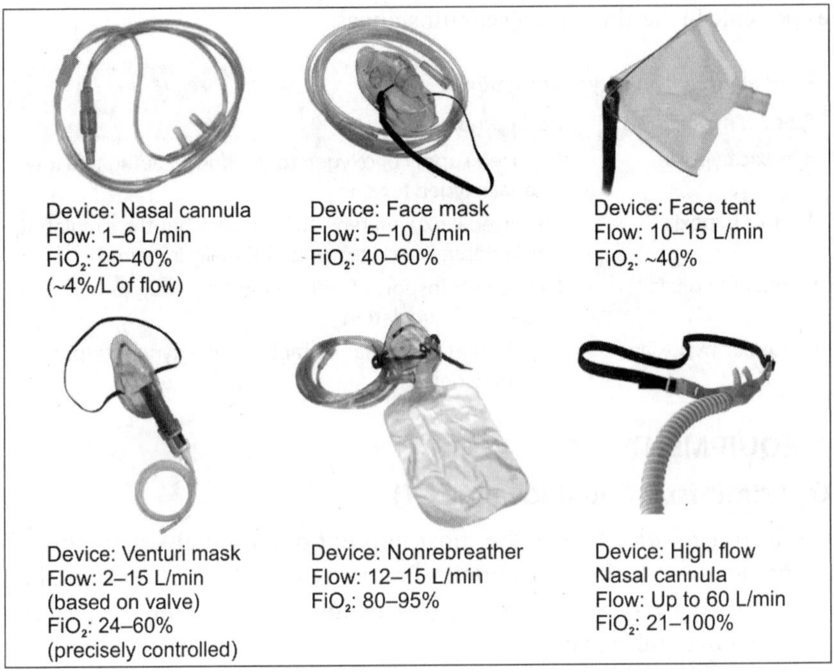

Fig. 1: *Oxygen delivery system:* Different devices.

- *Nonrebreathing masks* can supply 100% oxygen to the patient at a greater LPM flow rate because they contain a reservoir bag attached to the mask that is accessed by inhalation and used to fill the mask through a one-way valve **(Fig. 1)**. The mask also has ports on either side for exhalation. An add-on to an oxygen delivery system that increases oxygen concentration and, thus, administration percentage is a reservoir bag. The patient may obtain a higher concentration of oxygen by decreasing the amount of gas inhaled that is composed of atmospheric oxygen by permitting the collection of 100% O_2 in a reservoir bag.

- *High-flow nasal cannula (HFNC)* is a nasal cannula that may humidify oxygen and have flow rates higher than the patient's inspiratory pressure. With this configuration, 100% FiO_2 can be delivered without compromising the patient's capacity to speak, eat, and other oral functions. Moreover, HFNC can be employed to prolong apnea episodes prior to intubation.
- *Continuous positive airway pressure (CPAP)* is a mask that provides the patient with constant positive pressure.
- *Bilevel positive airway pressure, or BiPAP,* is a positive pressure administered through a mask with different levels for the inhale and exhale.
- *Bag valve mask devices,* also known as BVMs, are manually operated masks that are used for oxygen delivery at higher levels in patients who are unable to breathe on their own.
- *Ventilators* are devices that breathe via an endotracheal tube or tracheostomy for a patient. Positive pressure oxygen delivery can be titrated to meet the needs of the patient and applied to the ventilator.

SUMMARY

Oxygen therapy in the ICU is used to treat patients with respiratory failure, hypoxemia, or other conditions causing low oxygen levels. It aims to maintain adequate oxygen saturation (SpO_2) and prevent hypoxia, targeting SpO_2 between 92–96%, or 88–92% for patients with chronic lung diseases like chronic obstructive pulmonary disease. Various delivery methods include nasal cannulas, face masks, high-flow nasal cannulas, and mechanical ventilation for more severe cases.

Monitoring includes pulse oximetry and arterial blood gas analysis to assess oxygen and carbon dioxide levels. While essential for improving oxygenation, prolonged or high-concentration oxygen therapy can lead to complications like oxygen toxicity, hypercapnia, or lung damage (e.g., barotrauma). Careful titration is important to balance oxygen needs and minimize risks, particularly in conditions like acute respiratory distress syndrome. As patients recover, the goal is to wean off oxygen therapy gradually.

SUGGESTED READING

1. Grensemann J, Fuhrmann V, Kluge S. Oxygen Treatment in Intensive Care and Emergency Medicine. Dtsch Arztebl Int. 2018;115(27-28):455-62.
2. Young PJ, Frei D. Oxygen therapy for critically Ill and post-operative patients. J Anesth. 2021;35(6):928-38.

CHAPTER

3 Noninvasive Ventilation in the Intensive Care Unit

Harsh Parikh

INTRODUCTION

Noninvasive ventilation (NIV) has become a cornerstone in managing respiratory failure in the intensive care unit (ICU). Unlike invasive mechanical ventilation (IMV), which requires intubation, NIV delivers positive pressure ventilation through a face mask or nasal interface, avoiding the complications associated with endotracheal intubation. This mode of respiratory support has gained widespread use for both acute and chronic respiratory failure, improving patient's outcomes and reducing the need for intubation and its associated risks.

DEFINITION

Noninvasive positive pressure ventilation involves the delivery of oxygen into the lungs via positive pressure without the need for endotracheal intubation. It is used in acute and chronic respiratory failure but requires careful monitoring and titration to ensure its success and avoid complications.

PHYSIOLOGICAL PRINCIPLES OF NONINVASIVE VENTILATION

Noninvasive ventilation operates by delivering pressurized air or oxygen to the patient's airways through a noninvasive interface, typically a mask. The primary modes of NIV used in ICU settings are continuous positive airway pressure (CPAP) and bilevel positive airway pressure (BiPAP). Noninvasive positive-pressure ventilation (NPPV) reduces the work of breathing through three different methods. By applying positive end-expiratory pressure (PEEP) through expiratory positive airway pressure (EPAP), NPPV allows the body to overcome the dynamic intrinsic PEEP threshold required to initiate a breath and increase lung compliance. By applying inspiratory positive airway pressure (IPAP), NPPV contributes a more significant portion of the transpulmonary pressure (TPP) required during inspiration, thus reducing the body's breathing work. The main physiological effects of NIV include:

Positive Pressure Ventilation

Noninvasive ventilation delivers positive pressure during both the inspiratory and expiratory phases of the respiratory cycle. In CPAP, a constant level of positive airway pressure is maintained throughout, while in BiPAP, IPAP is higher than EPAP. This assists ventilation by improving lung expansion and reducing the work of breathing.

Reduction in Work of Breathing

Noninvasive ventilation reduces the effort required for breathing by supporting inspiratory effort and improving ventilation. This can be particularly helpful in conditions where respiratory muscles are fatigued or when patients are hypercapnic.

Improved Gas Exchange

By providing a greater volume of oxygenated air and removing carbon dioxide (CO_2) more efficiently, NIV enhances oxygenation and CO_2 clearance. The pressure helps to keep the alveoli open, promoting better gas exchange across the lung parenchyma and reducing atelectasis.

Reduction in Afterload and Preload

Noninvasive ventilation can reduce the work of the heart by decreasing venous return (preload) and lowering the resistance against which the heart has to pump (afterload). This can be particularly beneficial in patients with congestive heart failure (CHF) or cardiogenic pulmonary edema, where reducing the workload of the heart is a key therapeutic goal.

INDICATIONS

Absolute Indications

- Noninvasive ventilation for acute or acute-on-chronic respiratory acidosis secondary to chronic obstructive pulmonary disease (COPD) exacerbation where pH ≤7.35.
- Noninvasive ventilation is the prevention of endotracheal intubation and mechanical ventilation in a patient that is not immediately deteriorating.
- Noninvasive ventilation or CPAP for cardiogenic pulmonary edema.

Relative Indications

- Early NIV for immunocompromised patients with acute respiratory failure (ARF)
- Postoperative ARF

- As palliation to dyspneic patients in the setting of terminal cancer or other terminal conditions
- Chest trauma patients with ARF
- Prevention of postextubation respiratory failure in high-risk patients

Others

- Chronic stable COPD with hypercapnia
- Obesity hypoventilation syndrome
- Obstructive sleep apnea (OSA)
- Respiratory failure secondary to neuromuscular disease, and
- Restrictive thoracic disorders

CONTRAINDICATIONS FOR NONINVASIVE VENTILATION

Absolute Contraindications

- Facial trauma/burns
- Fixed upper airway obstruction
- Active vomiting
- Respiratory or cardiac arrest and hemodynamic instability
- Severe acidosis-metabolic or respiratory

Relative Contraindications

- A recent facial, upper airway, or upper gastrointestinal (GI) tract surgery
- Inability to protect the airway
- Life-threatening hypoxemia
- Medical or hemodynamic instability (hypotensive shock, myocardial infarction requiring intervention, and uncontrolled ischemia or arrhythmias)
- Altered mental status/agitation
- Bowel obstruction
- Copious respiratory secretions
- Focal consolidation
- Undrained pneumothorax
- Severe comorbidity

BENEFITS OF NONINVASIVE VENTILATION

Noninvasive ventilation offers multiple benefits over invasive mechanical ventilation, making it a valuable tool in ICU management:

Reduced Need for Intubation

Noninvasive ventilation is effective in preventing intubation in many patients with respiratory failure, particularly those with COPD exacerbations and cardiogenic pulmonary edema. By avoiding intubation, patients are spared from the risks of endotracheal tube-related complications.

Lower Risk of Ventilator-associated Pneumonia

Because NIV avoids intubation, it reduces the incidence of ventilator-associated pneumonia (VAP), a serious and common complication of invasive mechanical ventilation. This is particularly important in immunocompromised patients.

Improved Patient's Comfort

Compared to invasive ventilation, NIV allows patients to remain awake, communicate, eat, and drink. This enhances patient's comfort and reduces the need for sedatives, promoting earlier mobility and engagement in recovery.

Shorter ICU Stay and Lower Mortality

Numerous studies have shown that NIV reduces ICU length of stay, shortens hospital admissions, and decreases mortality rates in appropriate patient populations.

LIMITATIONS AND CHALLENGES OF NONINVASIVE VENTILATION

Risk of Delayed Intubation

Noninvasive ventilation can mask the severity of respiratory failure, leading to delayed intubation in some cases. Clinicians must closely monitor patients to identify signs of NIV failure, such as worsening gas exchange, increasing respiratory rate, or deteriorating mental status.

Interface-related Discomfort

The mask interface used for NIV can cause discomfort, pressure sores, and air leaks. Proper mask fitting and use of skin protection can mitigate some of these issues, but patient's tolerance remains a challenge.

Limited Use in Severe Hypoxemia or Acute Respiratory Distress Syndrome

Patients with severe hypoxemic respiratory failure, especially those with acute respiratory distress syndrome (ARDS), may not respond adequately to NIV. If PaO_2/FiO_2 ratios remain low despite NIV, intubation and invasive mechanical ventilation may be necessary.

Limited Application in Certain Populations

Patients with altered mental status, agitation, or those who cannot cooperate with NIV may not be suitable candidates, limiting the use of this modality in some clinical scenarios.

MONITORING AND MANAGEMENT

- *Respiratory rate:* Increased respiratory rate or sustained tachypnea may indicate worsening respiratory failure.
- *Oxygenation:* Monitoring oxygen saturation (SpO_2) and arterial blood gases (ABGs) is essential to ensure adequate oxygenation and ventilation.
- *Work of breathing:* Observation of increased work of breathing, such as use of accessory muscles, should prompt reassessment of NIV effectiveness.
- Patient's comfort and mask fit.

USE OF NONINVASIVE VENTILATION IN ACUTE SETTING

- The first category is for patients with simple airway conditions, such as OSA, needing end-EPAP, or CPAP alone. The titration of pressure in this situation requires overcoming the collapsing pressure of the upper airway.
- The second category is for those with hypercapnic or mixed respiratory failures, such as those with acute exacerbation of COPD. We can use EPAP of 5 cmH_2O and add pressure support of 10–15 cmH_2O, which can be titrated based on response in reducing CO_2 (measured by ABG).
- A third category is when patients hospitalized with hypercapnic respiratory failure are associated with obesity or OSA. We have to prevent upper airway collapse while maintaining adequate ventilation. Here, we can apply sufficient EPAP to overcome the collapsing upper airway pressure and add pressure support between 10 and 15 cmH_2O to provide adequate ventilation and titrate based on ABG.

MONITORING

Once pH is normalized, the pressure support can be weaned off slowly to allow a slight decrease in hypercapnia. When monitoring to ensure adequate response to NPPV in the acute setting, the clinician must consider the subjective and physiologic responses of the patient. Patients likely to succeed on NPPV in the acute setting have a drop in their respiratory rate after 1–2 hours, a decrease in heart rate, and better ventilator synchrony. A blood gas should be drawn 1 hour after initiation of bilevel positive airway pressure (BPAP) as a decrease in pCO_2 and an increase in pH predict NPPV success. In addition to the parameters above, tidal volume and air leak must be closely monitored as these can contribute to treatment failure if not corrected. The patient's hemodynamics, including blood pressure and heart rate, must be monitored during treatment as intrathoracic pressure right ventricular afterload increases and right ventricular preload decreases. This is consistent with prior studies demonstrating reduced cardiac output after initiating NPPV.

WEANING

The patient should be assessed on an individual basis for suitability for weaning from NIV. After 24 hours, if the patient is improving, build periods of time off NIV during the day; continue oxygen therapy via nasal specs or venturi mask, and monitor for any signs of work of breathing (increased respiratory rate/decreased oxygen saturation, and increased use of accessory muscles).

If the patient shows signs of clinical deterioration during weaning, an ABG may be required and NIV is resumed.

Patient should have NIV overnight during weaning period. Wean off over 2–3 days. Consider use of NIV overnight if nocturnal hypoventilation is present.

SUMMARY

Start treatment as early as possible. When arterial pH is <7.35, and $PaCO_2$ is elevated, it indicates the presence of acute or acute-chronic hypercapnia respiratory failure, which requires admission to the ICU.

The first goal is to correct arterial pH in acute or chronic hypercapnia respiratory failure.

High-intensity pressure support is indicated in chronic hypercapnic respiratory failure with arterial $PaCO_2$of >51 mm Hg. It should be targeted to correct CO_2 toward normal or at least reduced by 20% from initial levels.

When OSA is suspected, the EPAP should be adjusted empirically (use the 10% rule of actual body weight) if no PAP titration was performed.

SUGGESTED READING

1. Antonelli M, Conti G, Rocco M, Bufi M, De Blasi RA, Vivino G, et al. A comparison of noninvasive positive-pressure ventilation and conventional mechanical ventilation in patients with acute respiratory failure. N Engl J Med. 1998;339(7):429-35.
2. Bellone A, Lascioli R, Raschi S, et al. Non-invasive pressure support ventilation vs. conventional oxygen supplementation in acute cardiogenic pulmonary edema: a randomized multicenter trial. Chest. 2005;128(4):3107-15.
3. Brochard L, Mancebo J, Wysocki M, Lofaso F, Conti G, Rauss A, et al. Noninvasive ventilation for acute exacerbations of chronic obstructive pulmonary disease. N Engl J Med. 1995;333(13):817-22.
4. Duan J, Han X, Bai L, et al. Noninvasive ventilation for acute respiratory failure in critically ill patients: a systematic review and network meta-analysis. Crit Care. 2020;24(1):1-13.
5. Frat JP, Thille AW, Mercat A, Girault C, Ragot S, Perbet S, et al. High-flow oxygen through nasal cannula in acute hypoxemic respiratory failure. N Engl J Med. 2015;372(23):2185-96.
6. Guérin C, Girard R, Chemorin C, De Varax R, Fournier G. Face mask noninvasive mechanical ventilation reduces the incidence of nosocomial pneumonia. Intensive Care Med. 1997;23(10):1024-32.

7. Keenan SP, Sinuff T, Burns KE, Muscedere J, Kutsogiannis J, Mehta S, et al. Clinical practice guidelines for the use of noninvasive positive-pressure ventilation and noninvasive continuous positive airway pressure in the acute care setting. Canadian Med Assoc J. 2011;183(3):E195-214.
8. Masip J, Roque M, Sánchez B, Fernández R, Subirana M, Expósito JA. Noninvasive ventilation in acute cardiogenic pulmonary edema: systematic review and meta-analysis. JAMA. 2005;294(24):3124-30.
9. Scala R, Pisani L. Noninvasive ventilation in acute respiratory failure: which recipe for success? Eur Respir Rev. 2018;27(149):180029.
10. Vital FM, Ladeira MT, Atallah ÁN. Non-invasive positive pressure ventilation (CPAP or bilevel NPPV) for cardiogenic pulmonary edema. Cochrane Database Syst Rev. 2013;5:CD005351.

CHAPTER

4 High-flow Nasal Cannula in Intensive Care Unit

Harsh Parikh

INTRODUCTION

High-flow nasal cannula (HFNC) has emerged as a vital respiratory support tool in the intensive care unit (ICU). HFNC delivers humidified and heated oxygen at flow rates higher than those of conventional oxygen therapy. It has been increasingly used as an alternative to traditional noninvasive ventilation (NIV) or mechanical ventilation in patients with respiratory failure, offering several physiological advantages such as reduced respiratory effort, improved oxygenation, and enhanced patient's comfort.

PHYSIOLOGICAL PRINCIPLES

High-flow nasal cannula provides oxygen at high-flow rates, typically ranging from 20 to 60 liters per minute (L/min). The air-oxygen mixture is heated to near body temperature and humidified, which prevents the drying of mucous membranes and allows for better tolerance at higher flow rates. The primary physiological benefits include:

Improved Oxygenation

High-flow nasal cannula delivers a more accurate and stable fraction of inspired oxygen (FiO_2), as it meets or exceeds the patient's inspiratory flow demand. This minimizes the dilution of oxygen with room air, leading to more efficient oxygen delivery and improved arterial oxygenation.

Reduction of Dead Space

The high-flow rate of HFNC washes out carbon dioxide from the upper airway dead space, reducing rebreathing and improving carbon dioxide clearance. This contributes to an overall reduction in respiratory effort and minute ventilation.

Positive Airway Pressure

While HFNC does not provide the same level of continuous positive airway pressure (CPAP) as conventional NIV, it creates a modest amount of positive end-expiratory pressure (PEEP), which helps to maintain airway patency and improve gas exchange. The degree of PEEP generated depends on flow rate and patient-specific factors such as mouth closure.

Humidification and Warming of Inspired Gases

Heated and humidified oxygen delivered by HFNC preserves mucociliary function and prevents airway dryness, which are common problems in traditional oxygen therapy. This promotes better secretion clearance and patient's comfort, contributing to improved compliance and tolerance over prolonged use.

CLINICAL INDICATIONS IN ICU

High-flow nasal cannula is primarily indicated in patients with acute type 1 respiratory failure, particularly in cases where supplemental oxygen via traditional methods like nasal cannula or mask is insufficient. The main indications in the ICU include:

Acute Hypoxemic Respiratory Failure

Patients with acute hypoxemic respiratory failure (AHRF), such as those suffering from pneumonia, acute respiratory distress syndrome (ARDS), or coronavirus disease 2019 (COVID-19), often benefit from HFNC. It improves oxygenation without the need for invasive mechanical ventilation and is often used early in the course of disease to prevent intubation.

Postextubation Support

High-flow nasal cannula can be used to prevent reintubation in patients at high risk for respiratory failure following extubation. By providing effective oxygenation and reducing respiratory work, HFNC may serve as a bridge to full recovery after mechanical ventilation.

Preoxygenation for Intubation

High-flow nasal cannula can provide continuous oxygenation during intubation procedures, a practice known as apneic oxygenation. This technique is particularly useful in critically ill patients who are at high risk of desaturation during intubation.

Acute Exacerbation of Chronic Respiratory Conditions

Patients with chronic obstructive pulmonary disease (COPD) or interstitial lung disease (ILD) experiencing acute exacerbations may benefit from HFNC, particularly when they have increased oxygen needs but do not require NIV or intubation.

BENEFITS

High-flow nasal cannula offers several advantages over traditional oxygen therapy and NIV:

Patient's Comfort

Unlike NIV masks, HFNC uses nasal prongs that are less restrictive, allowing the patient to talk, eat, and drink while receiving respiratory support. The humidified and warmed gas is better tolerated than dry, cold oxygen, improving overall patient's comfort and compliance.

Noninvasive Nature

High-flow nasal cannula is noninvasive and does not require a tight-fitting mask, reducing the risk of pressure sores, claustrophobia, and discomfort that are common with NIV. This allows patients to use it for prolonged periods without the risk of developing skin breakdown.

Reduced Work of Breathing

By decreasing inspiratory resistance and improving oxygen delivery, HFNC reduces the patient's work of breathing. This can delay or even avoid the need for mechanical ventilation in some patients with respiratory failure, reducing associated risks like ventilator-associated pneumonia (VAP).

Flexible Use

High-flow nasal cannula can be titrated easily to meet patient's needs by adjusting the flow rate and FiO_2. This flexibility allows clinicians to provide tailored oxygen support based on the patient's condition.

LIMITATIONS AND RISKS

Inability to Provide High Positive End-expiratory Pressure

High-flow nasal cannula delivers only a modest level of positive airway pressure, making it less effective in patients with conditions that require higher levels of PEEP, such as severe ARDS.

Risk of Delayed Intubation

There is a risk that HFNC may mask the severity of respiratory failure, leading to delayed intubation. Careful monitoring and the use of early warning criteria (such as worsening respiratory rate, increasing work of breathing, or falling oxygen saturation) are essential to avoid this complication.

High-flow Rates and Barotrauma

While the risk is low, there is a theoretical concern that high-flow rates could contribute to barotrauma in some patients. However, this is rare, especially at flow rates below 60 L/min.

Not Suitable for Hypercapnic Respiratory Failure

Although HFNC improves CO_2 clearance through dead space washout, it may not be sufficient in patients with severe hypercapnic respiratory failure, particularly in those with COPD exacerbations. NIV or mechanical ventilation may be more appropriate in these cases.

CLINICAL EVIDENCE

Studies have demonstrated the benefits of HFNC in managing critically ill patients:

FLORALI trial: This landmark trial showed that HFNC was superior to standard oxygen therapy and comparable to NIV in preventing intubation in patients with acute hypoxemic respiratory failure. HFNC also improved 90-day survival rates and patient's comfort.

Coronavirus disease 2019 and HFNC: During the COVID-19 pandemic, HFNC became a mainstay of treatment for patients with severe hypoxemia. Studies indicated that early use of HFNC reduced the need for intubation and improved survival rates. Only problem was that HFNC gave a false sense of security and sometimes delayed intubations.

Postextubation support: Clinical trials have found the HFNC to be beneficial in reducing the risk of reintubation in high-risk patients after extubation, particularly in patients with COPD or heart failure.

MONITORING AND MANAGEMENT IN ICU

Effective use of HFNC requires careful patient's monitoring to ensure that it is providing adequate respiratory support. Key parameters to monitor include:

Oxygen saturation (SpO_2): Maintain SpO_2 within target ranges, usually between 92 and 96%, depending on the patient's condition.

Respiratory rate: An increasing respiratory rate or sustained tachypnea may indicate worsening respiratory failure.

Work of breathing: Subjective assessment of increased work of breathing (e.g., use of accessory muscles and nasal flaring) should prompt reassessment of therapy.

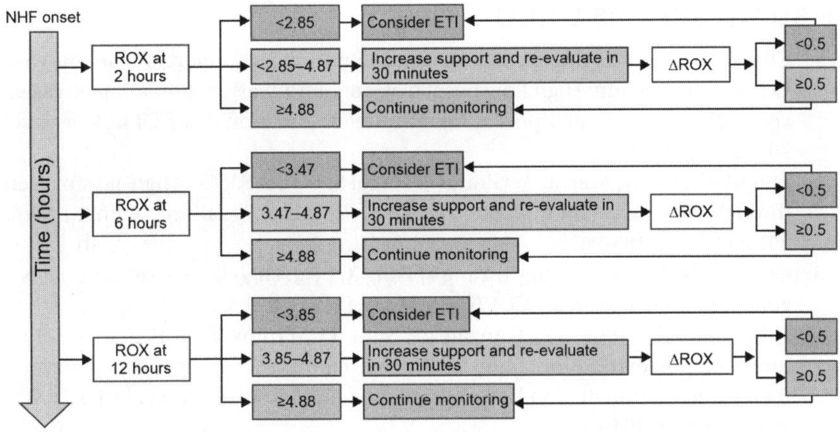

Fig. 1: Respiratory oxygenation (ROX) protocol for high-flow nasal cannula (HFNC) management. (ETI: endotracheal intubation; NHF: nasal high flow)

Arterial blood gases (ABGs): In patients with severe respiratory failure, ABG analysis may be necessary to evaluate oxygenation and ventilation status.

The respiratory oxygenation (ROX) index, combining SpO_2/FiO_2 and respiratory rate, can predict HFNC failure.

The formula is: $SpO_2/RR \times FiO_2$

Predictors of HFNC success include: If ROX ≥4.88 at 2, 6, and 12 hours after HFNC initiation, it was associated with a lower risk for intubation.

Predictors of HFNC failure include:

- ROX <2.85 at 2 hours
- ROX <3.47 at 6 hours
- ROX <3.85 at 12 hours

ROX score <3.85 is 100% predictive of failure at 12 hours for HFNC.

Respiratory oxygenation scores between 3.85 and 4.88 at 12 hours will need more frequent monitoring.

If parameters deteriorate, early escalation to noninvasive or invasive mechanical ventilation is required **(Fig. 1)**.

SUMMARY

High-flow nasal cannula has revolutionized the management of respiratory failure in the ICU, offering a comfortable, noninvasive alternative to traditional methods of oxygen therapy and ventilation. Its physiological benefits, patient's tolerance, and versatility make it an essential tool for critically ill patients. However, its use requires careful patient's selection and monitoring to avoid potential complications like delayed intubation. In the right clinical context, HFNC can significantly improve patient's outcomes and reduce the need for invasive interventions.

SUGGESTED READING

1. Chavez A, Bajwah S, Creagh-Brown B, et al. Respiratory support for patients with COVID-19 infection: High flow nasal oxygen, non-invasive ventilation, invasive ventilation, and extracorporeal membrane oxygenation. Curr Opin Crit Care. 2021;27(2):103-14.
2. Frat JP, Thille AW, Mercat A, Girault C, Ragot S, Perbet S, et al. High-flow oxygen through nasal cannula in acute hypoxemic respiratory failure. N Engl J Med. 2015;372(23):2185-96.
3. Geng S, Mei Q, Zhu C, Yang T, Yang Y, Fang X, et al. High flow nasal cannula is a good treatment option for COVID-19. Heart Lung. 2020;49(5):444-5.
4. Hernández G, Vaquero C, González P, Subira C, Frutos-Vivar F, Rialp G, et al. Effect of postextubation high-flow nasal cannula vs conventional oxygen therapy on reintubation in low-risk patients: A randomized clinical trial. JAMA. 2016;315(13):1354-61.
5. Nishimura M. High-flow nasal cannula oxygen therapy in adults: Physiological benefits, indication, clinical outcomes, and adverse effects. Respiratory Care. 2016;61(4):529-41.
6. O'Driscoll BR, Howard LS, Earis J, Mark V. British Thoracic Society guideline for oxygen use in adults in healthcare and emergency settings. Thorax. 2017;72(Suppl 1):ii1-ii90.
7. Papazian L, Corley A, Hess D, Fraser JF, Frat JP, Guitton C, et al. Use of high-flow nasal cannula oxygenation in ICU adults: A narrative review. Intensive Care Med. 2016;42(9):1336-49.
8. Roca O, Riera J, Torres F, Masclans JR. High-flow oxygen therapy in acute respiratory failure. Respir Care. 2010;55(4):408-13.
9. Spoletini G, Alotaibi M, Blasi F, Hill NS. Heated humidified high-flow nasal oxygen in adults: Mechanisms of action and clinical implications. Chest. 2015;148(1):253-61.
10. Zhu Y, Yin H, Zhang R, Wei J, et al. High-flow nasal cannula oxygen therapy vs conventional oxygen therapy and noninvasive ventilation in adults with acute hypoxemic respiratory failure: A systematic review and meta-analysis of randomized trials. Chest. 2020;158(3):964-79.

CHAPTER 5

Airway Management

Bindu Mulakavalupil

INTRODUCTION

Endotracheal intubation is a critical life-saving procedure. Airway management is a core skill essential for anesthesiologists and healthcare providers involved in resuscitation and acute care of patients.

DEFINITION

A *difficult airway* is defined as the clinical situation in which a conventionally trained anesthesiologist experiences difficulty with face mask ventilation of the upper airway, difficulty with tracheal intubation, or both.

A difficult airway is one for which a preintubation examination has identified attributes that are likely to make laryngoscopy, intubation, bag-mask ventilation (BMV), the use of an extraglottic device [EGD, e.g., combitube, laryngeal mask airway (LMA)], or surgical airway management more difficult than would be the case in an ordinary patient without those attributes. Identification of a difficult airway is a key component of the approach to airway management for any patient and is a key branch point on the main airway algorithm. The key reason for this is that, in general, one should not administer a neuromuscular blocking medication to a patient unless one has a measure of certainty that gas exchange can be maintained if laryngoscopy and intubation fail.

A *physiologically difficult airway* is one in which physiologic alterations in the patient increase the risk of cardiopulmonary complications during tracheal intubation and transition to positive pressure ventilation.

While either difficult BMV or difficult intubation occurs in approximately 5% of patients, a situation in which both BMV and intubation are difficult occurs concomitantly in much fewer patients. Of those, <1% of patients require a surgical airway for emergent management.

FAILED AIRWAY

The failed airway exists when either of the following conditions is met:

- Failure to maintain acceptable oxygen saturations during or after one or more failed laryngoscopic attempts [cannot intubate, cannot oxygenate (CICO)], *or*

- Three failed attempts at orotracheal intubation by an experienced intubator, even when oxygen saturation can be maintained.

Clinically, the failed airway presents itself in two ways, depending on the urgency created by the situation:

1. There is not sufficient time to evaluate or attempt a series of rescue options, and the airway must be secured immediately because of an inability to maintain oxygen saturation by BMV.
2. There is time to evaluate and execute various options because the patient is in a "*CICO*" situation.

HOW DO YOU ANTICIPATE DIFFICULT AIRWAY?

History

- History of oral, neck, or cervical spine surgery, or irradiation
- History of oral or neck tumor, cellulitis, or abscess
- History of neck or mandibular arthritis or other joint immobility
- Presentation because of oral, facial, neck, or cervical spine trauma
- Use of anticoagulants or presence of a coagulopathy

Focused physical examination: There are various clinical markers to identify difficult mask ventilation **(Table 1)**, difficult airway **(Table 2 and Box 1)**, difficult laryngoscopy **(Fig. 1)**, and difficult intubation **(Fig. 2)**.

TABLE 1: Difficult mask ventilation prediction (MOANS mnemonic).

M	Mask seal
O	Obesity/Obstruction
A	Aged (>55 years)
N	No teeth
S	Stiff lungs

TABLE 2: Difficult airway prediction (LEMON mnemonic).

L	Look externally
E	Evaluate 3-3-2 rule
M	Mallampati scale
O	Obstruction/Obesity
N	Neck mobility

BOX 1: Grading at direct laryngoscopy.

Grade 1: Full exposure of glottis (anterior + posterior commissure)
Grade 2: Anterior commissure not visualized
Grade 3: Epiglottis only
Grade 4: No glottic structure visible

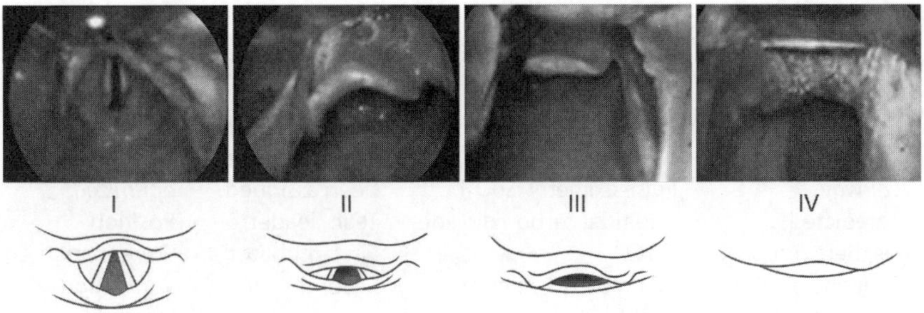

Fig. 1: Direct laryngoscopy grade.

Visible structures when patient opens mouth, protrudes tongue without help			
Samsoon and Young modification: Mallampati classification			
Increasing difficulty with intubation or mask ventilation			
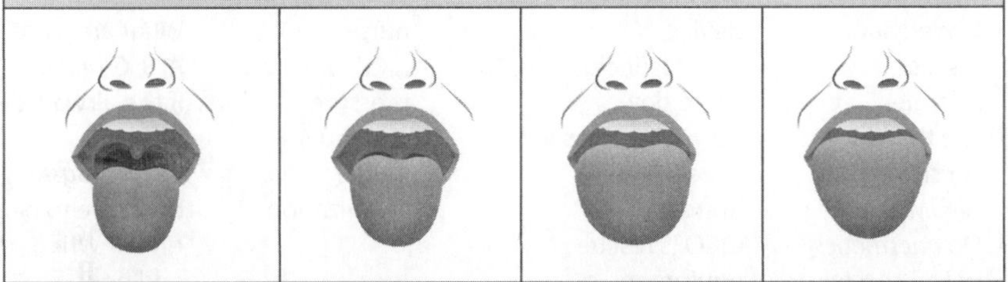			
• Soft palate • Fauces • Uvula • Tonsillar pillars	• Soft palate • Fauces • Uvula	• Soft palate • Fauces • Uvula	• None of the previous structures

Fig. 2: *Samsoon and Young modification:* Mallampati classification.

PREPARATION

It is essential to have a checklist for intubation so that important so as to reduce failure by compensating for potential limits of human memory and attention **(Table 3)**.

ROLE OF PREOXYGENATION

- Preoxygenation is the administration of oxygen to a patient prior to intubation to extend "the safe apnea time".
- The primary mechanism is "denitrogenation" of the lungs.
- In a healthy preoxygenated patient, the safe apnea time is up to 8 minutes.

Factors that decrease safe apnea time include:

- Critical illness
- Inadequate preoxygenation
- Obesity
- Pregnancy

TABLE 3: Checklist for preparation.

ICU intubation checklist			
Assess	***Equipment***	***Team***	***Plan***
• Is a *difficult airway* predicted? • Is there risk of *physiological compromise?* • Cardiovascular instability • Hypoxemia • Acidemia • Increased ICP • Aspiration • Underlying disease • Allergies • Are the *ICU consultant and ANUM* aware? • Do *anesthetics or ENT specialists* need to be contacted? Anesthetics the Alfred X44627	• Is *monitoring* ready? • Pulse oximetry (SpO_2) • End tidal carbon dioxide ($ETCO_2$) • BP (cycle q 1 minute if NIBP) • ECG • Is *equipment* checked and ready? • BVM with O_2 flowing • Airway adjuncts • Supraglottic airway device • ETT × 2 (including 1 size down) • Laryngoscopes × 2 (Direct/Video) • Bougie • CICO** rescue equipment • Suction • Stethoscope • Are *drugs and lines* ready? • IV checked and fluids on pumpset • Induction and paralytic drugs • Inopressors • Postintubation sedation	• Have *team roles* been assigned? • Team leader • First intubator* • Second intubator* • Airway assistant • CICO** rescuer • Drug administrator • Senior support nurse • ± Cricoid pressure • ± Manual in-line stabilization	• Is the patient *optimized*? • Position • Oxygenation • Ventilation • Hemodynamics • NGT suctioned • What are the *plans for anticipated physiological compromise?* • What are *plans A, B, C, and D* if the airway is difficult? • What *drugs/doses* are to be given? When and how? • Does anyone have *questions or concerns*?

*Two airway competent doctors *must* attend

**CICO = cannot intubate, cannot oxygenate—proceed to cricothyroidotomy

(ANUM: Associate Nurse Unit Manager; BP: blood pressure; BVM: bag-valve-mask; ECG: electrocardiogram; ETT: endotracheal tube; ICP: intracranial pressure; ICU: intensive care unit; IV: intravenous; NGT: nasogastric tube; NIBP: noninvasive blood pressure)

- Shunt physiology
- Airway occlusion
- Increased oxygen consumption
- Anemia.

DEVICES USED FOR PREOXYGENATION/APNEIC OXYGENATION

- O_2 nasal cannula 15 L/min
- High-flow nasal cannula (HFNC) 100/60

- Noninvasive ventilation (NIV)
- nonrebreathing mask (NRBM)
- Ambu (artificial manual breathing unit) bag with reservoir

INTUBATION IN A PATIENT WITH UNSTABLE CERVICAL SPINE

Any patient with suspected or confirmed unstable spine, place a stabilization device. During intubation, manual inline axial stabilization of the head and neck by an assistant is mandatory **(Fig. 3)**.

- Mask ventilation should be done with extreme caution.
- Cervical subluxation could occur during chin lift, jaw thrust, BMV and tracheal intubation as well as maneuvers such as head turning.

Tips for intubation in cervical injury:

- No cricoid pressure as causes posterior displacement of the cervical spine.
- Use video laryngoscope.
- Used bougie

POSITIONING

The head position should be optimized to get the best possible view of the vocal cords. The "sniffing position" has traditionally been considered the optimal position for direct laryngoscopy as it aligns the oral, pharyngeal, and laryngeal axes **(Fig. 4)**. This position is achieved by elevating the patient's head, extending the head at the neck, and aligning the ears horizontally with

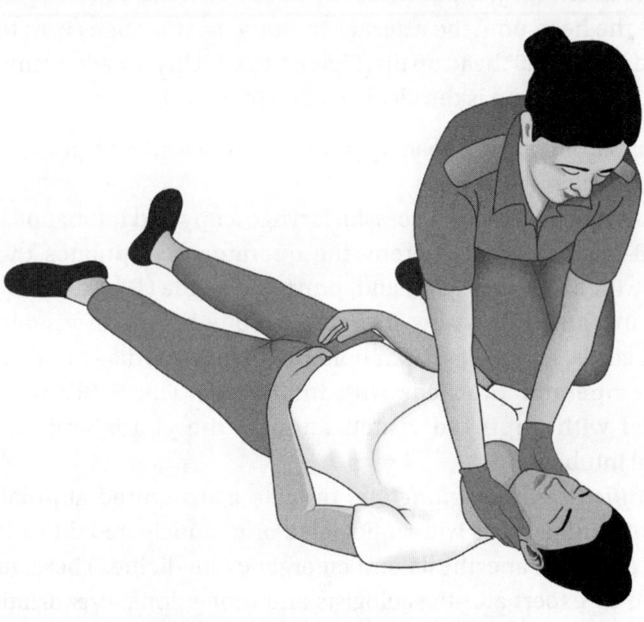

Fig. 3: Stabilization of cervical spine.

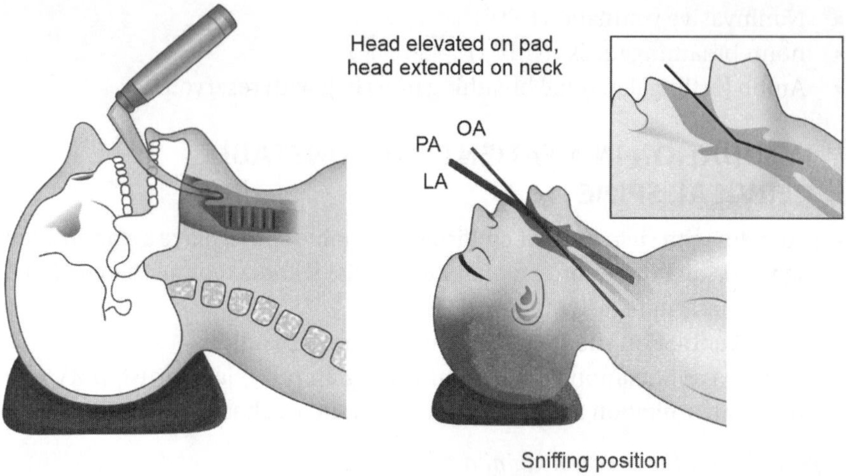

Fig. 4: Optimal positioning. (LA: laryngeal axis; OA: oral axis; PA: pharyngeal axis)

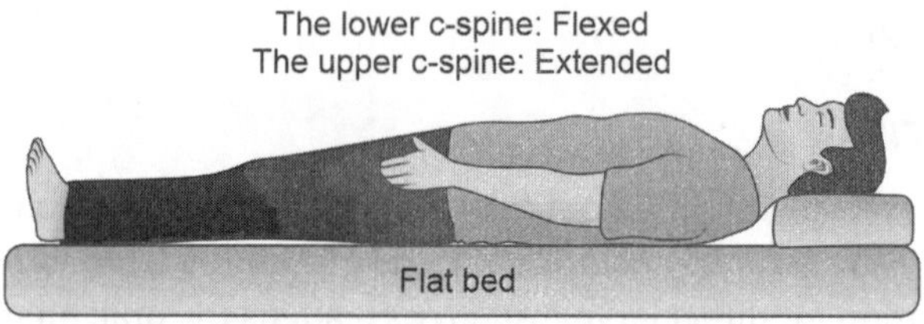

Fig. 5: Sniffing the morning air position.

the sternal notch **(Fig. 5)**. In morbidly obese patients, rolls may be utilized to elevate the head until the external auditory meatus aligns with the sternal notch and giving a 20° head up tilt **(Figs. 6A to C)**. This so called ramp position along with 25° head up is the ideal position in the ICU.

It has been found that 25° head up position has two advantages:
1. Preoxygenation is better.
2. Improved incidence of successful laryngoscopy and intubation.

B-U-R-P maneuver, whereby the operator manipulates the thyroid cartilage with his or her right hand, providing gentle (B)ackward, (U)pward, (R)ightward, and (P)ressure. If this technique results in visualization of the vocal cords, an assistant can hold the thyroid cartilage in that position while the operator proceeds with intubation. The BURP maneuver is associated with improved visualization of the glottis and subsequent successful intubation.

The *difficult airway guidelines* provide a structured approach to the management of patients with anticipated or unanticipated difficult airways, a critical aspect of anesthesia and emergency medicine. These guidelines, developed by expert anesthesiologists and professional organizations such as the Difficult Airway Society (DAS) guidelines, aim to improve safety

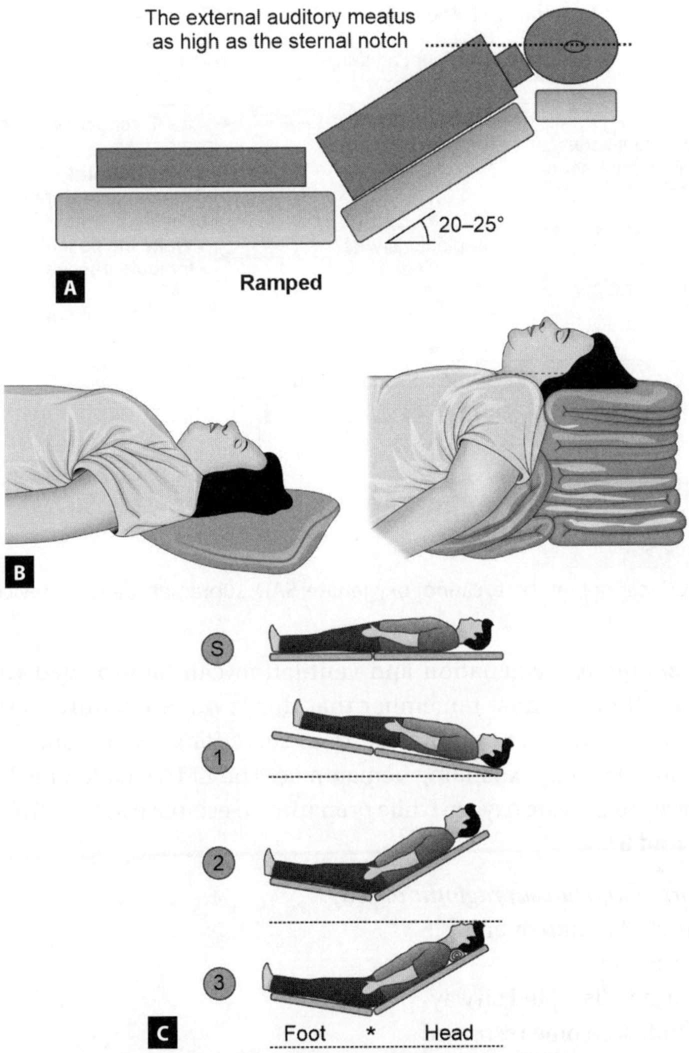

Figs. 6A to C: Ramped and 25° head up position.

and outcomes by offering clear protocols for identifying, planning for, and managing airway difficulties **(Flowcharts 1 and 2)**.

LARYNGEAL MASK AIRWAY

The LMA works by creating a seal over the larynx with a soft mask that allows for oxygen to be blown into the lungs, in a sense moving the bag-mask apparatus from the level of the mouth to the larynx.

The LMA is inserted "backward" into the posterior pharynx and then advanced while being rotated forward, seating the LMA in the hypopharynx. Once this is done, the cuff is inflated and bag ventilation can be performed.

Flowchart 1: Difficult Airway Society (DAS) guidelines.

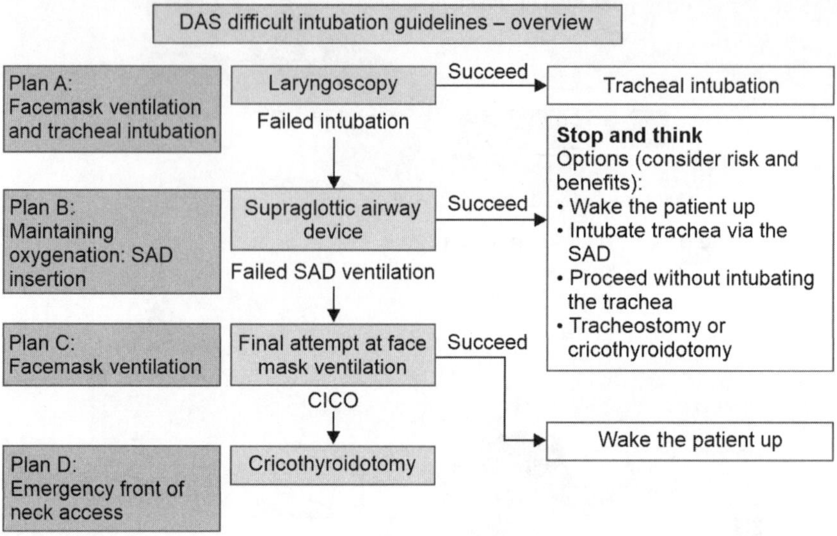

(CICO: cannot intubate, cannot oxygenate; SAD: supraglottic airway device)

Even if adequate oxygenation and ventilation can be provided with the LMA, the clinician must remember that this is not a definitive airway as the patient's airway is not protected from secretions, aspiration, blood, or mass lesions such as expanding hematomas. The LMA should only be used temporarily to provide oxygen while preparing to establish a definitive airway **(Figs. 7 and 8)**.

Predictors of difficult supraglottic airway:

- Restricted mouth opening
- Obstruction
- Distorted/disrupted airway
- Stiff lungs/c-spine restricted

NEEDLE CRICOTHYROTOMY

If the clinician is unable to perform tracheal intubation and cannot provide oxygen via the LMA, or mask front of neck access should be attempted and provided emergently via needle cricothyrotomy.

Predictors of Difficult Needle Cricothyroidotomy (Box 2)

- Previous surgery
- Obesity
- Radiation
- Trauma
- Hematoma.

Flowchart 2: All India Difficult Airway Association (AIDAA) guidelines for tracheal intubation in ICU.

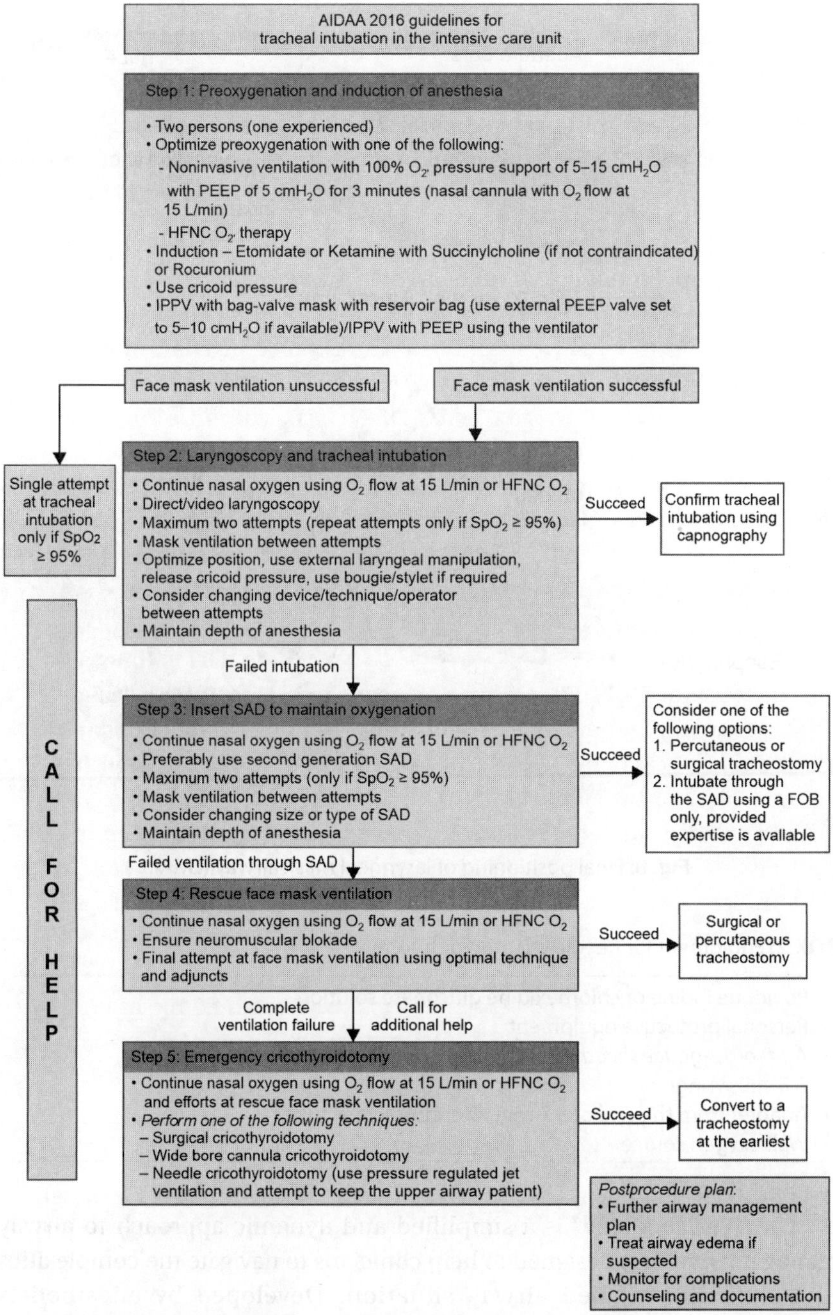

(FOB: fiberoptic bronchoscope; HFNC: high-flow nasal cannula; IPPV: intermittent positive pressure ventilation; O_2: oxygen; PEEP: positive end-expiratory pressure; SAD: supraglottic airway device; SpO_2: oxygen saturation)

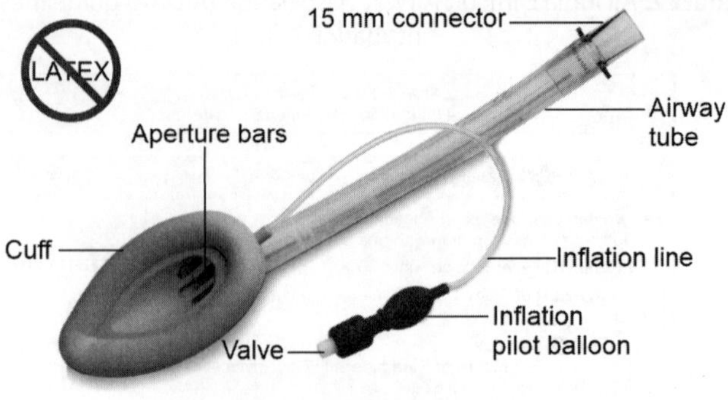

Fig. 7: Laryngeal mask airway.

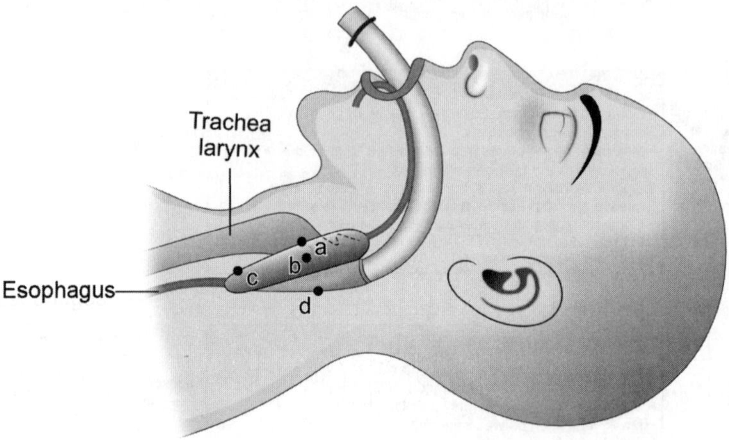

Fig. 8: Final positioning of laryngeal mask airway (LMA).

BOX 2: Equipment for needle cricothyroidotomy.

- Povidone iodine or chlorhexidine gluconate solution
- Personal protective equipment
- *A 14- or 12-gauge sheathed needle catheter:* 12-gauge is best
- A 3-mL syringe
- Adapter from the end of a 7-mm ID endotracheal tube
- Wall oxygen source

The *"Vortex Model"* is a simplified and dynamic approach to airway management that is designed to help clinicians to navigate the complexities of a difficult or failed airway situation. Developed by anesthetists Dr Nicholas Chrimes and Dr Peter Fritz, the Vortex model emphasizes rapid decision-making and coordinated use of available airway tools, prioritizing patient's oxygenation over fixation on any specific intubation technique **(Fig. 9)**.

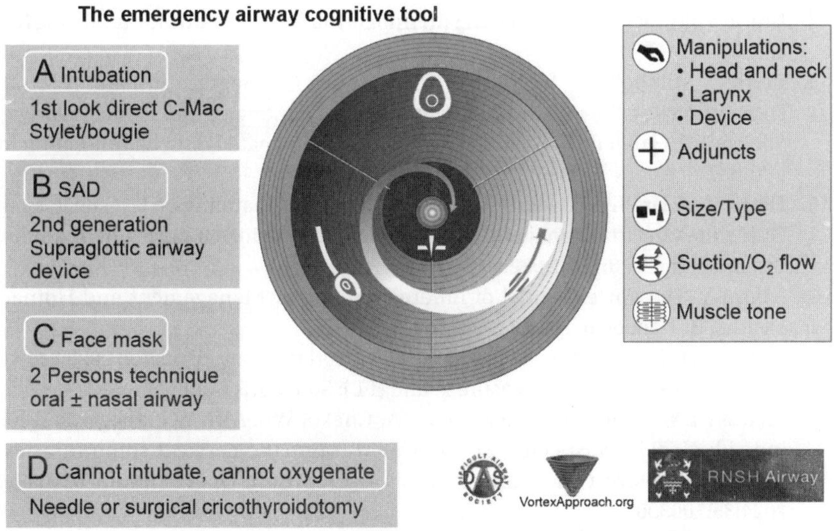

Fig. 9: The Vortex model of emergency airway management.
(SAD: supraglottic airway device)

At its core, the model provides a cognitive aid for managing airway crises by focusing on the simultaneous use of three nonsurgical airway techniques—(1) mask ventilation, (2) supraglottic airway devices (e.g., laryngeal mask airway), and (3) endotracheal intubation—while ensuring that providers maintain situational awareness and preparedness for a "cannot intubate, cannot oxygenate" (CICO) scenario, where surgical intervention might be necessary.

SUMMARY

A difficult airway occurs when securing or maintaining a patient's airway is challenging, particularly during intubation or ventilation. It can result from anatomical factors (e.g., obesity, facial trauma, airway tumors) or physiological limitations (e.g., limited neck mobility). Key assessment tools include the Mallampati classification and thyromental distance. Management involves preparing equipment (e.g., video laryngoscopes, supraglottic devices) and following algorithms like the ASA difficult airway algorithm. In severe cases, cricothyrotomy may be necessary. Failure to manage a difficult airway can lead to hypoxia, aspiration, airway trauma, or death, making early recognition and a systematic approach essential.

SUGGESTED READING

1. Apfelbaum JL, Hagberg CA, Connis RT, Abdelmalak BB, Agarkar M, Dutton RP, et al. 2022 American Society of Anesthesiologists Practice Guidelines for Management of the Difficult Airway. Anesthesiology. 2022;136:31-81.
2. Benumof JL. Laryngeal Mask Airway and the ASA Difficult Airway Algorithm. Anesthesiology. 1996;84:686-99.

3. Crawley SM, Dalton AJ. Predicting the difficult airway. BJA Education. 2015;15(5): 253-7.
4. Frerk C, Mitchell VS, McNarry AF, Mendonca C, Bhagrath R, Patel A, et al. Difficult Airway Society intubation guidelines working group. Difficult Airway Society 2015 guidelines for management of unanticipated difficult intubation in adults. Br J Anaesth. 2015;115(6):827-48.
5. Higgs A, McGrath BA, Goddard C, Rangasami J, Suntharalingam G, Gale R, et al. Guidelines for the management of tracheal intubation in critically ill adults. Br J Anaesth. 2018;120(2):323-52.
6. Lang SA. The Vortex Model of Emergency Airway Management and Human Factors. Br J Anaesth. 2016;117:el_14119.
7. McKenna P, Desai NM, Tariq A, Morley EJ. Cricothyrotomy. [Updated 2023 Feb 4]. In: StatPearls [Internet]. Treasure Island (FL): StatPearls Publishing; 2024.
8. Melesse DY, Tesema TT, Mekonnen ZA, Chekol WB. Airway management for individuals with suspected or confirmed traumatic cervical spine injuries: A comprehensive review and analysis. Periop Care Operat Room Manage. 2024;35:100390.
9. Myatra SN, Ahmed SM, Kundra P, Garg R, Ramkumar V, Patwa A, et al. The All India Difficult Airway Association 2016 guidelines for tracheal intubation in the Intensive Care Unit. Indian J Anaesth. 2016;60(12):922-30.
10. Myatra SN, Divatia JV, Brewster DJ. The physiologically difficult airway: an emerging concept. Curr Opin Anaesthesiol. 2022;35(2):115-21.
11. Rahiman SN, Keane M. Ramped Position: What the "Neck"! Chest. 2018;153(2): 567-8.

CHAPTER

6 Mechanical Ventilation

Harsh Parikh

INTRODUCTION

Mechanical ventilators push air during inspiration and release it during expiration, with a compressor, inspiratory valve, and expiratory valve.

INDICATION

The primary indications for invasive mechanical ventilation can be divided into the following categories:

- *Airway disease of compromise:*
  - Airway protection in a patient who is obtunded or has a dynamic airway, e.g., from trauma or oropharyngeal infection.
  - Airways obstruction is either proximal (e.g., angioedema) or distal (asthmatic bronchospasm or acute exacerbation of chronic obstructive pulmonary disease).
- *Hypoventilation:* Due to impaired drive, pump failure, or inability to exchange gases resulting in hypercapnic respiratory failure. The etiology can be divided into the following subcategories:
  - Impaired central drive (e.g., drug overdose)
  - Respiratory muscle weakness (e.g., muscular dystrophy and myositis)
  - Peripheral nervous system defects (e.g., Guillain-Barré syndrome or myasthenia crisis)
  - Restrictive ventilatory defects (e.g., chest wall trauma or disease or massive pneumothorax or effusion)
- *Hypoxemic respiratory failure:* Due to the inability to exchange oxygen or delivery to the peripheral tissues due to one of the following reasons:
  - Alveolar filling defects [e.g., pneumonia, acute respiratory distress syndrome (ARDS), or pulmonary edema]
  - Pulmonary vascular defects leading to ventilation-perfusion (V/Q) mismatch (massive pulmonary embolism or air emboli)
  - Diffusion defects (advanced pulmonary fibrosis)
- Increased ventilatory demand due to severe sepsis, shock, or severe metabolic acidosis.

TERMINOLOGY

- *Trigger:* The signal to start inspiration. It will open inspiratory valve and close expiratory valve. It is either ventilator triggered (after fix *time*) or patient triggered (sensed by *pressure* or *flow*).
- *Limit:* It implies that set limit cannot be overcome. It is either *flow* limited or *pressure* limited.
- *Cycling:* It is the signal that stops inspiration and start expiration. Inspiratory valve shuts after the set inspiratory *time* has elapsed or the set *volume* is delivered.
  - *Mandatory breath:* Triggered, limited, and cycled by ventilator.
  - *Assisted breath:* Triggered by patient, limited, and cycled by ventilator.
  - *Spontaneous breath:* Triggered and cycled by patient.

MODES

- Control modes (volume and pressure controlled) are for patients with high-dose sedatives/neuromuscular relaxants medicines, and severe disease. In this mode, ventilator will deliver *mandatory breath* irrespective of whether the patient will breathe or not. Ventilator will block any spontaneous breaths. It rests muscles of respiration. It needs high sedation/paralysis of respiratory muscle.
  - *Volume control ventilation (VCV):* Time triggered, flow limited, and volume cycled.

  Preset tidal volume is assured at a cost of potentially high-airway pressure.
  - *Pressure control ventilation (PCV):* Time triggered, pressure limited, and time cycled.

  Harmful high pressures are avoided at a cost of potentially hypoventilation.
- Assist control (A/C) mode (volume and pressure assist controlled) means that in addition to mandatory breath delivered by controlled mode, ventilator is capable of sensing patient's inspiratory effort and deliver *assisted breath.* It reduced work of breathing.
- Hyperventilation can occur if patient has increased respiratory rate.
- *Pressure support ventilation (PSV):* Patient triggered, pressure limited, and flow cycled.

  Patient initiates breath and ventilator delivers a *spontaneous breath* through preset inspiratory pressure to help to overcome airway resistance and keeps airways open. The patient controls the respiration rate, tidal volume, and minute ventilation. Tidal volume is variable and depends on lung compliance and resistance. If the patient does not begin a breath, no breaths are delivered. It is a weaning mode.

- *Other modes:*
  - Pressure-regulated volume control (PRVC) is a mode of ventilation in which the ventilator attempts to achieve set tidal volume at the lowest possible airway pressure.
  - *Synchronized intermittent mandatory ventilation (SIMV):* Patients can take own breaths with their own tidal volume between mechanically assisted breaths. It can lead to respiratory muscle fatigue. It is a weaning mode.
  - *Continuous positive airway pressure (CPAP):* Positive airway pressure provided during both inspiration and expiration. It is a weaning mode.

INITIAL SETTINGS

Table 1 shows initial ventilator setting in different clinical scenarios.

ALARMS OF VENTILATION

No alarm should be switched off without a problem being identified.

- *High pressure limit:* Limit set around 35–40 cmH_2O.
  It will be activated in secretion, coughing, gagging, patient fighting ventilator, condensate in tubing, kinked or compressed tubing, increased resistance (bronchospasm), and decreased compliance (pulmonary edema and pneumothorax).
- *Low pressure limit:* Set at 50% of patient's average minute ventilation.
  It will be activated in total or partial disconnect, endotracheal tube (ETT)/tracheal tube (TT) cuff leak, and total or partial extubation.
- *Apnea alarm:* Can be kept at 20 seconds.
  It will be activated in respiratory arrest, over sedation, and extubation of ET/TT tube.
- *Low O_2 concentration alarm:* When FiO_2 falls below set value. Indicates issue with O_2 supply.

ADDITIONAL CARE

- Once tracheal tube is placed properly, begin with manual ventilation with AMBU bag, place on mechanical ventilator after checking correct placement of ET tube.
- Check for the airway pressure, SO_2, end-tidal carbon dioxide ($ETCO_2$), blood pressure, and chest X-ray.
- Check arterial blood gas (ABG) after 15–20 minutes.
- Patient will be needed to start necessary sedation, antigastritis medicine, deep venous thrombosis (DVT) prophylaxis, eye care, mouth care, and infection control measure.
- Attach heat and moisture exchangers (HME) for humidification.

TABLE 1: Initial ventilator setting in different clinical scenarios.

Indication	*Mode*	*Respiratory rate (breaths/ minute)*	*Tidal volume (mL/kg of ideal body weight)*	*FiO_2 (wean as per ABG)*	*PEEP**	*Additional ventilator settings*	*Comments*
Airway protection	ACV, PCV, and PRVC	12–14	8–10	100%, target $SpO_2 > 92\%$	5	Pressure limit: 40, trigger-flow, peak flow rate: 60 L/min, I:E**: 1:1.5–2	Maintain till issue resolves
Asthma exacerbation	ACV	8–12	6–8	100%, target $SpO_2 > 92\%$	0–5	High peak flow rate, trigger-flow-2,I:E: 1:2–3	Monitor for auto PEEP, accept mild hypercarbia
COPD exacerbation	ACV	8–12	6–8	100%, target SpO_2—90%	0–5	High peak flow rate, trigger-flow, I:E: 1:2–3, trigger-flow: 2 L/min	Apply external PEEP to treat auto PEEP, accept mild hypercarbia
Pneumonia/ pulmonary edema	ACV/PRVC	16–24	6–8	100%	5–10 as per PaO_2	I:E: 1–1.5, trigger-flow-2 L/min	Secretion management
ALI/ARDS	ACV/PRVC	16–24	6	100%	5–15 as per PaO_2	I:E: 1:1, trigger-flow-2 L/min	Sedation, monitor for barotrauma
Postoperative	ACV/PRVC	10–16	8–10	100%	5	I:E: 1:1.5, trigger-flow-2	Rapid wean

*Positive end-expiratory pressure: PEEP is used to increase the functional residual capacity and keep open collapsable alveoli, thus reducing atelectatic trauma.
**Ratio of inspiratory time: expiratory time (I:E) ratio: In normal, spontaneous breath expiratory time is about twice as long as inspiratory time.
(ABG: arterial blood gas; ACV: assist control ventilation; ALI: acute lung injury; ARDS: acute respiratory distress syndrome; COPD: chronic obstructive pulmonary disease; PCV: pressure control ventilation; PEEP: positive end-expiratory pressure; PRVC: pressure-regulated volume control)

- Position of the patient at least 30° head up, with change of position every 2nd hourly bilaterally.
- Patient will be placed on air mattress to prevent pressure sore.
- Suctioning of ET/TT as and when needed with either closed suction system or blunt tip suction catheter with sterile precautions.

VENTILATOR MANIPULATION

When in any doubt about adequacy of mechanical ventilator, manually ventilate the patient with an AMBU bag with the maximum available O_2.

- *Hypoxemia:*
  - Increase fraction of inspired oxygen (FiO_2)
  - Increase positive end-expiratory pressure (PEEP)
  - Increase inspiratory time
- *Hypercarbia:*
  - Increase respiratory rate
  - Increase tidal volume
  - Reduce dead space of circuit
- *Anxious patient:* Properly sedate/paralyze the patient.

COMPLICATIONS

- Ventilator-induced lung injury (VILI)—in ARDS patient, ventilator leads to inflammation through barotrauma/volutrauma.
- *Auto-PEEP:* Air trapping in lung. In severe asthma/COPD patient. It can be reduced by prolong expiratory time.
- *Hypotension and low cardiac output:* Through reduced venous return and reduced left ventricular (LV) filling.
- *Prevention of ventilation-associated infection (VAP):* Any new lung infection after 48 hours of starting mechanical ventilator. It can be prevented by following VAP bundle.
- *Diaphragm atrophy:* Due to controlled ventilation. Early weaning should be done to prevent it.
- *Impaired mucociliary motility:* Due to positive pressure ventilation will lead to VAP.
- *Pneumothorax/subcutaneous emphysema:* Due to barotrauma.

PREVENTION OF VENTILATION-ASSOCIATED INFECTION

- Insert ET/TT with subglottic suction catheter
- Keep cuff pressure around 25 cmH_2O
- Head up position 30°
- Peptic ulcer prophylaxis
- Good oral hygiene with chlorhexidine
- Daily sedation assessment and spontaneous breathing trial

- Deep vein thrombosis (DVT) prophylaxis
- Change of position 2nd hourly each side.

WEANING OF VENTILATOR

- Weaning is the process of liberation from, or discontinuation of, mechanical ventilatory support.
- *Weaning can be considered once:*
    - The underlying process necessitating mechanical ventilation is resolving.
    - PaO_2/FiO_2 >150 on FiO_2 <40% and PEEP <5 cmH_2O
    - pH >7.25
    - Hemodynamic stable
    - Able to initiate an inspiratory effort
    - Awake and alert
    - Core temperature <38°C
    - Hb >7 g/dL

Classification of weaning by duration:

- "Simple"—ventilator discontinued after the first assessment.
- "Difficult"—ventilator discontinued from 2 to 7 days after initial assessment.
- "Prolonged"—ventilator discontinued in >7 days after initial assessment.

FIRST RISK ASSESSMENT CHECKLIST: TOLERANCE FOR SPONTANEOUS BREATHING TRIAL (FLOWCHART 1)

Spontaneous breathing for 30 minutes through ventilator with "flow trigger" mode rate set to 0, PSV set to 0, PEEP 5 cmH_2O, or a T-piece trial.

The following seven items are checked to judge the successful spontaneous breathing trial (SBT).

1. Respiratory rate (RR) >35 breaths/min for 5 minutes or more
2. Rapid shallow breathing index (RSBI) >100 cycles/min/L [RSBI—ratio of respiratory rate to tidal volume (f/VT)]
3. SaO_2 < 90% for 5 minutes or more
4. Heart rate (HR) >120 beats/min, or sustained increase 20% greater than baseline.
5. Systolic blood pressure <90 mm Hg or >180 mm Hg for 5 minutes or more
6. Emergence of a chest pain or a new electrocardiogram change
7. Dyspnea, increased anxiety, and diaphoresis

Next, judge the patients' eligibility for extubation if they do not meet at least one of these seven criteria. If they meet at least one of these seven criteria, they are rested on mechanical ventilation until the next morning and rechecked the next day.

Flowchart 1: First risk assessment checklist: Tolerance for spontaneous breathing trial (SBT).

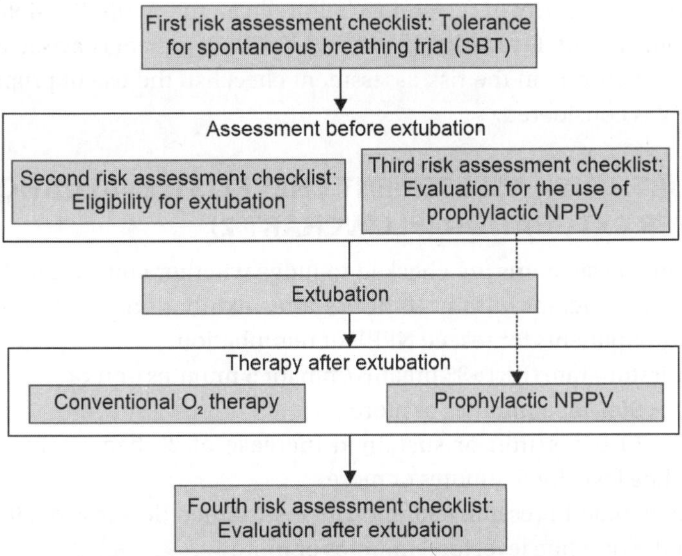

(NPPV: noninvasive positive-pressure ventilation)

SECOND RISK ASSESSMENT CHECKLIST: ELIGIBILITY FOR EXTUBATION

The following seven items are checked to judge the eligibility of patients for extubation.

1. No severe disturbance in level of consciousness (e.g., ability to protect the airway)
2. Presence of cough reflex
3. Presence of gag reflex
4. Stable cardiovascular system (e.g., HR <120 beats/min, no ischemic changes on electrocardiogram; and no severe cardiac arrhythmia)
5. Respiratory rate <35 breaths/min
6. Rapid shallow breathing index <100 breaths/min/L
7. Presence of cuff leak

Patients are extubated if they satisfy all of the above criteria. If they do not, mechanical ventilation is continued, and items in this checklist are rechecked the next day.

THIRD RISK ASSESSMENT CHECKLIST: EVALUATION FOR THE USE OF PROPHYLACTIC NONINVASIVE POSITIVE-PRESSURE VENTILATION

The following three items are checked for the use of prophylactic noninvasive positive-pressure ventilation (NPPV).

1. Age >65 years
2. Cardiac failure as the reason for intubation
3. Increased severity of respiratory failure [e.g., the Acute Physiology and Chronic Health Evaluation (APACHE) II >12]. If patients have at least one of three criteria in the risk assessment checklist, the use of prophylactic NPPV is considered.

FOURTH RISK ASSESSMENT CHECKLIST: EVALUATION AFTER EXTUBATION (FLOWCHART 2)

The following six items are checked to judge whether conventional oxygen therapy is sufficient within 48 hours after extubation and to judge the eligibility of patients for rescue NPPV or reintubation.

1. Respiratory rate (RR) >35 breaths/min for 5 minutes or more
2. SpO_2 < 90% for 5 minutes or more
3. HR >120 beats/min or sustained increase of 20 beats/min over the baseline level for 5 minutes or more
4. Systolic blood pressure <90 mm Hg or sustained decrease of 30 mm Hg over the baseline level for 5 minutes or more

Flowchart 2: Difficult Airway Society (DAS) extubation guidelines: "At risk" algorithm.

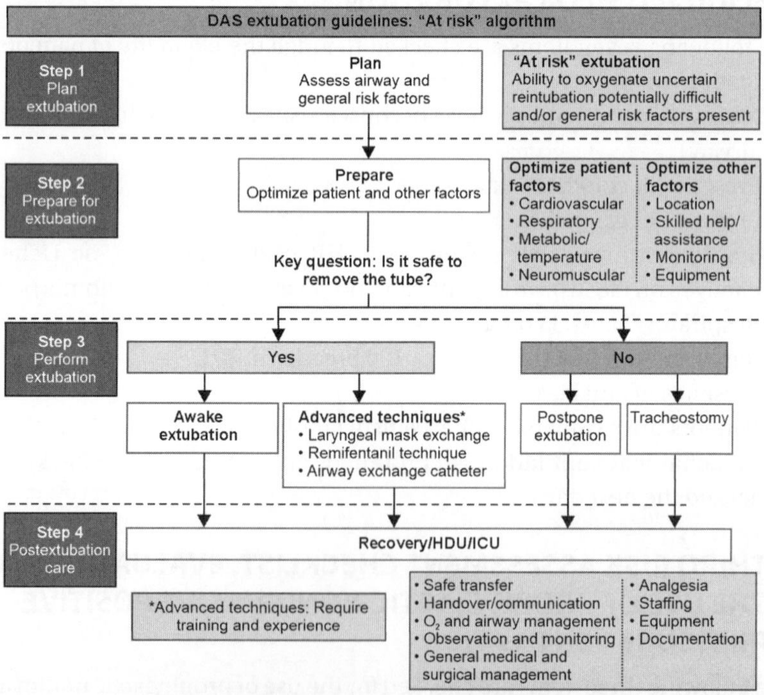

(HDU: high dependency unit; ICU: intensive care unit)

5. Chest pain or electrocardiographic abnormalities (emergence of ischemic changes or arrhythmia)
6. Dyspnea, increased anxiety, and diaphoresis.

Patients who meet at least one of these six criteria are adjudged as requiring ventilatory assistance. Eligibility and contraindications for rescue use of NPPV are evaluated. Rescue NPPV is initiated if indicates; if not, tracheal intubation is performed.

MANAGEMENT TO AVOID DELAYED WEANING

Optimize Respiratory Muscle Power

- Nutrition
- Avoid neuromuscular blocking drugs, decrease steroid use and other contributors to critical illness—induced weakness.
- Encourage spontaneous breathing but avoid exhaustion.
- Normal electrolytes
- Normal functional residual capacity (FRC)
- Physiotherapy

Decrease Respiratory Work

- Sit up
- *Decrease respiratory demand:*
    - *Decrease CO_2:* Treat pyrexia, treat agitation, avoid overfeeding, and minimize dead space.
    - Correct metabolic acidosis.
- *Decrease resistance:* Large, short diameter ETT, treat disease, and decrease work of breathing (WOB).
- *Increase compliance:* Treat lung disease; decrease abdominal distension (chest wall factors are not usually reversible.).

Optimize Ventilatory Drive

- Stop sedation.
- Consider causes from the brain to the neuromuscular junction.

Increase Oxygenation and Carrying Capacity

- Sit up and avoid atelectasis.
- Correct anemia.
- Correct acid-base disturbance (shift in Hb-O_2 dissociation curve).

Address Cardiac Dysfunction

- Removal of positive pressure ventilation (PPV) may unmask left ventricular (LV) dysfunction.
- Treat ischemia.

Address Sputum Clearance

- Treat infection, chest physiotherapy, suction, and bronchoscopy.
- Mucolytics are controversial.

SUMMARY

A mechanical ventilator fully or partially substitutes the ventilatory work done by the patient.

All modes of mechanical ventilation help to ventilate and oxygenate patients, supporting gas exchange until the underlying abnormality resolves.

Mechanical ventilation setting must be done as per disease.

Alarm must be set before initiating mechanical ventilation.

Prevention of secondary infection should be practiced from beginning of mechanical ventilation.

Mechanical ventilation should be weaned as per standard protocol.

SUGGESTED READING

1. Hickey S, Giva A. (2023). Mechanical Ventilation. National Library of Medicine. [online] Available from: https://www.ncbi.nlm.nih.gov/books/NBK539742/ [Last accessed July, 2024].
2. Isakow W. Initial Ventilator Setup. In: Kollef M (Ed). The Washington Manual of Critical Care, 3rd edition. Gurugram, Haryana: Wolters Kluwer India Pvt Ltd.; 2018. pp. 47-53.
3. Kapadia F, Sharma R, Jare J. Mechanical Ventilation. In: Chaudhary D, Dixit S, Govil D (Eds). ISCCM Textbook of Critical Care Medicine. New Delhi: Jaypee Brothers Medical Publishers (P) Ltd.; 2023. pp. 217, 222.
4. Nickson C. (2019). Weaning from Mechanical Ventilation. Life in the Fastlane. [online] Available from https://litfl.com/weaning-from-mechanical-ventilation/ [Last accessed July, 2024].
5. Nitta K, Okamoto K, Imamura H, Mochizuki K, Takayama H, Kamijo H, et al. A comprehensive protocol for ventilator weaning and extubation: a prospective observational study. J Intensive Care. 2019;7:50.

SECTION 3

Pulmonary Disorders

CHAPTER

7

Community-acquired Pneumonia

Poorva Dilip Magarkar

INTRODUCTION

Community-acquired pneumonia (CAP) is defined as an acute infection of lung parenchyma acquired outside hospital or healthcare facilities. It is one of the leading causes of hospitalization and death in all age groups. Its causes include bacteria, viruses, fungi, and parasites. Patients with underlying illnesses such as chronic obstructive pulmonary disease (COPD), tobacco smoking, Alzheimer's disease, diabetes, alcoholics, cystic fibrosis, and immune system problems have an increased risk of developing pneumonia.

ETIOLOGY

The pathogens causing CAP can be classified as:

- *Typical agents: Streptococcus pneumoniae, Haemophilus influenzae, Moraxella catarrhalis, Staphylococcus aureus,* Group A Streptococci, anaerobes, and gram-negative organisms.
- *Atypical agents: Legionella, Mycoplasma, Chlamydia pneumoniae,* and respiratory viruses: Severe acute respiratory syndrome coronavirus 2 (SARS-CoV-2) [Coronavirus disease 2019 (COVID-19)], influenza A and B, rhinovirus, respiratory syncytial virus, human metapneumovirus, adenovirus 4 and 7, and parainfluenza virus.
- *Other rare CAP pathogens:*
  - Viruses:
    - Coxsackievirus
    - Echovirus
    - Other coronaviruses [Middle East respiratory syndrome (MERS)-CoV, SARS]
    - Hantavirus
    - Epstein–Barr virus
    - Cytomegalovirus
    - Herpes simplex virus
    - Human herpesvirus 6
    - Varicella-zoster virus
    - Metapneumovirus

- Bacteria:
  - *Chlamydophila psittaci* (psittacosis)
  - *Coxiella burnetii* (Q fever)
  - *Francisella tularensis* (tularemia)
- Mycobacteria:
  - *Mycobacterium* tuberculosis
  - Nontuberculous mycobacteria (uncommon)
- Endemic fungi (cause subacute or chronic pneumonia):
  - *Pneumocystis jirovecii*
  - *Aspergillus* species
  - *Mucorales* species
  - *Histoplasma* species
  - *Cryptococcus* species
  - *Blastomyces* species
  - *Coccidioides* species

- *Parasites: Strongyloides stercoralis, Toxoplasma gondii*

PATHOPHYSIOLOGY

Pathogens reach the alveoli by means of microaspiration (aspiration of small quantity of oropharyngeal secretions), inhalation, macroaspiration (aspiration of a large quantity of oropharyngeal or gastric contents), or hematogenous spread. If pathogens overcome the alveolar defense mechanisms, they will multiply and will cause tissue injury and damage the lung. The local and systemic inflammatory responses constitute a physiologic response to lung infection. In some patients, the initial systemic inflammatory response can become dysregulated and cause tissue injury and organ dysfunction.

SYMPTOMS AND SIGNS

Symptoms include malaise, fever, chills, rigor, cough, shortness of breath, and chest pain. Cough is usually productive in older children and adults and dry in infants, young children, and older adults. Dyspnea usually is mild and exertional. Chest pain is pleuritic and is adjacent to the infected area. Pneumonia may present as upper abdominal pain due to lower lobe infection causing irritation of the diaphragm. Gastrointestinal symptoms nausea, vomiting, and diarrhea are also common.

Symptoms vary at the extremes of age and immunocompromised patients. Infection in infants may manifest as nonspecific irritability and restlessness. In older adults, the infection may manifest as confusion, slowing of activities, and obtundation. Fever can be absent.

Pneumonia can cause acute decompensation of underlying chronic illness like congestive heart failure, which confound the presentation and result in delay for diagnosis and treatment.

Characteristic pulmonary findings on physical examination include the following: Tachypnea, rales heard over the involved lobe or segment, increased tactile fremitus, bronchial breath sounds, and egophony, if consolidation is present. Decreased tactile fremitus, and dullness on chest percussion may result from parapneumonic effusion or empyema.

DIAGNOSIS AND EVALUATION

Historical clues and physical examination findings may suggest a causative pathogen, but the symptoms and clinical signs are not sufficient to reliably differentiate the exact etiologic agent. Therefore, additional testing are necessary to identify the pathogen and to optimize therapy.

Routine diagnostic workup include the following:

- Complete blood count
- Renal function tests
- Serum electrolytes
- Liver function test
- C-reactive protein (CRP)
- *Blood culture:* Especially important in immunodeficient patients.
- Sputum culture
- *Urinary antigens:* Available for *Streptococcus pneumoniae* and *Legionella*.
- *Polymerase chain reaction (PCR):* Commercially available PCR assays can detect most important respiratory viruses and atypical bacteria.
- *Bronchoscopy:* Useful in immunocompromised host.
- *Thoracentesis:* Usually not required in uncomplicated parapneumonic effusion. If it fails to resolve or gets infected and develops into fibropurulent stage which requires drainage.
- *Open lung biopsy:* It is the last resort in patients who deteriorate and etiology is unclear or in patients with failure of treatment.
- *Imaging:*
    - *Chest X-ray (CXR):* Presence of a new infiltrate.
    - *Computed tomography thorax:* It is the gold standard. It gives accurate information about lung parenchyma and mediastinum which helps in diagnosis and also about complications. It helps exclude other noninfectious diagnosis such as atelectasis, pulmonary infarction, interstitial lung disease, and tumor that may appear similar on CXR. Identifies fungal pneumonia or pneumonia caused by mycobacteria.
    - *Ultrasound:* It has good sensitivity of 94% and specificity of 96% in the diagnosis of pneumonia. But, it has slow learning curve and there is interoperator variability.

CRITERIA TO ASSESS SEVERITY OF COMMUNITY-ACQUIRED PNEUMONIA

Objective criteria are required to stratify the patient for management such as outpatient versus inpatient. These criteria do not replace the clinical judgment. Multiple scoring systems are available to assess the severity of CAP **(Table 1)**.

TREATMENT (TABLES 2 TO 4)

Adequate empiric antimicrobial therapy for CAP includes coverage for *S. pneumoniae* and atypical bacterial pathogens.

TABLE 1: Multiple scoring systems to assess the severity of CAP.

Pneumonia severity index (PSI): It consists of 20 variables. PSI is complex and requires several laboratory assessments. Patients are categorized into five strata (I–V) with increasing risk of mortality	• *Class (I–III):* Mortality is <1% • *Class IV:* 9% mortality • *Class V:* 27% mortality • *PSI I–II:* Can be treated at home • *PSI III:* Needs to be observed in emergency room till further decision • *PSI IV–V group:* Recommended for hospitalization
CURB-65: Proposed by the British Thoracic Society (BTS) to predict mortality Scores with mortality rate (%): • Score 0: 0.7% • Score 1: 3.2% • Score 2: 3% • Score 3: 17% • Score 4: 41.5% • Score 5: 57%	• C: Confusion • U: Urea >7 mmol/L (= BUN >19 mg/dL) • R: Respiratory rate ≥30 breaths/min • Blood pressure: Systolic pressure <90 mm Hg or diastolic pressure ≤60 mm Hg • 65: age ≥65 years • Score range from 0 to 5. Require ICU admission, if CURB-65 score = 4 or 5
The CRB-65	Simplified version of CURB-65 does not include blood urea. Applicable for outpatient clinics
SMART-COP: Score of 3 or more points identifies 92% of those who will require intensive respiratory support	• Systolic arterial pressure <90 mm Hg • Multilobar involvement on chest X-ray (CXR) • Albumin level <35 g/L • Respiratory rate—50 years and younger: ≥25 breaths/min, older than 50 years: ≥30 breaths/min • Tachycardia (≥125 beats/min) • New onset confusion • *Oxygen level:* 50 years and younger: PaO_2 <70 mm Hg • Oxygen saturation ≤93%, or PaO_2/FiO_2 ratio <333 • *Older than 50 years:* PaO_2 <60 mm Hg, oxygen saturation ≤90%, or PaO_2/FiO_2 ratio <250 • Arterial pH <7.35

Contd...

Contd...

IDSA/ATS criteria for severe CAP: Includes major and minor criteria. One major plus three minor signifies patient has severe CAP	*Major criteria:* • Dependence on mechanical ventilation • Septic shock that requires vasopressors *Minor criteria:* • Respiratory rate >30 breaths/min • PaO_2/FiO_2 ratio <250 • Multilobar infiltrates • Confusion/disorientation • Uremia (BUN level >20 mg/dL) • Leukopenia (WBC count <4,000 cells/mm^3) • Thrombocytopenia (platelet count <100,000 cells/mm^3)
	Hypothermia (core temperature <36°C)
	Hypotension requiring aggressive fluid resuscitation

(ATS: American Thoracic Society; BUN: blood urea nitrogen; CAP: community-acquired pneumonia; IDSA: Infectious Diseases Society of America; WBC: white blood cell)

TABLE 2: Initial treatment strategies for outpatients with community-acquired pneumonia.

Without comorbidities or risk factors	*With comorbidities such as diabetes, chronic heart, lung, liver, or renal disease, alcoholism, malignancy or asplenia*
• Amoxicillin 1 g three times daily (strong recommendation, moderate quality of evidence) • Doxycycline 100 mg twice daily (conditional recommendation, low quality of evidence) • Macrolide (azithromycin 500 mg on first day then 250 mg daily or clarithromycin 500 mg twice daily or clarithromycin extended release 1,000 mg daily) only in areas with pneumococcal resistance to macrolides <25% (conditional recommendation, moderate quality of evidence)	• *Combination therapy:* – Amoxicillin/clavulanate 500 mg/125 mg three times daily, *or* amoxicillin/clavulanate 875 mg/125 mg twice daily, *or* 2,000 mg/125 mg twice daily, *or* a cephalosporin (cefpodoxime 200 mg twice daily or cefuroxime 500 mg twice daily) – Macrolide (azithromycin 500 mg on first day then 250 mg daily), clarithromycin (500 mg twice daily or extended release 1,000 mg once daily) (strong recommendation, moderate quality of evidence for combination therapy), *or* doxycycline 100 mg twice daily (conditional recommendation, low quality of evidence for combination therapy) • *Monotherapy:* – Respiratory fluoroquinolone (levofloxacin 750 mg daily, moxifloxacin 400 mg daily, or gemifloxacin 320 mg daily) (strong recommendation, moderate quality of evidence)

TABLE 3: Nonsevere inpatient pneumonia.

Standard regimen	• *Combination therapy:* β-lactam (ampicillin + sulbactam 1.5–3 g every 6 hours, cefotaxime 1–2 g every 8 hours, ceftriaxone 1–2 g daily, or ceftaroline 600 mg every 12 hours) and macrolide (azithromycin 500 mg daily or clarithromycin 500 mg twice daily) (strong recommendation, high quality of evidence) • *Monotherapy:* Respiratory fluoroquinolone (levofloxacin 750 mg daily, moxifloxacin 400 mg daily) (strong recommendation, high quality of evidence)
Prior respiratory isolation of MRSA	*MRSA coverage needed:* Obtain cultures/nasal PCR to confirm need for therapy or de-escalation vancomycin (15 mg/kg every 12 hours, adjust based on levels) or linezolid (600 mg every 12 hours)
Prior respiratory isolation of *Pseudomonas aeruginosa*	• *P. aeruginosa* coverage needed • Obtain cultures to confirm need for therapy or de-escalation • Piperacillin-tazobactam (4.5 g every 6 hours), cefepime (2 g every 8 hours), ceftazidime (2 g every 8 hours), imipenem (500 mg every 6 hours), meropenem (1 g every 8 hours), or aztreonam (2 g every 8 hours)
Recent hospitalization and parenteral antibiotics and locally validated risk factors for MRSA	• Withhold MRSA coverage unless culture results are positive • Add coverage if PCR is positive and obtain cultures and withhold empiric therapy against MRSA, if rapid testing is negative
Recent hospitalization and parenteral antibiotics and locally validated risk factors for *P. aeruginosa*	Obtain cultures but start coverage for *P. aeruginosa* only if culture are positive

(MRSA: methicillin-resistant *Staphylococcus aureus;* PCR: polymerase chain reaction)

Treatment recommendations contain multiple antibiotic options without any preference order. The choice between these options requires a risk-benefit assessment for each individual patient and local epidemiological data.

Initial treatment strategies for inpatients with community-acquired pneumonia are given in **Tables 3 and 4**.

In patients with severe CAP or sepsis, antibiotics should be given within the first hour of onset of hypotension to reduce mortality.

The recommended duration of therapy is 5–7 days in patients with good clinical response such as the absence of fever for >48–72 hours, not requiring supplemental oxygen, and resolution of tachycardia, tachypnea, or hypotension. A 14-day therapy with macrolide or doxycycline will treat tularemia pneumonia or psittacosis. A 5-day therapy with oseltamivir is recommended for all patients who test positive for the influenza virus.

TABLE 4: Severe inpatient pneumonia.

Standard regimen	• β-lactam (ampicillin + sulbactam 1.5–3 g every 6 hours, cefotaxime 1–2 g every 8 hours, ceftriaxone 1–2 g daily, or ceftaroline 600 mg every 12 hours) and macrolide (azithromycin 500 mg daily or clarithromycin 500 mg twice daily) (strong recommendation, high quality of evidence) • β-lactam (ampicillin + sulbactam 1.5–3 g every 6 hours, cefotaxime 1–2 g every 8 hours, ceftriaxone 1–2 g daily, or ceftaroline 600 mg every 12 hours) and levofloxacin 750 mg daily or moxifloxacin 400 mg daily
Prior respiratory isolation of MRSA	• MRSA coverage needed • Obtain cultures/nasal PCR to confirm need for therapy or de-escalation vancomycin (15 mg/kg every 12 hours, adjust based on levels) or linezolid (600 mg every 12 hours)
Prior respiratory isolation of *Pseudomonas aeruginosa*	• *P. aeruginosa* coverage needed • Obtain cultures to confirm need for therapy or de-escalation • Piperacillin-tazobactam (4.5 g every 6 hours), cefepime (2 g every 8 hours), ceftazidime (2 g every 8 hours), imipenem (500 mg every 6 hours), meropenem (1 g every 8 hours), or aztreonam (2 g every 8 hours)
Recent hospitalization and parenteral antibiotics and locally validated risk factors for MRSA	Add MRSA coverage and obtain nasal PCR and cultures
Recent hospitalization and parenteral antibiotics and locally validated risk factors for *P. aeruginosa*	Add coverage for *P. aeruginosa* and obtain cultures

(MRSA: methicillin-resistant *Staphylococcus aureus;* PCR: polymerase chain reaction)

Prolonged therapy is indicated in patients with certain bacterial pathogens *Pseudomonas* (14–21 days), *S. aureus* (7–21 days), or *Legionella pneumonia* (14 days), a delayed response, and for complications such as empyema, lung abscess, or necrotizing pneumonia. Patients should be assessed on daily basis and treatment should be switched from intravenous (IV) to oral when they are improving clinically, stable hemodynamically, and are able to take oral medications.

Antiviral therapy is indicated for select viral pneumonias. For influenza, oseltamivir 75 mg orally twice a day or zanamivir 10 mg inhaled twice a day started within 48 hours of symptom onset. It is given for 5 days to reduce the duration and severity of symptoms in patients who develop influenza infection. In hospitalized patients with confirmed influenza infection, observational studies suggest benefit even 48 hours after symptom onset.

Follow-up X-rays are generally not recommended in patients whose pneumonia resolves clinically as expected. Resolution of radiographic abnormalities lag behind clinical resolution by several weeks. CXR to be considered in patients whose symptoms that do not resolve or that worsen over time.

COMMUNITY-ACQUIRED METHICILLIN-RESISTANT *STAPHYLOCOCCUS AUREUS*

This is an important cause of CAP with high mortality. Community-acquired methicillin-resistant *Staphylococcus aureus* (CA-MRSA) carries Panton-Valentine leukocidin (*PVL*) gene which is responsible for exotoxin production which promotes invasiveness and rapid progression of disease. It is usually preceded by "flu-like" illness or necrotizing skin infection. Patient presents with hemoptysis, diarrhea, vomiting, tachycardia, tachypnea, and hypotension. It is often complicated by severe necrotizing pneumonia, staphylococcal shock syndrome. Cavitation, pneumothorax, jaundice, empyema, acute renal failure, and pericarditis like complications are common in post-MRSA pneumonia. On investigations, they have multilobar infiltrates on CXR, effusions, and cavitation, leukopenia, markedly elevated CRP, creatinine kinase, and gram-positive cocci on sputum Gram stain.

Current evidence suggests linezolid as a drug of choice for CA-MRSA pneumonia as it suppresses exotoxin production. Clindamycin also suppress toxin production but there is emergence of resistance. Daptomycin cannot be used for CA-MRSA pneumonia because it is inactivated by lung surfactant. Depending upon the extent of infection, duration of treatment varies between 7 and 21 days. Cavitating pneumonia and lung abscess needs treatment for several weeks. Newer drugs such as ceftaroline (a fifth-generation cephalosporin) and ceftobiprole, and quinupristin-dalfopristin are available for CA-MRSA but evidence is scarce.

NONRESPONDING PNEUMONIA

It is a condition in which inadequate clinical response is observed despite antibiotic treatment. Patterns observed in nonresponding pneumonia (NRP) are:

- *Progressive NRP:* It is a clinical deterioration in patient's condition leading to acute respiratory failure and/or septic shock, within first 72 hours of admission.
- *Persistent NRP:* Absence of or delay in achieving clinical stability.
- *Nonresolving or slow resolving pneumonia:* Persistence of pulmonary infiltrates for >30 days after initial pneumonia.

Risk factors should be assessed for delayed resolution such as age, comorbidities, pneumonia severity, and specific pathogens. Following considerations should be kept in mind when pneumonia fails to resolve with usual treatment.

- Wrong identification of causative organism
- Correct organism but inappropriate antibiotic and dose
- Loculated infection (empyema)
- Resistant organisms
- Development of nosocomial pneumonia
- *Reconsider the etiology:* Tuberculosis, actinomyces or *Nocardia* species, polymicrobial
- *Metastatic infection:* Endocarditis, meningitis, septic arthritis, or deep abscess like splenic or renal abscess
- Obstruction (lung cancer, foreign body), postobstructive pneumonia
- Noninfectious causes
- *Concurrent infection:* Intravascular catheter, urinary, abdominal, and skin infections, particularly in ICU patients.

ROLE OF CORTICOSTEROIDS

The glucocorticoids used in the treatment of CAP is evolving, with recent evidence showing benefit of survival among severe CAP patients (who had been admitted to the ICU and had received mechanical ventilation) and who are at high risk for respiratory failure, treated with hydrocortisone at a dose of 200 mg daily initially, followed by a tapering dose. Glucocorticoids should be avoided in patients with influenza or aspergillus pneumonia.

PREVENTION OF COMMUNITY-ACQUIRED PNEUMONIA

The CAP may be prevented by treating underlying illnesses which increase its risk, by smoking cessation, and by vaccination. A vaccine against *S. pneumoniae*, available for adults, is recommended for healthy individuals over 65 and all adults with COPD, heart failure, diabetes mellitus, alcoholics, cirrhosis, increased risk of meningitis, or who have had a splenectomy. There are two vaccines available: PPSV 23 and PCV 13. In addition, vaccines against influenza and COVID-19, should be administered according to current Advisory Committee on Immunization Practices recommendations.

SUMMARY

Community-acquired pneumonia is one of the most common infection and is an important cause of morbidity and mortality. Disease presentation varies from a mild illness which can be managed as an outpatient to a severe illness requiring treatment in the intensive care unit. Diagnosing early and determining the appropriate level of care is important for improving outcome. Appropriate antibiotic stewardship principles, optimal antimicrobial selection, dosage, and duration will help to minimize resistance and adverse effects.

SUGGESTED READING

1. Metlay JP, Waterer GW, Long AC, Anzueto A, Brozek J, Crothers K, et al. Diagnosis and Treatment of Adults with Community-acquired Pneumonia. An Official Clinical Practice Guideline of the American Thoracic Society and Infectious Diseases Society of America. Am J Respir Crit Care Med. 2019;200(7):e45-67.
2. Regunath H, Oba Y. Community-Acquired Pneumonia. In: StatPearls [Internet]. Treasure Island (FL): StatPearls Publishing; 2024.
3. Thomas M File Jr, Ramirez JA. Community-acquired pneumonia. N Engl J Med. 2023;389(7):632-41.

CHAPTER 8

Acute Respiratory Distress Syndrome

Poorva Dilip Magarkar

INTRODUCTION

Acute respiratory distress syndrome (ARDS) has been widely recognized as a major clinical problem worldwide, with a high morbidity and mortality burden. ARDS was first described by Ashbaugh and Petty in 1967. It is recognized >50 years ago, and its definition has evolved over time **(Table 1)**, with a recent suggestion expanded to include intubated and nonintubated patients.

NEW DEFINITION

Three categories of ARDS are created to expand the current definition and retains essential components of the Berlin definition with minor modifications. The current time frame for the diagnosis of ARDS is retained. In addition, to chest radiography or computed tomography (CT), ultrasound accepted as a modality for identifying signs of loss of lung aeration consistent with (noncardiogenic) pulmonary edema or lung consolidation, especially when chest radiography or CT is not available. Ultrasound can be reliable, if the trained operator detects bilateral consolidations and noncardiogenic pulmonary edema, especially in resource-limited areas. This definition has created three categories of ARDS according to oxygenation, to expand the current definition **(Table 2)**.

PATHOGENESIS

The pathophysiology of ARDS is complex. Injury to both layers of the alveolar-capillary barrier is typical and contributes to the characteristic physiological abnormalities. Alveolar epithelial cells are of two types: Type I cells make up 90% of the alveolar epithelium, are injured easily. Damage to type I cells allows increased entry of fluid into the alveoli and decreased clearance of fluid from the alveolar space. Type II cells have important functions, the production of surfactant, ion transport, and proliferation and differentiation into type I cells after injury. Damage to type II cells results in impaired production of surfactant leading to decreased compliance and alveolar collapse.

Injury ranges from epithelial activation with expression of adhesion molecules and activation of proinflammatory and procoagulant pathways,

TABLE 1: Berlin criteria of AECC definition and Kigali modification.

	AECC definition	*Berlin criteria*	*Kigali modification of Berlin criteria*
Timing	Acute onset	Within 1 week of a known clinical insult or new or worsening respiratory symptoms	Within 1 week of a known clinical insult or new or worsening respiratory symptoms
Oxygenation	PaO_2/FiO_2 ≤200 mm Hg (defined as acute lung injury if ≤300 mm Hg)	• *Mild:* PaO_2/FiO_2 >200 ≤300 mm Hg • *Moderate:* PaO_2/FiO_2 >100 ≤200 mm Hg • *Severe:* PaO_2/FiO_2 ≤100 mm Hg	SpO_2/FiO_2 ≤315
PEEP requirement	None	Minimum 5 cmH_2O PEEP by invasive mechanical ventilation (noninvasive acceptable for mild ARDS)	No PEEP requirement, consistent with AECC definition
Chest imaging	Bilateral infiltrates seen on frontal chest radiograph	Bilateral opacities not fully explained by effusions, lobar/lung collapse or nodules by chest radiograph or CT	Bilateral opacities not fully explained by effusions, lobar/lung collapse or nodules by chest radiograph or ultrasound
Origin of edema	Pulmonary artery wedge pressure <18 mm Hg when measured or no evidence of left atrial hypertension	Respiratory failure not fully explained by cardiac failure or fluid overload (need objective assessment, such as echocardiography, to exclude hydrostatic edema)	Respiratory failure not fully explained by cardiac failure or fluid overload (need objective assessment, such as echocardiography, to exclude hydrostatic edema)

(AECC: American-European Consensus Conference; ARDS: Acute respiratory distress syndrome; CT: computed tomography; PEEP: positive end-expiratory pressure)

TABLE 2: Three categories of acute respiratory distress syndrome (ARDS).

	Nonintubated ARDS	*Intubated ARDS*	*Modified definition for resource-limited settings*
Oxygenation	PaO_2/FIO_2 <300 mm Hg *or* SpO_2/FIO_2 <315 (if SpO_2 <97%) on HFNO with flow >30 L/min or NIV/CPAP with at least 5 cmH_2O PEEP	• *Mild:* 200 < PaO_2/FiO_2 <300 mm Hg *or* 235 < SpO_2/FiO_2 <315 (if SpO_2 <97%) • *Moderate:* 100 < PaO_2/FiO_2 <200 mm Hg or 148, SpO_2/FiO_2 <235 (if SpO_2 <97%) • *Severe:* PaO_2/FiO_2 <100 mm Hg or SpO_2/FiO_2 <148 (if SpO_2 <97%)	• SpO_2/FiO_2 <315 (if SpO_2 <97%) • Neither PEEP nor minimum flow rate of oxygen is required for diagnosis in resource-limited settings

(CPAP: continuous positive airway pressure; HFNO: high flow nasal oxygen; NIV: noninvasive ventilation)

injury to intercellular junctions leading to increased permeability, necrosis of epithelial cells with denuding of the alveolar basement membrane. Damage to epithelial barrier, facilitates alveolar flooding and impairs the transport of fluid. Disease-associated molecular patterns are released into the airspace, amplifying proinflammatory signaling. There is also shedding of anticoagulant molecules and the release of tissue factor which favor intra-alveolar fibrin and hyaline membrane formation. Also, there is a shedding of anticoagulant molecules on the endothelial surface such as thrombomodulin and the endothelial protein C receptor, and upregulation of procoagulant molecules favoring microvascular thrombus formation.

Both local and systemic acute inflammation are prominent features of ARDS contributing to lung epithelial and endothelial injury. Neutrophils migrate from the lung vasculature into the alveoli and release a variety of mediators, reactive oxygen species, proteases, and proinflammatory lipid-derived mediators such as prostaglandins and leukotrienes, interleukin-1-β, interleukin-18. Macrophage pattern recognition receptors bind disease-associated [damage-associated molecular patterns (DAMPs)] or pathogen-associated molecular patterns (PAMPs) and activate macrophages leading to the release of proinflammatory cytokines and neutrophil chemoattractants such as interleukin-8.

Three phases of ARDS identified on histopathology are as follows:

1. *Exudative phase:* Occurs immediately and lasts approximately 3–7 days. This phase is characterized by diffuse alveolar damage leading to filling of alveoli with edema and cellular debris. This results in reduced alveolar ventilation, intrapulmonary shunting, and reduced lung compliance with increased work of breathing requiring mechanial ventilatory support.
2. *Proliferative phase:* Starts 7–14 days after the initial insult and overlaps with exedutive phase and lasts for another 2–3 weeks. There is a repair of damaged epithelium/endothelium, restoration of barrier function, and proliferation of fibroblasts, clearing of alveolar edema and debris, improving gas exchange.
3. *Fibrotic phase:* Occurs in some patients as chronic inflammation sets in leading to fibrosis of alveoli after 2–3 weeks. Develop progressive interstitial and alveolar fibrosis, with large emphysematous bullae which are prone to rupture, and prolonged ventilator dependency with increased morbidity and mortality.

CAUSES

Direct Causes

- Pneumonia
- Aspiration
- Inhalational injuries

- Blunt pulmonary trauma
- Near drowning
- Fat embolism
- *Drug toxicities/overdoses:* Narcotics, tricyclic antidepressants, chemotherapeutic agents, amiodarone.

Indirect Causes

- Sepsis
- Severe trauma
- Large volume blood transfusion
- Pancreatitis
- Reperfusion after cardiopulmonary bypass.

PATHOPHYSIOLOGIC CONSEQUENCES

- *Refractory hypoxemia and shunt:* Occurs due to flooding of the alveolar space, alveolar collapse due to increase surface tension, noncardiogenic pulmonary edema due to leaky alveolar-capillary membrane. All these lead to a mismatched ventilation/perfusion (V/Q) as blood flowing through capillaries in the collapsed alveoli cannot take part in gas exchange.
- *Decreased lung compliance:* Loss of surfactant and alveolar flooding makes the alveolar spaces very stiff, resulting in noncompliant lungs. In late stages of ARDS, fibrosis also decreases the compliance.
- *Pulmonary hypertension:* Develops due to hypoxic pulmonary vasoconstriction and local production of endothelin-1 and thromboxane A2. Formation of microthrombi and macrothrombi in pulmonary vessels and remodeling of arterial, venous, and lymphatic circulation, leads to decrease in cross-section of the lumens due to deposition of fibrin and collagen. Pulmonary hypertension can lead to further hypoxia by right-to-left shunting across a patent foramen ovale and end-organ hypoperfusion due to right ventricular failure leading to reduced cardiac output.

DIFFERENTIAL DIAGNOSIS

- Pulmonary hemorrhage
- Near drowning
- Drug reaction
- Acute interstitial pneumonitis (Hamman–Rich syndrome)
- Differentiation syndrome (retinoic acid syndrome)
- Acute hypersensitivity pneumonitis
- Transfusion-related acute lung injury (TRALI)
- Acute eosinophilic pneumonia
- Reperfusion injury
- Leukemic infiltration

- Cardiogenic edema
- Exacerbation of interstitial lung disease
- Organizing pneumonia
- Bilateral pneumonia
- Disseminated malignancy

WORKUP

The ARDS is a clinical diagnosis, and no specific laboratory abnormalities are noted beyond the expected disturbances in gas exchange and radiographic findings. In general, clinical evaluation and routine chest radiography are sufficient in patients with ARDS. However, CT scanning may be indicated as it is more sensitive than plain chest radiography in detecting pulmonary interstitial emphysema, pneumothoraces and pneumomediastinum, pleural effusions, cavitation, and mediastinal lymphadenopathy. Patients should undergo 2D echocardiography for the purpose of screening and to know the presence and severity of right ventricular dysfunction.

The ARDS Clinical Trials Network studied pulmonary artery catheter versus central venous catheter guided fluid therapy after initial resuscitation to know the difference in mortality. The study found no difference in mortality, ventilator days, intensive care unit (ICU) days, or need for pressors or dialysis. The pulmonary artery catheter group had twice as many catheter-related complications.

Bronchoscopy may be considered in patients with an uncertain diagnosis as there is a risk of losing alveolar recruitment.

TREATMENT

Prevention is the key treatment. It aims to correct the underlying cause whilst avoiding further injury to lung injury and carrying out best supportive care. Patients are mechanically ventilated, guarded against fluid overload with diuretics, and given nutritional support until improvement is seen.

Noninvasive Ventilation/High Flow Nasal Cannula

Noninvasive ventilation/high flow nasal cannula have a potentially useful role in a patient with mild ARDS. They should not be used if PaO_2/FiO_2 is <150 mm Hg. It should be used in selected, less severely ill patients, with close monitoring to help improve oxygenation.

Invasive mechanical ventilation: Mechanical ventilation should be initiated electively in following situations.

- Worsening respiratory fatigue
- Worsening hypercarbia
- Persistent hypoxemia

The mechanical ventilation protocol is based upon the concept of "baby lung" with only about a third of the alveoli remaining open and takes part in gas exchange. Respiratory compliance correlates well with the remaining normally aerated lung tissue. Thus, compliance truly measures the volume of baby lung. The ARDS lung is divided into three zones: a nonrecruitable zone, in the bases, an injured but recruitable midzone, and a spared though potentially overdistended zone in the apices. The appropriate ventilatory strategy can open up or recruit these shut alveoli in dependent region.

The landmark ARMA trial demonstrated a 22% relative reduction in mortality when tidal volumes of 6 mL/kg of predicted body weight (PBW) were used rather than traditional volumes of 12 mL/kg.

INITIAL VENTILATOR SETTINGS

Initially, the following setting needs to be decided:

- *Mode:* Volume control ventilation or pressure control as the starting mode. There is no substantial evidence suggesting the superiority of one mode over the other.
- *Tidal volume (TV):* Calculate ideal body weight (IBW): Male IBW = 50 + 2.3 [height (inches) – 60]; female IBW = 45.5 + 2.3 [height (inches) – 60]; initial tidal volume 8 mL/kg IBW, reduce TV by 1 mL/kg intervals every 2 hours until TV = 6 mL/kg IBW.
- *FiO_2 and positive end-expiratory pressure (PEEP):* Initial FiO_2 should be kept high and PEEP 5–10 cmH_2O to keep oxygen saturation >90%. In severe and diffuse ARDS, start with a higher PEEP of 10–12. FiO_2 should be titrated down subsequently to achieve PaO_2 = 55–80 mmHg or SpO_2 = 88–95%
- Plateau pressure (P_{plat}) <30 cmH_2O to reduce the risk of barotrauma. If P_{plat} is >30 cmH_2O, decrease TV by 1 mL/kg steps (minimum 4 mL/kg IBW). If P_{plat} is <30 cmH_2O and breath stacking occurs, one may increase TV in 1 mL/kg IBW increments (to a maximum of 8 mL/kg) as long as P_{plat} is <30 cmH_2O.
- *Inspiratory flow or inspiratory time or I:E ratio:* Set the inspiratory flow rate to achieve goal of inspiratory expiratory ratio of 1:1.0–1.3.
- *Acidosis management:* pH <7.30. If pH is 7.15–7.30, increase respiratory rate (RR) until pH is >7.30 or $PaCO_2$ is <25 mm Hg (maximum RR = 35); If pH is still <7.15, $NaHCO_3$ is considered. If pH is >7.45, decrease RR if possible.
- *Sedation neuromuscular blockade:* It is usually mandatory in patients receiving lung protective ventilation. Deep sedation is preferred in the initial stages to improve synchrony, to prevent ventilator-induced lung injury (VILI), especially with neuromuscular blockade.

All patients should be administered with neuromuscular agents for the first 48 hours. Restricted fluid strategy is recommended.

RESCUE METHODS FOR CRITICAL HYPOXEMIA IN SEVERE ARDS

When oxygenation is inadequate despite the maximum ventilatory support, or when patients require unacceptable levels of FiO_2 or airway pressure, rescue measures are required.

Recruitment maneuver (RM): Recruitment maneuver is application of a high level of sustained airway pressure to open up the collapsed and potentially recruitable alveoli and then apply appropriate PEEP to prevent the collapse of the recruited alveoli. There is still insufficient evidence to use recruitment maneuvers routinely and electively in all patients of severe ARDS. Recent adjuvant radiotherapy trial (ART) has shown increased mortality. So, it should be used only with caution in selected patients. Patient with early diffuse ARDS are generally good recruiters, but patients with late ARDS (>1 week) and focal ARDS generally do not respond well to recruitment. Following methods are commonly used.

- *Sustained inflation:* Keep the patient in continuous positive airway pressure (CPAP) mode and deliver 40 cmH_2O pressure for up to 30 seconds at FiO_2 of 1.0.
- *Stepwise recruitment maneuver or decremental PEEP method:* In this approach, both plateau pressure and PEEP are gradually increased with the driving pressure kept constant at 15 cmH_2O. After the recruitment, the PEEP is kept high (e.g., 20–25 cmH_2O) and is then gradually decreased in 2 cmH_2O decrement. Compliance is measured at each step, to get the best compliance. After identifying the PEEP at which the best compliance or oxygenation is maintained, the recruitment maneuver is applied again. After this second recruitment, PEEP is set 2 cm above the PEEP level identified with the best compliance.
- Patient in put on pressure control mode FiO_2 of 1.0. Inspiratory pressure 40–50 cmH_2O, PEEP 20–30 cmH_2O, RR 8–20/min, Inspiratory time 1-3 seconds for duration of 1–2 minutes.

Prone positioning: Prone position alters the physiology of gas exchange and lung mechanics and thus results in improved oxygenation.

- Reduces ventral-dorsal transpulmonary pressure difference.
- Improved ventilation and recruitment of the previously dependent dorsal lung via regional changes in chest wall mechanics and reduced lung compression by the heart and mediastinum.
- Gravitational distribution of perfusion toward the better ventilated previously ventral lung.

- Improves ventilation perfusion mismatch and shunt.
- Improves bronchial drainage.
- Reversal of acute cor pulmonale.
- More homogeneous ventilation.

Prone ventilation started as soon as possible. Each prone session of 16–20 hours duration to be given in a day. To be stopped only when improvement in oxygenation (P/F >150 with PEEP <10 and FiO_2 <0.6) persists over next 4 hours after supining. The PROSEVA study group showed improvement in oxygenation and significant reduction in mortality with prone ventilation.

Extracorporeal membrane oxygenation (ECMO): ECMO is a technique where blood is removed from patient and passed through artificial biomembrane which functions to oxygenate blood and remove CO_2 from blood and then return it back to patient. In case of isolated respiratory failure, venovenous ECMO is used. In case of associated circulatory failure, venoarterial ECMO is used.

Inhaled pulmonary vasodilators: Inhaled nitric oxide and epoprostenol are commonly pulmonary vasodilators. They promote pulmonary vasodilatation and blood flow to ventilated areas of lungs and divert blood away from poorly ventilated areas of lung thus improving ventilation perfusion mismatch and oxygenation. They can be used as transient measure in patient with refractory hypoxemia due to severe pulmonary hypertension. They have no mortality benefit.

High frequency oscillatory ventilation (HFOV): Type of ventilation which combines high respiratory rate (>180 breaths/min) with tidal volumes as low as anatomical dead space. HFOV at present is not recommended for use in adult ARDS as OSCAR and OSCILLATE trials failed to demonstrate any mortality benefit.

Airway pressure release ventilation (APRV): This mode allows patients to breathe spontaneously while receiving high airway pressure with an intermittent pressure release. APRV has some small supporting trial evidence but is yet to be evaluated in a large multicenter trial.

ROLE OF CORTICOSTEROIDS IN ACUTE RESPIRATORY DISTRESS SYNDROME

Several questions about corticosteroids remain unanswered. The optimal regimen remains unknown. Steroids may only be effective, if given early, before the inflammatory process has caused irreversible damage to the alveoli. Further research is needed to determine the appropriate formulation, dose, timing, and course of therapy to better guide. Glucocorticoids are generally avoided in patients with less severe ARDS or those with persistent ARDS beyond 14 days.

Apart from these measures, as in other ICU patients, nutrition plays an important role. The enteral route is safer, and has no effect with immunomodulatory nutrition. Deep vein thrombosis (DVT) prophylaxis to be added. Care must also be taken to prevent pressure sores.

SUMMARY

Despite advances in critical care, ARDS has high morbidity and mortality. Those who survive may have a poor quality of life. There is no way to prevent the condition despite knowing many risk factors for ARDS. Besides restricting fluids in high-risk patients, close monitoring for hypoxia is important. Outcome improves if hypoxia is identified early. ARDS sequelae make returning to a normal life challenging for patients who survives. As measured by functional testing, there is an almost near-complete return of pulmonary capacity for many survivors.

SUGGESTED READING

1. Bein T, Grasso S, Moerer O, Quintel M, Guerin C, Deja M, et al. The standard of care of patients with ARDS: ventilatory settings and rescue therapies for refractory hypoxemia. Intensive Care Med. 2016;42(5):699.
2. Combes A, Hajage D, Capellier G, Demoule A, Lavoué S, Guervilly C, et al. Extracorporeal membrane oxygenation for severe acute respiratory distress syndrome. N Engl J Med. 2018;378(21):1965-71.
3. Confalonieri M, Salton F, Fabiano F. Acute respiratory distress syndrome. Eur Respir Rev. 2017;26(144):160116.
4. Diamond M, Peniston HL, Sanghavi DK, Mahapatra S. Acute respiratory distress syndrome. In: Stat*Pe*arls [Internet]. Treasure Island (FL): StatPearls Publishing; 2024.
5. Grasselli G, Calfee CS, Camporota L, Poole D, Amato MBP, Antonelli M, et al. ESICM guidelines on acute respiratory distress syndrome: definition, phenotyping and respiratory support strategies. Intensive Care Med. 2023; 49(7):727-59.
6. Matthay MA, Arabi Y, Arroliga AC, Bernard G, Bersten AD, Brochard LJ, et al. A new global definition of acute respiratory distress syndrome. Am J Respir Crit Care Med. 2024;209(1):37-47.
7. Writing Group for the Alveolar Recruitment for Acute Respiratory Distress Syndrome Trial (ART) Investigators; Cavalcanti AB, Suzumura ÉA, Laranjeira LN, Paisani DM, Damiani LP, Guimarães HP, et al. Effect of lung recruitment and titrated PEEP versus low PEEP on mortality in patients with acute respiratory distress syndrome: a randomízed clinical trial. JAMA. 2017;318(14):1335-45.
8. Zhao L, Su F, Zhang N, Wu H, Shen Y, Liu H, et al. The impact of the new acute respiratory distress syndrome (ARDS) criteria on Berlin criteria ARDS patients: a multicenter cohort study. BMC Med. 2023;21(1):456.

CHAPTER 9

Severe Asthma

Poorva Dilip Magarkar

INTRODUCTION

Asthma is a heterogeneous disease, usually characterized by chronic airway inflammation. It is defined by the history of respiratory symptoms, such as wheeze, shortness of breath, chest tightness, and cough, that vary over time and in intensity, together with variable expiratory airflow limitation. Asthma exacerbations can be life-threatening and it is defined as episodes characterized by progressive increase in symptoms of shortness of breath, cough, wheezing, chest tightness, or progressive decrease in lung function, i.e., change from patients' usual status that is sufficient to require change in the treatment. Exacerbation can be the first presentation or occur with the preexisting asthma. Status asthmaticus is defined as a prolonged severe episode of asthma that is unresponsive to initial standard therapy, that may lead to respiratory failure. The episodes may be rapid onset developed within hours or progress during several hours to days.

TRIGGERS FOR ASTHMA EXACERBATION

- Viral respiratory tract infections
- Poor adherence to treatment
- Exercise
- Outdoor air pollution
- Gastroesophageal reflux disease
- Chronic sinusitis
- Environmental allergens
- Use of aspirin, β-blockers
- Tobacco smoke
- Obesity
- Emotional factors or stress

PATHOPHYSIOLOGY

The pathological process begins with the inhalation of an irritant or an allergen, which due to bronchial hypersensitivity, leads to airway inflammation and causes an increase in mucus production. This leads to a significant increase in airway resistance, which is most pronounced on expiration.

Airway obstruction occurs due to:
- Inflammatory cell infiltration
- Mucus hypersecretion with mucus plug formation
- Smooth muscle contraction

CLINICAL ASSESSMENT OF SEVERE ASTHMA EXACERBATIONS (TABLE 1)

Rapid evaluation of the patient is essential, focusing on key points of the history such as duration of symptoms, inciting exposures, medication use, and previous history of severe attacks.

Analysis of arterial blood gases is important as it usually reveals mild hypoxemia, hypocapnia, and respiratory alkalosis. As the severity of obstruction increases, $PaCO_2$ first normalizes and subsequently increases because of patient's exhaustion, inadequate alveolar ventilation, and increase in physiologic dead space. In severe, advanced stage disease, metabolic (lactic) acidosis may coexist. Lactic acidosis may be explained by high dose of parenteral β-adrenergic agonists; increased work of breathing resulting in anaerobic metabolism of the muscles and overproduction of lactic acid; coexisting profound tissue hypoxia; the

TABLE 1: Evaluation points of severe asthma exacerbations.

	Mild	*Moderate*	*Severe*	*Imminent respiratory arrest*
Breathlessness	Walking	Talking	At rest	
Talks in	Sentences	Phrases	Words	
Respiratory rate	Increased	Increased	>30/min	
Alertness	May be agitated	Usually agitated	Usually agitated	Drowsy or confused
Accessory muscle use	Usually not	Usually	Usually	Paradoxical thoracoabdominal moment
Wheezing	Often end expiratory	Loud	Usually loud	Absent
Heart rate	100	100–120	>120	Bradycardia
Pulsus paradoxus	Absent <10 mm Hg	May be present 10–25 mm Hg	Often present >25 mm Hg	Absent may suggest fatigue
PEF	>80%	60–80%	<60%	
PaO_2	Normal	>60 mm Hg	<60 mm Hg	
$PaCO_2$	<45 mm Hg	<45 mm Hg	>45 mm Hg	

(PEF: peak expiratory flow)

presence of intracellular alkalosis; and decreased lactate clearance by the liver because of hypoperfusion.

Chest radiographs in the majority of patients will be normal but chest radiographic examination is necessary to exclude complications. Complete blood counts may be appropriate in patients with fever and/or purulent sputum.

Airway obstruction and expiratory airflow limitation leading to insufficient expiratory time results in air trapping, dynamic hyperinflation (DHI), and persistent positive end-expiratory pressure (PEEP) also referred to as intrinsic PEEP. This increases the work of breathing while simultaneously placing the diaphragm at a mechanical disadvantage resulting in increased O_2 consumption and CO_2 production. DHI affects cardiovascular function due to increased intrathoracic pressure leading to decreased cardiac output, compromising blood flow to respiratory muscles leading to fatigue.

TREATMENT

Severe exacerbations are life-threatening. Treatment requires careful assessment and close monitoring. The immediate management should begin with assessment of A (airway), B (breathing), and C (circulation). Look for altered mentation and a silent chest.

- *Oxygen:* Via nasal cannulae or face mask to maintain SpO_2 >92%
- *Inhaled bronchodilators:* Mainstay of treatment. Start short-acting β2 agonist (SABA), a short-acting antimuscarinic agent (SAMA), and oral or intravenous corticosteroid. Salbutamol (2.5–5 mg) by jet nebulization every 20 minutes for three doses, and ipratropium bromide in a dose of 0.5 mg by jet nebulization every 20 minutes for three doses. After the initial doses of nebulization, salbutamol (2.5–5 mg) should be continued every 1–4 hours and ipratropium bromide (500 µg) every 4–6 hours, based on the clinical response. Intravenous β2-agonists are no more effective. Long-acting β2-agonists to be continued as add-on therapy in hospitalized patient and in outpatient setting. If nonavailability of nebulizer, use four puffs of salbutamol meter dose inhalers (MDI) through a spacer device.
- *Steroids:* Steroids started early, especially when the response to initial bronchodilator therapy is poor. They decrease inflammatory response and upregulate β-receptors. Both oral and intravenous steroids are equally effective and the doses recommended are 1 mg/kg. Prednisolone or 100 mg every 6th hourly hydrocortisone or 0.5–1 g/kg methylprednisolone in once daily or divided doses. Earlier the steroid, better the outcome and less relapse. Their average duration of onset of action is 6–12 hours. Taper after 36–48 hours, depending on clinical response.
- *Magnesium sulfate:* 2 g over 20 minutes can be tried in refractory cases, although its role is unproven.

TABLE 2: Initial ventilator settings.

Parameters	*Settings*
Mode	Volume control
Tidal volume	6–8 mL/kg
Respiratory rate	10–12 breaths/min
Minute ventilation	6–8 L/min
I:E ratio	1:3 up to 1:5
Inspiratory flow	60–70 L/min
Waveform	Square
PEEP	5 cmH_2O
P_{plat}	<30 cmH_2O
FiO_2	Titrate to keep SpO_2 >90%

(PEEP: positive end expiratory pressure; I:E: inspiratory: expiratory)

- *Antibiotics:* Routine use is not recommended as the most common cause for exacerbation is a viral infection. Justified only if patients have fever, purulent sputum, or if there is evidence of pneumonia.
- *Ventilatory support:* The goal of management is to unload the respiratory muscles, correct hypoxemia, adequate ventilation, and minimize lung injury, particularly from DHI, while treating the underlying airway inflammation and bronchoconstriction **(Table 2)**.

Noninvasive ventilation (NIV): The use of NIV is controversial in mild-moderate exacerbations. If attempted, patients to be selected carefully and closely monitored. Similarly, the evidence for HFNC in this setting is still debatable.

Invasive ventilation: Indications for intubation and ventilation are impending respiratory arrest from fatigue, altered sensorium that interferes with appropriate therapy, cardiac arrest, and respiratory arrest.

Large endotracheal tube (ETT) to be used as it will reduce airflow resistance and facilitate ventilation, may facilitate procedures if necessary (e.g., bronchoscopy). Aggressive bag-mask ventilation should be avoided as it will rapidly precipitate severe gas-trapping and may cause pneumothorax and hypotension.

A lung protective and permissive hypercapnia strategy should be employed. Individualized PEEP (iPEEP) should be monitored by an end-expiratory hold maneuver. The iPEEP is equal to total PEEP minus set PEEP. The goal should be to maintain iPEEP <20 cmH_2O. This can be achieved by reducing the respiratory rate (not below 10–14 breaths/min) or decreasing the tidal volume (6–8 mL/kg). Increasing the flow rate (≥100 L/min) or square waveform has minimal impact on DHI once the minute ventilation has been limited. Hypotension due to DHI may be managed by temporary disconnection of ventilator circuit from ETT. Sedation and neuromuscular blockade may be used to prevent patient ventilator dyssynchrony and avoided as infusion to prevent critical illness polymyoneuropathy **(Figs. 1 and 2)**. Once there is DHI, work of breathing, gas exchange, and need for sedation improve, patient can be put on spontaneous ventilation mode.

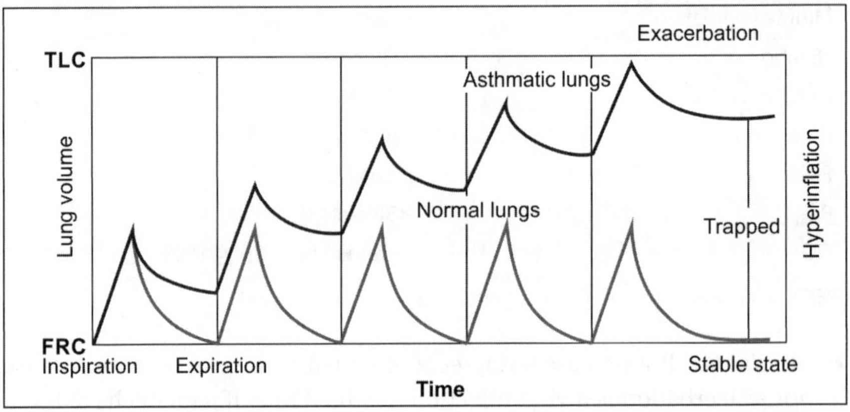

Fig. 1: Dynamic hyperinflation (Volume time) scalar.
(FRC: functional residual capacity; TLC: total lung capacity)

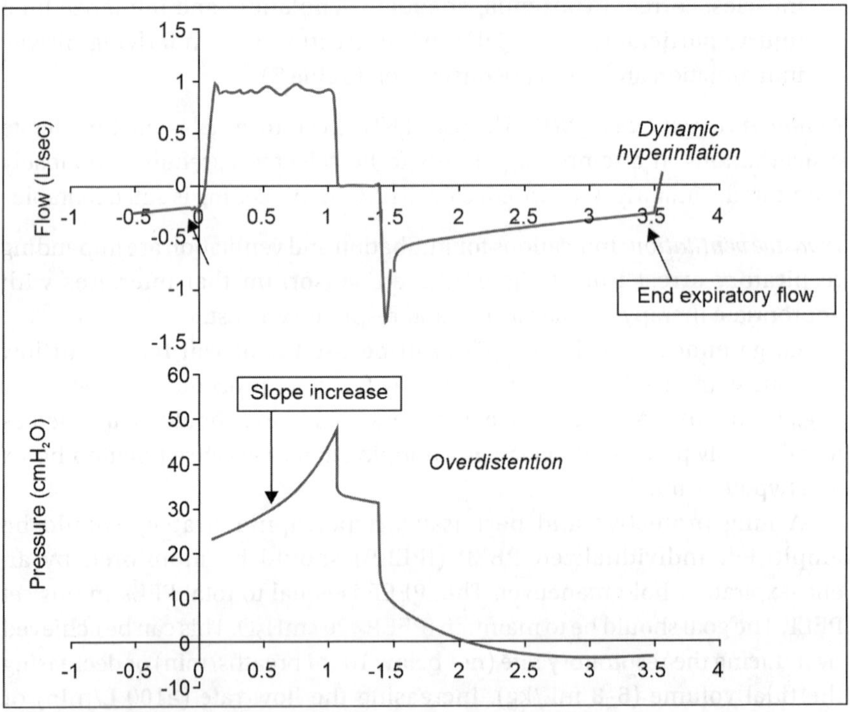

Fig. 2: Dynamic hyperinflation (Flow-time, pressure-time) scalar.

RESCUE THERAPIES

- *Heliox:* Mixture of helium (He) and oxygen (O_2) mixed in a ratio of He: O_2–70:30. Use is based on the decreased density of heliox compared with air resulting in more laminar rather than turbulent airflow, thus decreasing work of breathing. Data suggest improved delivery of aerosolized bronchodilators (albuterol), when given with heliox rather than oxygen, but no significant difference in bronchospasm relief.
- *Intravenous ketamine:* Tried in treatment of refractory asthma because of its bronchodilatory properties. It is administered as bolus dose of 0.5–1 mg/kg followed by infusion of 2 mg/kg/h.
- *Adrenaline*: It reduces bronchial mucosal edema by its vasoconstrictive action. It has bronchodilatory effect by decreasing the parasympathetic tone. Adrenaline is given subcutaneously and can be used in patients who do not tolerate or respond to nebulized medications.
- *Methylxanthines:* Not recommended for initial treatment. They have increased incidence of adverse effects when used in combination with SABA. Aminophylline may be used, loading dose of 5–6 mg/kg is followed by a continuous infusion of 0.6 mg/kg/h.
- *Intravenous leukotriene inhibitors:* Role of leukotriene antagonist is more applicable in asthma exacerbation secondary to aspirin or nonsteroidal anti-inflammatory drugs (NSAIDs).
- *Inhalational anesthetic agents:* For refractory cases, inhaled anesthetics (sevoflurane, isoflurane, and halothane) have been used. They exert bronchodilatory properties by action on bronchial smooth muscle via calcium-dependent channels and by attenuating cholinergic tone. The dose titrated according to clinical response.
- *Bronchoscopic removal of impacted mucus:* Can be used to remove impacted mucus to improve ventilation.
- *Extracorporeal life support:* Extracorporeal carbon dioxide removal ($ECCO_2R$) as well as extracorporeal membrane oxygenation (ECMO) can be used for severe respiratory acidosis that is refractory to maximal medical and ventilator management. Evidence for routine extracorporeal life support (ECLS) use is still lacking for now.
- *Intravenous β2 agonist:* Routine use of parenteral β2 agonist are no longer recommended due to increased side effects.

SUPPORTIVE THERAPY

Deep vein thrombosis prophylaxis and stress ulcer prophylaxis are mandatory in these patients. Adequate nutrition support should be given.

SUMMARY

As a result of the ongoing inflammatory processes asthma patients experience exacerbations irrespective of their disease severity, phenotype, or despite optimal guideline-directed treatment. The identification of patients at risk for severe exacerbations is important. Patient's education and written plans of management, control of triggering factors, and comorbid conditions, monitoring asthma control, and pulmonary function and optimal pharmacotherapy are needed to prevent and/or decrease exacerbations.

SUGGESTED READING

1. Abrams D, Brodie D. Emerging indications for extracorporeal membrane oxygenation in adults with respiratory failure. Ann Am Thorac Soc. 2013; 10(4):371-7.
2. Global initiative for asthma. (2024). Global strategy for asthma management and prevention. [online] Available from www.ginasthma.org [Last accessed July, 2024].
3. Kostakou E, Kaniaris E, Filiou E, Vasileiadis I, Katsaounou P, Tzortzaki E, et al. Acute severe asthma in adolescent and adult patients: current perspectives on assessment and management. J Clin Med. 2019;8(9):1283.
4. Reddel HK, Bacharier LB, Bateman ED, Brightling CE, Brusselle GG, Buhl R, et al. Global Initiative for Asthma Strategy 2021: executive summary and rationale for key changes. Eur Respir J. 2021;59(1):2102730.

CHAPTER

10 Acute Exacerbation of Chronic Obstructive Pulmonary Disease

Poorva Dilip Magarkar

INTRODUCTION

Chronic obstructive pulmonary disease (COPD) is a heterogeneous lung condition characterized by chronic respiratory symptoms (dyspnea, cough, and sputum production) due to abnormalities of the airways (bronchitis, bronchiolitis) and/or alveoli (emphysema) that cause persistent, often progressive, airflow obstruction (GOLD's 2023 report).

Acute exacerbation of chronic obstructive pulmonary disease (AECOPD) is a purely clinical diagnosis. An exacerbation of COPD (ECOPD) is defined as an event characterized by increased dyspnea and/or cough and sputum that worsens in 14 days which may be accompanied by tachypnea and/or tachycardia and is often associated with increased local and systemic inflammation caused by infection, pollution, or other insult to the airways (GOLD's 2023 report). Other acute events, such as decompensated heart failure, pneumonia, and pulmonary embolism, can mimic or aggravate an ECOPD. Severity of COPD is based on spirometry, symptoms assessed by the modified Medical Research Council (mMRC) or the COPD assessment test (CAT) questionnaires, and the frequency of exacerbations **(Fig. 1)**.

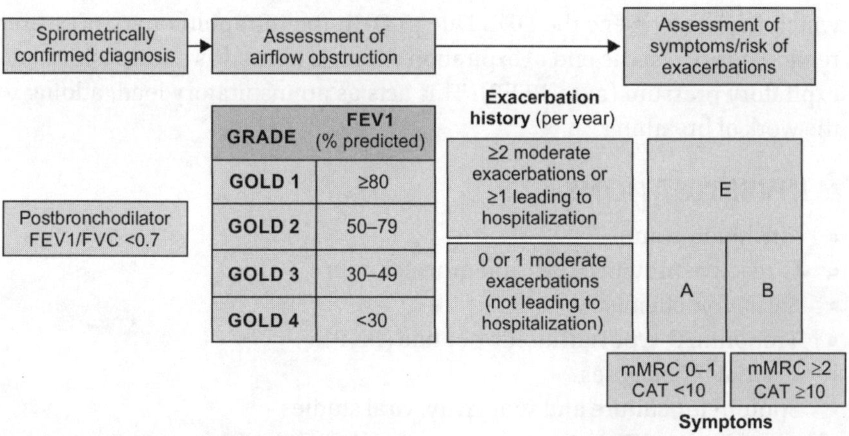

Fig. 1: The Global Initiative for Chronic Obstructive Lung Disease (GOLD) ABE assessment tool. (CAT: COPD assessment test; FEV: forced expiratory volume; FVC: forced vital capacity; mMRC: modified Medical Research Council)

RISK FACTORS AND ETIOLOGY FOR COPD EXACERBATION

One-third of COPD exacerbations do not have identifiable cause.

- History of prior exacerbations
- Smoking and air pollution
- History of hospitalizations for AECOPD
- Advanced age
- Duration of underlying COPD
- Presence of comorbidities such as cardiac disease, diabetes mellitus, pulmonary hypertension, etc.
- Infectious etiologies—*Respiratory viral infections*: Rhinovirus, respiratory syncytial virus, influenza, parainfluenza, adenovirus, coronavirus, and human metapneumovirus. *Bacterial infections: Haemophilus influenzae, Moraxella catarrhalis, Streptococcus pneumoniae*, etc.
- Noninfectious etiologies: Myocardial ischemia, pulmonary embolism, congestive heart failure, aspiration, gastroesophageal reflux disease (GERD), etc.

PATHOPHYSIOLOGY

The COPD patients have expiratory flow limitation (EFL) due to airway narrowing and airway inflammation leading to insufficient time for expiration and it causes air trapping. During exercise or increased demand, inspired tidal volume increases, EFL causes an increase in end expiratory lung volume and dynamic hyperinflation (DHI). During exacerbation, bronchospasm and mucosal edema cause increase in airways resistance and worsen DHI. DHI reduces the compliance of the respiratory system, alter pulmonary hemodynamics, reduces hypoxic drive, alveolar hypoventilation, leading to deterioration of ventilation-perfusion (V/Q) mismatch and respiratory failure. The patient become tachypneic, have rapid shallow breathing pattern which further worsens the DHI. Due to DHI, the intrapulmonary pressures remain positive at the end of expiration which is termed as auto-positive end expiratory pressure (auto-PEEP). This acts as an inspiratory load, adding to the work of breathing.

INVESTIGATIONS

- Full blood count
- C-reactive protein (CRP) and procalcitonin
- Serum biochemistry
- Troponin/B-type natriuretic peptide (BNP)
- Arterial blood gases
- Sputum for culture and sensitivity, viral studies
- Chest X-ray (CXR), computed tomography (CT) scan
- Echocardiography
- Electrocardiogram (ECG)

MANAGEMENT

Signs such as tachycardia, tachypnea, wheezing, and accessory muscle use support diagnosis of AECOPD. Patients may have leukocytosis with positive sputum cultures, respiratory viral panels, or blood cultures. Arterial blood gas (ABG) can be useful in detecting worsening hypercarbia ($PaCO_2$ >50 mm Hg) or hypoxemia (PaO_2 <60 mm Hg). Chest radiographs can be used to detect etiologies for dyspnea.

Initial management of AECOPD includes assessment and stabilization of airway, maintaining breathing, and assisting the circulation. Monitoring of oxygen saturation with pulse oximetry should be initiated immediately in addition to monitoring other vital signs. These patients require nebulized bronchodilators, oxygen titrated to arterial saturation of 88–92%, corticosteroids, antibiotics, and at times noninvasive ventilation (NIV) also.

- *Oxygen therapy:* Should be instituted after assessing ABG and SpO_2, should be maintained between 88 and 92%.
- *Bronchodilators:*
    - *Beta-2 agonists:* Salbutamol 2.5–5 mg nebulization every 2–4 hours. Efficacy of metered dose inhaler is as good as nebulizers when used with spacers. In acute emergencies continuous nebulization is given for first hour. Inhaled bronchodilators are superior to systemic bronchodilators.
    - *Anticholinergics:* Used along with beta-2 agonists. Ipratropium bromide in a dose of 0.5 mg by jet nebulization every 20 minutes for three doses.
    - After the initial doses of nebulization, salbutamol (2.5–5 mg) should be continued every 1–4 hours and ipratropium bromide (500 μg) every 4–6 hours, based on the clinical response.
    - *Steroids:* Steroids speed up recovery by improving forced expiratory volume 1 (FEV1) and forced vital capacity (FVC), reduce hospital stay, reduce chance of treatment failure, and decrease the chance of recurrent hospitalization. Oral corticosteroids are preferred, as parenteral corticosteroids have not demonstrated benefit but should be considered in patients with poor oral intake. Dose of 40 mg prednisolone for 5 days is recommended.
    - *Antibiotics:* Initial broad-spectrum coverage based on local antimicrobial resistance patterns is appropriate. Cultures, respiratory viral panel, can often help narrow coverage after 48 hours. β-lactam with β-lactamase inhibitor combination (amoxicillin and clavulanic acid), or third generation cephalosporin such as ceftriaxone or cefotaxime is preferred. If *Pseudomonas* infection is suspected, chest imaging suggestive of bronchiectasis, use of broad-spectrum antibiotics within the past 3 months, chronic systemic glucocorticoid use cefepime, ceftazidime, or piperacillin-tazobactam [4.5 g

TABLE 1: Initial ventilator settings.

Parameters	*Settings*
Mode	Volume control
Tidal volume	6–8 mL/kg
Respiratory rate	10–12 breaths/min
Minute ventilation	6–8 L/min
I:E ratio	1:3 up to 1:5
Inspiratory flow	60–70 L/min
Waveform	Square
PEEP	5 cmH_2O
P_{plat}	<30 cmH_2O
FiO_2	Titrate to keep SpO_2 >90%

(I:E: inspiratory: expiratory; PEEP: positive end expiratory pressure)

intravenous (IV) 6 hourly] should be given. The duration of antibiotic therapy is generally 5–7 days, can vary according to severity of disease and clinical response.

- *Magnesium sulfate:* It potentially increases bronchodilatory action (increases FEV1) of inhaled β-2 agonists, when used alongside, it can be considered on case-to-case basis. Dose of magnesium sulfate is 1.5–2 g intravenously over 20 minutes.

- *Noninvasive ventilation* **(Table 1)***:* Indicated in hypercapnic respiratory failure with pH <7.35. It is beneficial in AECOPD, as it lowers the rate of intubation, shortens hospital stay, and decreases mortality. It optimizes oxygenation and reduces CO_2 by effectively unloading the respiratory muscles, it increases tidal volumes, reduces respiratory rates, decreases intrinsic PEEP, and thus diaphragmatic work of breathing.

  Explain the procedure to the patient, select appropriate interface oral, nasal, full facemask or helmet, select machine either NIV or intensive care unit (ICU) ventilator. Spontaneous or spontaneous timed mode (ST) is selected on NIV ventilator. On conventional ventilators, NIV mode is used. Inspiratory positive airway pressure (IPAP) and expiratory positive airway pressure (EPAP) settings are titrated to effect. Start with low settings, IPAP of 6–8 cmH_2O and EPAP of 2–4 cmH_2O. The difference between IPAP and EPAP should be at least 4 cmH_2O and titrated according to tidal volume. In ICU ventilators, PEEP is equal to the selected EPAP, and pressure support is selected over PEEP [Pressure support (PS) = IPAP – EPAP]. Increase EPAP by 1–2 cmH_2O till inspiratory efforts are sensed and a breath is triggered. Inability of machine to sense patient effort suggests major leak or presence of auto-PEEP. IPAP is increased stepwise 1–2 cmH_2O till adequate minute ventilation is achieved with no major leak. Pressure points on the nasal bridge, paranasal regions are padded. After the patient gets accustomed to the flow, the mask is then strapped on with harness.

Serial ABG should be measured after initiation of NIV. A lack of improvement in symptoms or worsening hypercarbia, respiratory acidosis, or hypoxemia on ABG suggests the need for intubation and invasive mechanical ventilation.

- *Invasive ventilation*: Indications are threatened airway (gurgling secretions), multiorgan failure (cardiogenic/septic shock), patient worsening despite optimized bilevel positive airway pressure (BiPAP)/ high-flow nasal cannula (HFNC) support, and respiratory/cardiac arrest.

Sedation is often needed to ensure synchrony. The patient should not be ventilated to a normal $PaCO_2$, but instead to a normal pH and baseline $PaCO_2$. Large endotracheal tube (ETT) to be used as it will reduce airflow resistance and facilitate ventilation, may facilitate procedures if necessary (e.g., bronchoscopy). Aggressive bag-mask ventilation should be avoided as it will rapidly precipitate severe gas-trapping.

DYNAMIC HYPERINFLATION

Due to severe airflow limitation adequate amount of air cannot be expelled out and some amount of air remains trapped in alveoli during expiration. This results in the development of auto-PEEP or intrinsic PEEP, which worsens the breathing difficulty and increases work of breathing. Auto-PEEP increases end expiratory lung volumes and pushes diaphragm down, which makes it at anatomical disadvantage for effective contraction. The diaphragm has to generate enough negative pressure to overcome auto-PEEP and produce further negative pressure to cause airflow. Auto-PEEP increases intrathoracic pressure, reduces venous return, increases right ventricular afterload reducing left ventricular (LV) preload in series leading to hypotension, pulseless electrical activity (PEA), and cardiac arrest.

Ventilator graphics provides clues to the presence of auto-PEEP. On flow time scalar, the inspiration will start, even before the expiration is completed and flow reaches the baseline. The flow volume loop will show the amount of volume at the end of expiration as the next breath is initiated **(Figs. 2A and B)**.

Auto-PEEP can be optimized by treating bronchospasm, secretions, and other reversible causes. Decrease respiratory rate (RR) and inspiratory: expiratory (I:E) ratio (1:3–1:5), application of PEEP, 80% of intrinsic PEEP. If patient is hypotensive, disconnect circuit from ETT and observe.

If patient requires invasive ventilation, should be kept mechanically ventilated for at least ~24 hours to give rest to diaphragm. Bronchospasm and diaphragmatic fatigue generally decreases after 36–48 hours. European Respiratory Society and American Thoracic Society (ERS and ATS) suggest NIV for early weaning in patients of COPD.

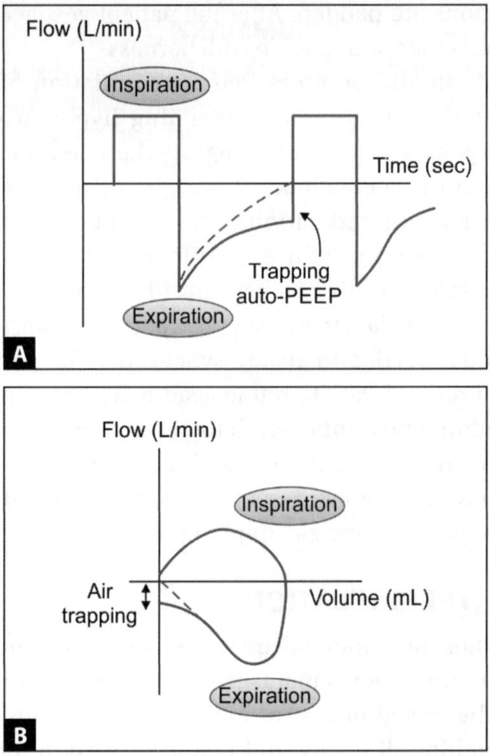

Figs. 2A and B: Ventilator graphics. (PEEP: positive end-expiratory pressure)

Extracorporeal life support: Extracorporeal carbon dioxide removal ($ECCO_2R$) as well as extracorporeal membrane oxygenation (ECMO) can be used for severe respiratory acidosis that is refractory to maximal medical and ventilator management.

SUPPORTIVE THERAPY

Oxidative stress and hypoxia can cause endothelial dysfunction, leading to thrombotic events. Deep vein thrombosis prophylaxis and stress ulcer prophylaxis are mandatory in these patients. Adequate nutritional support should be given.

After recovery from an exacerbation COPD, prevention of another exacerbation is important, in both the short and the long term. Pulmonary rehabilitation may prevent future exacerbation. Interventions likely to prevent exacerbations are pneumococcal vaccination, combination inhaler therapy with an inhaled corticosteroid (ICS)/long-acting β-agonist (LABA), and long-acting muscarinic antagonist (LAMA), and patient education. Nutrition counseling should be done.

SUMMARY

Chronic obstructive pulmonary disease is a chronic illness that can be periodically exacerbated by acute worsening of symptoms characterized by increased dyspnea, cough, sputum production and sputum purulence. Accurate assessment of patients with AECOPD is key to reducing the impact of disease severity and prescribing the correct treatment. The mainstays treatment are bronchodilators and systemic glucocorticoids. Respiratory support in the form of oxygen therapy, noninvasive positive pressure ventilation may be required to treat hypoxemia and hypercapnia. Patient education generally improves outcomes in AECOPD.

SUGGESTED READING

1. Ahmed SM, Athar M. Mechanical ventilation in patients with chronic obstructive pulmonary disease and bronchial asthma. Indian J Anaesth. 2015;59(9):589-98.
2. CDC. Pneumococcal Vaccination: who and when to vaccinate. [online] Available from https://www.cdc.gov/vaccines/vpd/pneumo/hcp/who-when-to-vaccinate.html [Last accessed July, 2024].
3. Crisafulli E, Barbeta E, Ielpo A, Torres A. Management of severe acute exacerbations of COPD: an updated narrative review. Multidiscip Respir Med. 2018;13:36.
4. India State-Level Disease Burden Initiative CRD Collaborators. The burden of chronic respiratory diseases and their heterogeneity across the states of India: the Global Burden of Disease Study 1990-2016. Lancet Glob Health. 2018;6(12):e1363-74.
5. Leuppi JD, Schuetz P, Bingisser R, Bodmer M, Briel M, Drescher T, et al. Short-term vs conventional glucocorticoid therapy in acute exacerbations of chronic obstructive pulmonary disease: the REDUCE randomized clinical trial. JAMA. 2013;309(21):2223-31.
6. Terry PD, Dhand R. The 2023 GOLD Report: Updated Guidelines for Inhaled Pharmacological Therapy in Patients with Stable COPD. Pulm Ther. 2023;9(3):345-57.
7. Venkatesan P. GOLD COPD report: 2023 update. Lancet Respir Med. 2023;11(1):18.
8. Walters JA, Tan DJ, White CJ, Gibson PG, Wood-Baker R, Walters EH, et al. Systemic corticosteroids for acute exacerbations of chronic obstructive pulmonary disease. Cochrane Database Syst Rev. 2014;2014(9):CD001288.

CHAPTER

11 Acute Pulmonary Embolism

Poorva Dilip Magarkar

INTRODUCTION

Pulmonary embolism (PE) is defined as occlusion in the pulmonary arterial tree, preventing blood flow, distal to the occlusion. PE is generally caused by thrombosis in a systemic blood vessel, usually in a deep vein of the lower limb. Intensive care unit (ICU) patients typically have multiple risk factors for PE.

PATHOPHYSIOLOGY

About 70–80% of PEs begin as thrombi in the deep veins of the lower extremities or pelvis. Thrombus formation is facilitated by three factors (the Virchow triad): (1) Venous stasis, (2) hypercoagulability, and (3) endothelial injury. Intravascular thrombosis occurs whenever the natural anticoagulation system is overwhelmed by procoagulant factors. Risk factors contributing to deep vein thrombosis (DVT) are given in **Table 1**.

Inherited coagulation disorders can rarely be responsible alone for the occurrence of DVT/PE. The thrombus formed in the deep veins of the leg can dislodge and travel to and occlude pulmonary vasculature, causing increased pulmonary vascular resistance (PVR) by mechanical obstruction and due to the reflex vasospasm and release of vasoconstrictor substances. Depending upon the size of the thrombus, pulmonary vascular compromise, underlying cardiopulmonary reserve, the right ventricular (RV) dysfunction, heart failure, and even shock can develop. The occluding thrombus leads to dead space ventilation, hypoxemia (worsens vasoconstriction), reduced diffusion capacity, and V/Q mismatch. Increased RV pressure overload along with increased myocardial oxygen demand can also result in RV ischemia and infarction, further worsening RV dysfunction and cardiac output **(Fig. 1)**.

CLINICAL PRESENTATION

The symptoms and signs of acute PE are all nonspecific. PE is suspected in a patient with dyspnea, chest pain, presyncope or syncope, or hemoptysis. Hemodynamic instability is a rare but important clinical presentation,

TABLE 1: Risk factors of deep vein thrombosis.

Strong risk factors	*Moderate risk factors*	*Weak risk factors*
Fracture of lower limb	Arthroscopic knee surgery	Bed rest >3 days
Hospitalization for heart failure or atrial fibrillation/ flutter (within previous 3 months)	Autoimmune diseases	Diabetes mellitus
Hip or knee replacement	Blood transfusion	Arterial hypertension
Major trauma	Central venous lines, intravenous catheters and leads	Immobility due to sitting (e.g., prolonged car or air travel)
Myocardial infarction (within previous 3 months)	Chemotherapy	Increasing age
Previous VTE	Congestive heart failure or respiratory failure	Laparoscopic surgery (e.g., cholecystectomy)
Spinal cord injury	• Erythropoiesis-stimulating agents • Hormone replacement therapy, in vitro fertilization, oral contraceptive therapy, postpartum period • Infection (specifically pneumonia, urinary tract infection, and HIV) • Inflammatory bowel disease • Cancer (highest risk in metastatic disease) • Paralytic stroke • Superficial vein thrombosis • Thrombophilia	• Obesity • Pregnancy • Varicose veins

(HIV: human immunodeficiency virus; VTE: venous thromboembolism)

as it indicates central or extensive PE. Dyspnea may be acute and severe in central PE, often mild and transient in small peripheral PE. Chest pain is a frequent symptom, caused by pleural irritation due to emboli causing pulmonary infarction. Central PE can have angina like chest pain. Signs of RV pressure overload may be present in case of larger emboli such as raised jugular venous pressure (JVP), tender hepatomegaly, parasternal heave, loud P2, and murmur of tricuspid regurgitation (TR). Other examination findings include calf swelling, tenderness, erythema, palpable cords, pedal edema, rales, and decreased breath sounds.

DIAGNOSIS

Management of PE depends upon early diagnosis to decide appropriate reperfusion and anticoagulant therapy to reduce mortality and morbidity.

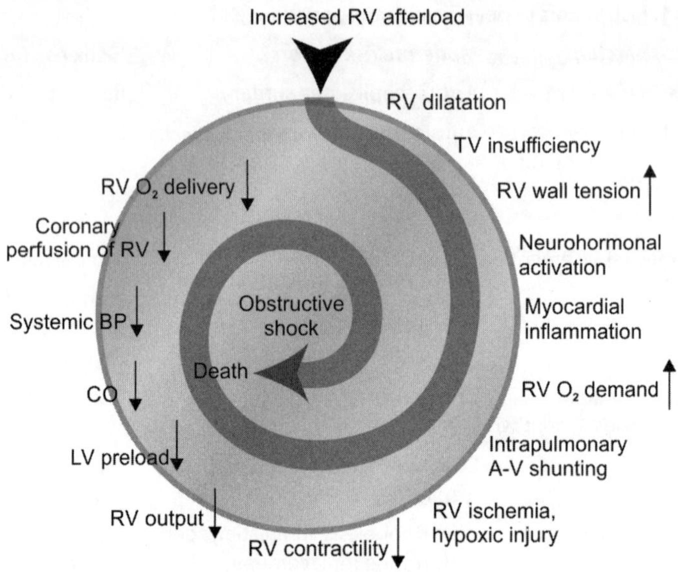

Fig. 1: Right ventricular (RV) dysfunction. (BP: blood pressure; CO: cardiac output; LV: left ventricular; TV: tricuspid valve)

Standard diagnostic strategies for PE consist of three steps: Evaluating clinical probability, D-dimer testing when indicated, and chest imaging if indicated. The first step of the diagnostic strategy is estimating the clinical probability of PE as low, moderate, or high. Two structured scores are validated for identifying the clinical probability of PE: Wells score and revised Geneva score **(Table 2)**.

- *Arterial blood gas (ABG) analysis*: Widened alveolar-arterial gradient for oxygen, respiratory alkalosis, and hypocapnia are commonly seen.
- *B-type natriuretic peptide (BNP) and proBNP*: Markers of RV dysfunction and reflect the severity of RV dysfunction in acute PE.
- *Troponin:* Serum troponin I and T levels are beneficial prognostically and are linked to clinical deterioration and death after PE.
- *D-dimer:* D-dimer levels are elevated in plasma, whenever there is an acute thrombotic process. A normal D-dimer level makes acute PE or DVT unlikely. But positive predictive value of elevated D-dimer levels is low, D-dimer testing is not useful for confirmation of PE. The use of age-adjusted cutoffs may improve the performance of D-dimer testing in the elderly. The formula is age (years) × 10 μg/L for patients >50 years of age.
- *Electrocardiography (ECG):* The most common ECG findings in PE are tachycardia and nonspecific ST-segment T-wave changes, S1Q3T3 pattern, RV strain, and new right bundle branch block.

TABLE 2: Scores for identifying clinical probability of PE.

Revised Geneva score		***Wells score***	
Variable	***Points***	***Variable***	***Points***
Predisposing factors		*Predisposing factors*	
Age >65 years	+1		
Previous DVT or PE	+3	Previous DVT or PE	+1.5
Surgery or fracture within 1 month	+2	Recent surgery or immobilization	+1.5
Active malignancy	+2	Cancer	+1
Symptoms		*Symptoms*	
Unilateral lower limb pain	+3		
Hemoptysis	+2	Hemoptysis	+1
Clinical signs		*Clinical signs*	
Heart rate		Heart rate	
75–94 beats/min		>100 beats/min	+1.5
±95 beats/min	+5		
Pain on lower limb deep vein at palpitation and unilateral edema	+5 +4	Clinical signs of DVT	+3
		Clinical judgement	
		Alternative diagnosis less likely than PE	+3
Clinical probability	***Total***	***Clinical probability (3 levels)***	***Total***
Low	0–3	Low	0–1
Intermediate	4–10	Intermediate	2–6
High	±11	High	±7
		Clinical probability (2 levels)	***Total***
		PE unlikely	0–4
		PE likely	>4

(DVT: deep vein thrombosis; PE: pulmonary embolism)

- *Chest radiograph:* Chest X-ray (CXR) **(Fig. 2)** is usually normal or show nonspecific abnormalities such as atelectasis or effusion. It helps to rule out alternative diagnoses.
- *Fleischner sign:* Enlarged pulmonary artery.
- *Hampton's hump:* Peripheral wedge of airspace opacity and implies lung infarction.
- *Westermark sign:* Regional oligemia and highest positive predictive value.
- *Knuckle sign:* Abrupt tapering or cutoff of a pulmonary artery secondary to an embolus.
- *Palla sign:* Enlarged right descending pulmonary artery.

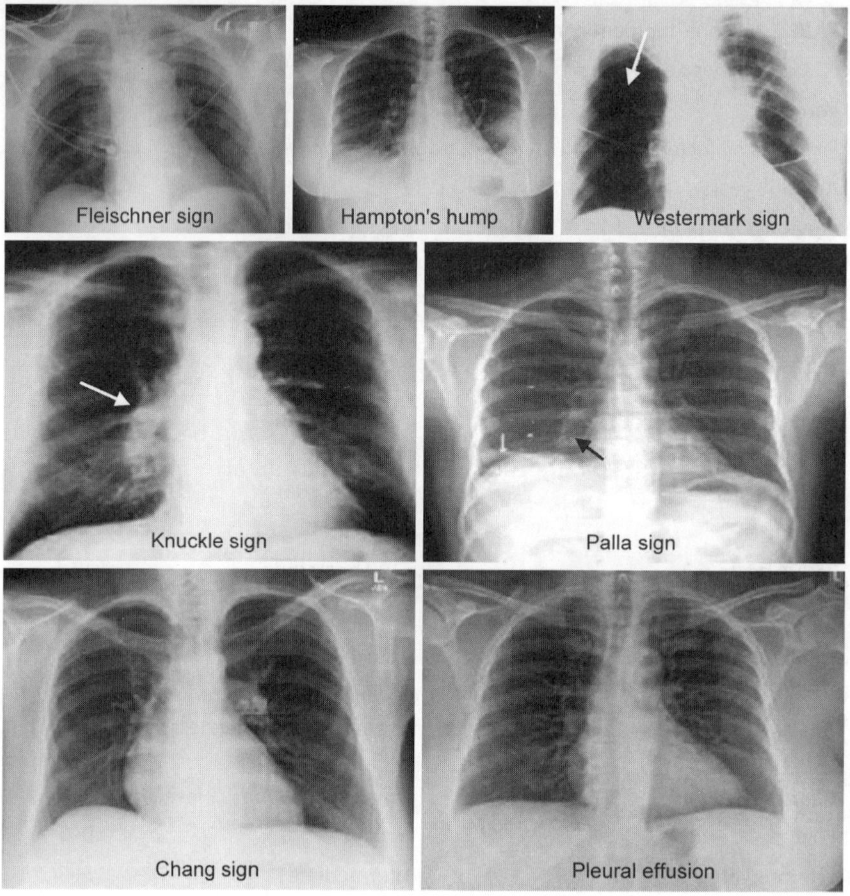

Fig. 2: Chest X-ray.

- *Chang sign:* Dilated right descending pulmonary artery with sudden cutoff, and in some cases pleural effusion evident.
- *Computed tomographic pulmonary angiography (CTPA):* Gold standard for the diagnosis of PE. It has an excellent accuracy in diagnosing PE. CT scan showing right pulmonary thrombus with RV enlargement (RV/LV ratio >1) suggestive of massive PE. It allows appropriate visualization of the pulmonary arteries down to the subsegmental level.
- *Lung scintigraphy:* V/Q scanning is mostly performed for patients in whom computed tomography pulmonary angiogram (CTPA) is contraindicated or inconclusive, or when additional testing is needed. A normal chest radiograph is usually required before V/Q scanning.
- *Pulmonary angiography:* In pulmonary angiography, contrast is injected via a catheter introduced into the right heart under fluoroscopy, which was the gold standard in the past for the diagnosis of PE, presents like

intraluminal filling defects, and as amputation of a pulmonary arterial branch. Thrombi as small as 1–2 mm within the subsegmental arteries can be visualized by digital subtraction angiography.

- *Magnetic resonance angiography (MRA):* Due to low availability, inconclusive MRA scan, and low sensitivity, MRA is not in usual clinical practice to diagnose PE.
- *Echocardiography:* It may demonstrate intracardiac, main pulmonary artery, and its main branches clots, RV enlargement, and signs of RV dysfunction. The pulmonary ejection acceleration time (measured in the RV outflow tract) <60 ms with a peak systolic tricuspid valve gradient <60 mm Hg ("60/60" sign), or McConnell sign (with depressed contractility of the RV free wall compared to the RV apex), is suggestive of PE. An RV/LV diameter ratio 1.0 or more and tricuspid annular plane systolic excursion (TAPSE) <16 mm are associated with unfavorable prognosis **(Figs. 3A to H)**.

Compression ultrasonography (CUS): PE originates from a lower limb DVT in a majority of patients, and rarely from upper-limb DVT. In the setting of suspected PE, CUS can be limited to a simple four point examination bilateral groin and popliteal fossa. The only validated diagnostic criterion for DVT is incomplete compressibility of the vein, which indicates the presence of a clot, whereas flow measurements are unreliable.

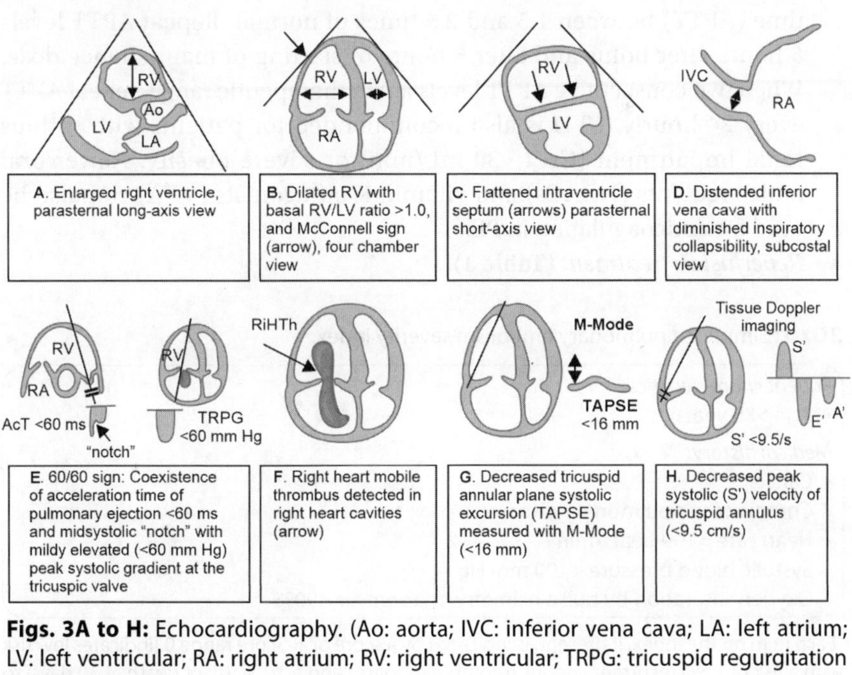

Figs. 3A to H: Echocardiography. (Ao: aorta; IVC: inferior vena cava; LA: left atrium; LV: left ventricular; RA: right atrium; RV: right ventricular; TRPG: tricuspid regurgitation peak gradient)

TREATMENT

Patients diagnosed with PE should be stratified according to their risk for in-hospital mortality (low, intermediate, or high risk) when selecting therapy. The simplified PE severity index (sPESI) is a 6-item score that classifies patients with PE **(Box 1)**.

- *The supportive measures:* Supplemental oxygen is indicated in patients with oxygen saturation <90%. Mechanical ventilation noninvasive or invasive should be utilized in unstable patients. RV failure should be treated with judicious use of crystalloids ≤500 mL over 15–30 minutes, vasopressors norepinephrine, 0.2–1.0 μg/kg/min and inotropes dobutamine, 2–20 mg/kg/min and if needed mechanical circulatory support venoarterial extracorporeal membrane oxygenation (ECMO) can be employed.
- *Anticoagulation*: Low-molecular-weight heparin (LMWH) or fondaparinux or unfractionated heparin (UFH) can be used for anticoagulation in acute PE. *Enoxaparin:* 1 mg/kg subcutaneously (SC) twice a day. *Fondaparinux: Weight <50 kg*—5 mg SC once a day, *weight 50–100 kg*—7.5 mg SC once a day, and *weight >100 kg*—10 mg SC once a day. Use of UFH is largely restricted to patients with overt hemodynamic instability or imminent hemodynamic decompensation in whom primary reperfusion treatment will be necessary. Bolus infusion of 80 units IU/kg followed by 18 units IU/kg, keeping activated partial thromboplastin time (APTT) between 1.5 and 2.5 times of normal. Repeat APTT levels 6 hours after bolus and after 6 hours of starting of maintenance dose. When two consecutive APTT levels are in therapeutic range, repeat APTT every 24 hourly. UFH is also recommended for patients with serious renal impairment [CrCl <30 mL/min] or severe obesity. Newer oral anticoagulants (NOACs) and vitamin K antagonists (VKA) can also be used for anticoagulation in PE.
- *Reperfusion treatment* **(Table 3)**

BOX 1: Simplified pulmonary embolism severity index.

Patient characteristics:[a]
- Age >80 years

Medical history:
- Cancer
- Chronic cardiopulmonary disease
- Heart rate >109 beats/min
- Systolic blood pressure <100 mm Hg
- Oxygen saturation by pulse oximetry on room air <90%

[a]Each item on the index, if present, is indicated by a score of 1. Score range 0 (indicates low risk with a risk of 1.5% recurrent venous thromboembolism and a 1.1% risk of death at 30 days) to 6 (score greater than 0 indicates intermediate or high risk with a 10% risk of death at 30 days).

TABLE 3: Reperfusion therapy.

Molecule	*Regimen*
rtPA	100 mg over 2 hours C.6 mg/kg over 15 minutes (maximum dose 50 mg)[a]
Streptokinase	250,000 IU as a loading dose over 30 minutes, followed by 100,000 IU/h over 12–24 hours *Accelerated regimen:* 1.5 million IU over 2 hours
Urokinase	4,400 IU/kg as a loading dose over 10 minutes, followed by 4,400 IU/kg/h over 12–24 hours *Accelerated regimen:* 3 million IU over 2 hours

[a]Sometimes used in extreme hemodynamic instability such as cardiac arrest.
(rtPA: recombinant tissue plasminogen activator)

- *Systemic thrombolysis:* Leads to faster improvements in pulmonary obstruction, pulmonary artery pressure (PAP), and pulmonary vascular resistance (PVR) in patients with PE, reduction in RV dilation. The greatest benefit is observed when treatment is initiated within 48 hours of symptom onset, but thrombolysis can still be useful who have had symptoms for 6–14 days. Patients with high-risk PE, defined as the presence of cardiogenic shock, thrombolysis has significant reduction in mortality and recurrent PE. Use in intermediate risk PE is controversial, thrombolysis was associated with a significant reduction in the risk of hemodynamic decompensation or collapse, but it also showed an increased risk of severe bleeding.
- *Invasive treatment (surgical embolectomy or percutaneous mechanical thrombectomy):* It is indicated when thrombolytic therapy is contraindicated and where hemodynamic status does not improve with medical treatment **(Box 2)**. Mechanical reperfusion is based on the insertion of a catheter into the pulmonary arteries via the femoral route and used for mechanical fragmentation, thrombus aspiration, or a pharmacomechanical approach combining mechanical or ultrasound fragmentation of the thrombus with in situ reduced-dose thrombolysis.

- *Vena cava filters:* These trap the emboli and prevent them from entering the pulmonary circulation. Filters are indicated in patients who have an absolute contraindication to anticoagulants, and in patients with recurrent venous thromboembolism (VTE) despite anticoagulation. Retrievable filters are preferred, such that once the contraindication has resolved, the filter can be removed.

The aim of anticoagulation after acute PE is to complete the treatment of the acute episode and prevent recurrence of VTE over the long-term. Therapeutic anticoagulation for ≥3 months is recommended for all patients with PE. Extended oral anticoagulation of indefinite duration should be considered for patients with a first episode of PE and no identifiable risk

BOX 2: Contraindications to fibrinolysis.

Absolute:
- History of hemorrhagic stroke or stroke of unknown origin
- Ischemic stroke in previous 6 months
- Central nervous system neoplasm
- Major trauma, surgery, or head injury in previous 3 weeks
- Bleeding diathesis
- Active bleeding

Relative:
- Transient ischemic attack in previous 6 months
- Oral anticoagulation
- Pregnancy or first postpartum week
- Noncompressible puncture sites
- Traumatic resuscitation
- Refractory hypertension (systolic blood pressure >180 mm Hg)
- Advanced liver disease
- Infective endocarditis
- Active peptic ulcer

factor. For patients with PE and cancer, extended anticoagulation (beyond the first 6 months) should be considered for an indefinite period or until the cancer is cured.

A timely diagnosis of PE is crucial because of the high associated mortality and morbidity, which may be prevented with early treatment.

SUMMARY

Acute pulmonary embolism is a common condition with a variable presentation, making the diagnosis challenging. It must be differentiated from other cardiopulmonary conditions presenting with similar symptoms to ensure accurate diagnosis and management. Coordination among the interprofessional team members to diagnose and manage acute pulmonary embolism, enhance the care of patients. By combining patient presentation, clinical suspicion, and scoring systems, diagnosis may be streamlined and unnecessary treatment can be minimized.

SUGGESTED READING

1. Kahn SR, de Wit K. Pulmonary Embolism. N Engl J Med. 2022;387(1):45-57.
2. Kasturi S. Current concepts in the diagnosis and management of pulmonary embolism. Int J Clin Med. 2021;12(3):115-29.
3. Konstantinides SV, Meyer G, Becattini C, Bueno H, Geersing GJ, Harjola VP, et al. ESC scientific document group (2020). 2019 ESC Guidelines for the diagnosis and management of acute pulmonary embolism developed in collaboration with the European Respiratory Society (ERS). Eur Heart J. 2020;41(4):543-603.
4. Meyer G, Vieillard-Baron A, Planquette B. Recent advances in the management of pulmonary embolism: focus on the critically ill patients. Ann Intensive Care. 2016;6(1):19.

SECTION

4 Cardiovascular Diseases

CHAPTER

12 Hemodynamic Monitoring

Poorva Dilip Magarkar

INTRODUCTION

Shock is defined as a life-threatening acute circulatory failure, which leads to either failure of oxygen delivery or its utilization by the tissues. Shock can be caused by a single pathology or a combination of different disease processes. Shock, unless identified and corrected promptly, may lead to multiorgan failure and death.

Hemodynamic monitoring forms an integral part of critically ill patient's management. The main goal is to assess cardiovascular system and its response to tissue oxygen demands. Therapeutic measures include fluid resuscitation, vasopressors, or inotropic agents. This monitoring includes several different techniques, each with its own advantages and disadvantages, and may range from invasive to less and noninvasive techniques, calibrated or noncalibrated.

Those who are unstable, or at risk of instability, should receive an arterial line for continuous invasive blood pressure measurement and regular analysis of arterial blood gases (ABGs). When initial resuscitation fails to improve the hemodynamic status, advanced hemodynamic monitoring will be required to guide further management.

Most common intervention for any shock is volume expansion. The rationale is to increase the cardiac output (CO) and oxygen delivery to tissue. The response to a fluid challenge is complicated. Due to varying shapes the Frank-Starling curve could take depending on the ventricular systolic function; volume expansion can lead to either a significant or a negligible increase in stroke volume (SV) and CO after fluids. The gold standard for assessing fluid responsiveness is to perform a fluid challenge which involves the infusion of a specific amount of intravenous fluid to assess ventricular preload reserve and subsequent hemodynamic effects. Fluid responsiveness is conventionally defined as >10–15% increase in SV in response to a fluid challenge. Fluid responsiveness depends on dynamic interaction between intravascular volume, vascular tone, and ventricular function.

STATIC HEMODYNAMIC ASSESSMENT

Several studies have demonstrated poor predictive value of these static indices.

- *Capillary refill time (CRT):* Press the nailbed of patient's finger (second or third finger) between thumb and index finger so that the blood is pushed out. Do this for 5 seconds and count the number of seconds it takes for the color of the nailbed to return to the original color. CRT >3.5 seconds indicates poor peripheral perfusion. CRT is one of the first parameters to normalize during resuscitation
- *Central venous pressure (CVP) monitoring:* CVP is used as a marker of preload, an index of intravascular volume status. It is influenced by the volume status, myocardial contractility, afterload, and intrathoracic and intra-abdominal pressures. Hence, the CVP can be confusing and at the same time difficult to interpret. CVP does not predict fluid responsiveness and should not be used to guide fluid administration. Data might suggest that extreme CVP values can help to guide fluids responsiveness whereas intermediate values cannot.
- *Pulmonary capillary wedge pressure:* Measured by catheterization of pulmonary artery. Pulmonary artery occlusion pressure (PAOP) is a better estimate of left ventricular end-diastolic pressure (LVEDP) than CVP. It is a poor predictor of fluid responsiveness. Even left ventricular end-diastolic volume (LVEDV) cannot be used for this purpose because the relationship between left ventricular filling and LVEDV is dependent on heart cavities characteristics and inotropic state, which are different between individuals and at different stages of illness.
- *Intra-arterial pressure waveform analysis* ***(Fig. 1)****:* Besides real-time recording of arterial pressure, other hemodynamic interpretations can be made. Systolic blood pressure variations (swing in the waveform) seen

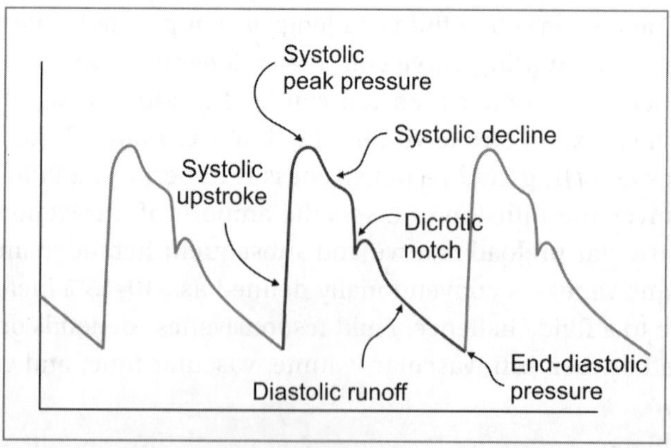

Fig. 1: Intra-arterial pressure waveform.

during hypovolemia. Steep slope of upstroke means good contractility and vice versa. Area under the curve represents the SV. Position of the dicrotic notch, low indicates low systemic vascular resistance and high indicates high afterload. Slope of the descent, steep indicates low systemic vascular resistance (SVR).

- *Arterial blood gas analysis:* The normal lactate ranges from 0.5 to 2 mmol/L and rise >2 mmol/L is significant. Hyperlactatemia is a prognostic marker in shock states. Lactate normalization within first 6 hours of resuscitation is the strongest independent predictor of survival. Lactate levels should be used along with the clinical scenario and also serial measurements of lactate have more value than a single measure.
- *Base deficit (BD):* It is derived from ABG and correlates with the need for crystalloid resuscitation, need for urgent blood transfusion in hypovolemic shock and also with mortality.
- *Mixed (SvO_2) and central venous ($ScvO_2$) oxygen saturation:* One of the early goals for resuscitation in sepsis patients. Low $ScvO_2$ suggests poor tissue hypoperfusion and patients should be evaluated to determine the cause of shock and guide further therapy. A high $ScvO_2$ may indicate impaired oxygen utilization by the tissues. Trials showed no mortality benefit in resuscitation targeting venous $ScvO_2$ >70%.
- *Central venous-arterial CO_2 gradient ($PcvaCO_2$):* Venous-to-arterial carbon dioxide gradient can be used to assess the adequacy of CO. An increased $PcvaCO_2$ gradient can suggest ischemic hypoxia at tissues due to inadequate CO. Values <6 mm Hg correlate with a high cardiac index, improved microcirculatory perfusion, and values >6 mm Hg indicate impaired perfusion.
- *The venous-arterial CO_2 to arterial-venous O_2 ratio ($Cv\text{-}aCO_2/Ca\text{-}vO_2$ ratio):* Oxygen consumption (VO_2) and CO_2 production (VCO_2) are directly proportional to CO and their respective arterial-to-venous and venous-to-arterial content differences. $Cv\text{-}aCO_2/Ca\text{-}vO_2$ ratio >1.0 could suggest the presence of anaerobic metabolism. Could anticipate lactate increase during early stages of shock.
- *Global end-diastolic volume index (GEDVI)/extravascular lung water index (EVLWI)/pulmonary vascular permeability index (PVPI):* These tests are used to differentiate between cardiogenic and noncardiogenic pulmonary edema and fluid therapy can be implemented appropriately. The normal values for GEDVI (600–800 mL/m^2), EVLWI (12 mL/kg), and PVPI ≤2 should be kept in mind to deliver fluid therapy in critically-ill patients.
- *Echocardiography:* Patients with left ventricular (LV) systolic dysfunction are at higher risk of fluid overload and need closer monitoring during fluid resuscitation. In patients with a grossly dilated right ventricle (RV)

with RV systolic dysfunction, fluid administration can lead to overdistension of the RV, and precipitate RV ischemia due to the increased wall tension. The ratio of E to é correlates well with LV-filling pressures. An E/é ratio of >15 suggests elevated LV-filling pressures. Estimate of RV and LV end-diastolic area, as surrogates for end-diastolic volume (EDV), can be used for fluid responsiveness.

DYNAMIC HEMODYNAMIC MONITORING

These tests are based on the principle of inducing short-term changes in cardiac preload, using heart-lung interactions, by infusion of small volumes of fluid, and to observe the effect on CO. Dynamic indices should be preferred over static indices to predict fluid responsiveness.

- *Pulse pressure variation (PPV):* PPV is defined as percentage change in pulse pressure (difference between systolic and diastolic pressure) during a single respiratory cycle. It is calculated as:

  $$PPV = [(\text{Pulse pressure}_{max} - \text{Pulse pressure}_{min})/\text{Pulse pressure}_{mean}] \times 100$$

  It is a reliable predictor in ventilated patients with regular cardiac rhythms. The median threshold of the PPV is 12% (interquartile range 10–13%) with a sensitivity of 88% and a specificity of 89% **(Fig. 2)**.
- *Stroke volume variation (SVV):* SVV is the percentage change in SV during a single respiratory cycle. It is calculated a-s:

  $$SVV = [(\text{Stroke volume}_{max} - \text{Stroke volume}_{min})/\text{Stroke volume}_{mean}] \times 100\%$$

  An SVV >10–12% predict fluid responsiveness with high sensitivity and specificity **(Fig. 2)**.

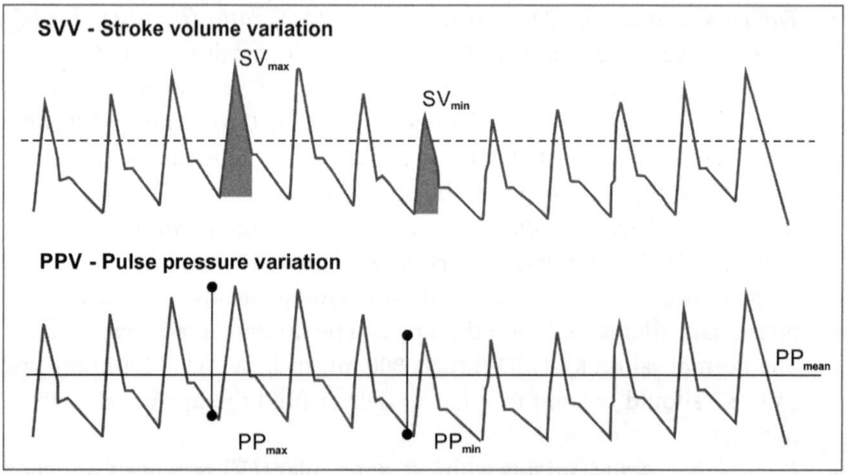

Fig. 2: Pulse pressure variation and stroke volume variation.

TABLE 1: Conditions where pulse pressure and stroke volume variations are less reliable.

False positive	*False negative*
Right heart failure	Low tidal volume
Raised intra-abdominal pressure	Low lung compliance
Spontaneous breathing	High respiratory rate
Cardiac arrhythmias	Open chest

During positive pressure ventilation, insufflation decreases preload of the right ventricle, causing decrease in preload of the left ventricle. If left ventricular SV changes in response to cyclic positive pressure ventilation, indicates that both ventricles are preload dependent **(Table 1)**.

- *Inferior vena cava assessment:* The principle behind this is also based on heart-lung interactions. The changes in intrathoracic pressure induced by mechanical ventilation induce some variations in the vena cava in close proximity to the heart when the central blood volume is low. Respiratory variations in superior vena cava (SVC) and inferior vena cava (IVC) diameters can easily be estimated by echocardiography **(Figs. 3A and B)**.

  During controlled mechanical ventilation, IVC diameter is maximum during inspiration. The respiratory variations in the diameter of the IVC are used to calculate the IVC distensibility index. A cutoff value of ≥18% reliably predicts fluid responsiveness.

  IVC distensibility index

  $= [(\text{IVC diameter}_{max} - \text{IVC diameter}_{min})/\text{IVC diameter}_{min}] \times 100$

  Fluid responsiveness assessed in spontaneously breathing patients by calculating the IVC collapsibility index. The optimal cutoff ranges between 40 and 48%.

  IVC collapsibility index

  $= [(\text{IVC diameter}_{max} - \text{IVC diameter}_{min})/\text{IVC diameter}_{max}] \times 100$

- *Superior vena cava assessment:* During the respiratory cycle under mechanical ventilation, SVC collapses with the increase in intrathoracic pressure which is reversed to IVC changes. SVC can be visualized on transesophageal and on transthoracic echocardiography by experienced sonographers. A variation in SVC >37–39% is predictive of fluid responsiveness.

  SVC collapsibility index

  $= [(\text{SVC diameter}_{max} - \text{SVC diameter}_{min})/\text{SVC diameter}_{min}] \times 100$

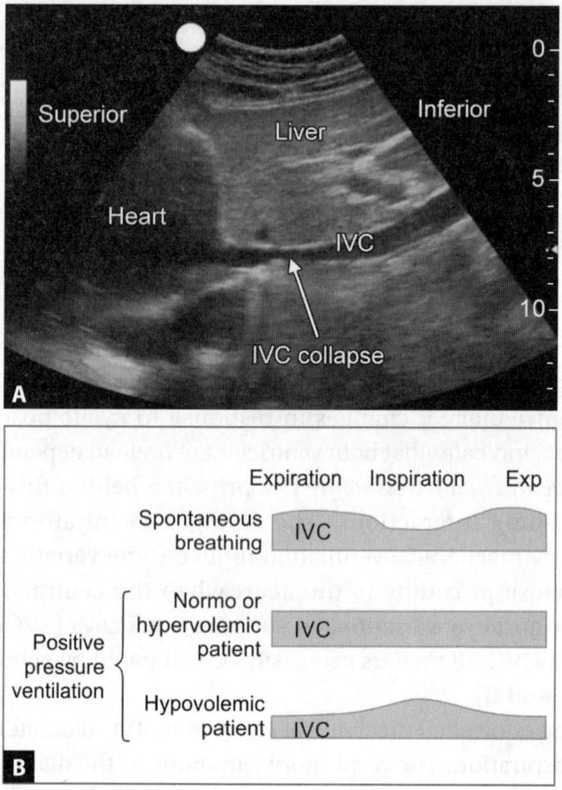

Figs. 3A and B: Echocardiography. (IVC: inferior vena cava)

- *Passive leg raising (PLR) test:* The transition from the semirecumbent position to a position where lower limbs are raised to 45° and the trunk is horizontal, induces the transfer of venous blood from the lower limbs and also from the splanchnic territory, toward the cardiac cavities. Perform the test by changing the bed position, not by raising the patient's legs manually. A PLR test was equivalent to about 300 mL of fluid challenge, but this is only an average value, this volume is variable depending on the patient circumstances. The diagnostic threshold found was 10% increase in CO. The PLR test can be used in spontaneous breathing, low tidal volume (Vt) ventilation and low lung compliance, and cardiac arrhythmias. A real-time measurement of CO is needed. Esophageal Doppler and pulse wave contour analysis can be used. If the ventilation conditions are stable, changes in end-tidal carbon dioxide are proportional to changes in CO. If end-tidal carbon dioxide value increased by >5% or 2 mm Hg during the PLR test, fluid responsiveness could be reliably predicted **(Fig. 4)**.

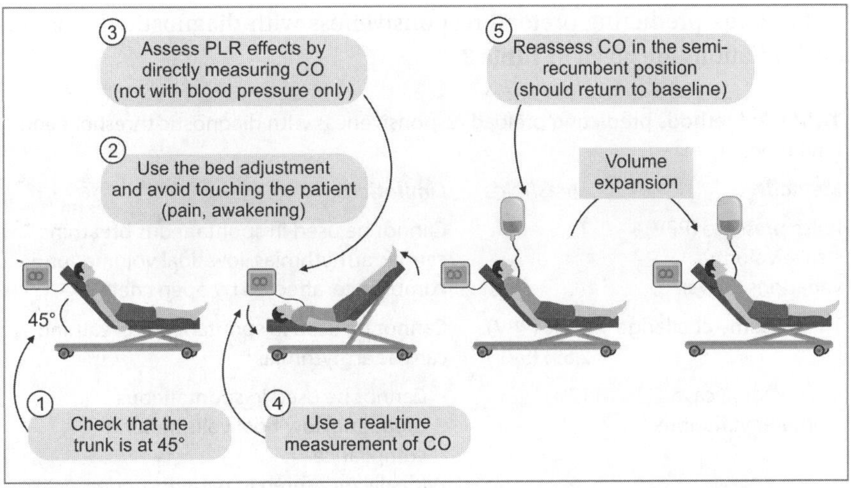

Fig. 4: Passive leg raising test. (CO: cardiac output; PLR: passive leg raising)

- *Fluid challenge (FC):* At least 4 mL/kg crystalloid be given over 5–10 minutes for performing fluid-challenge test. A positive response to FC would imply a 10–15% increase in SV or CO.
- *Mini-fluid challenge:* Consist of infusing 100–150 mL of fluids over 1–2 minutes and measuring the response of CO or one of its surrogate. The threshold for variation of CO after a mini-fluid challenge is small 5% on average, thus it requires a very precise technique to measure CO during the test.
- *Tidal volume challenge:* PPV and SVV are not reliable in case of low Vt ventilation. The test involves transiently increasing Vt from 6 to 8 mL/kg predicted body weight (PBW) for 1 minute and observing the change in PPV/SVV (ΔPPV_{6-8}) from baseline (PPV_6) to that at 8 mL/kg PBW (PPV_8). A ΔPPV_{6-8} >3.5% and ΔSVV_{6-8} >2.5% predict fluid responsiveness with high accuracy.
- *End-expiratory occlusion test (EEOT):* The test consists of interrupting the ventilator at end-expiration for 15–30 seconds and assessing the changes in CO. During this, inspiration is prevented, thereby preventing an increase in the intrathoracic pressure, resulting in increase in the venous return, and thus preload and right ventricular SV in fluid responsive patients. An increase in CO of >5% after an EEOT predicts fluid responsiveness. This test is like giving a mini auto fluid challenge. This test is more reliable when used with a continuous CO monitoring.
- *Aortic velocity time integral (VTI):* Helps in identifying the underlying etiology of shock. Normal values in adult patients at rest are between 18 and 22 cm, lower values are an index of reduced CO.

Methods predicting preload responsiveness with diagnostic threshold and limitations are given in **Table 2**.

TABLE 2: Methods predicting preload responsiveness with diagnostic threshold and limitations.

Method	*Threshold*	*Limitations*
Pulse pressure (PPV)/ stroke volume variations (SVVs)	12%	Cannot be used in spontaneous breathing, cardiac arrhythmias, low tidal volume/lung compliance, affected by open chest
Tidal volume challenge	3.5% (PPV), 2.5% (SVV)	Cannot be used in spontaneous breathing, cardiac arrhythmias
Inferior vena cava diameter variations	12%	• Cannot be used in spontaneous breathing, low tidal volume/lung compliance • Ideally measured in patients under controlled ventilation • A higher cutoff for IVC distensibility (50%) may be considered in patients with spontaneous breathing
Superior vena cava diameter variations	36%	• Requires performing transesophageal Doppler • Cannot be used in case of spontaneous breathing, low tidal volume/lung compliance
Passive leg raising	1%	• Requires a direct measurement of cardiac output • May be affected by raised intra-abdominal pressure • Contraindicated in cases of raised ICP and unstable spine injury
End-expiratory occlusion test	5%	• Cannot be used in nonintubated patients • Cannot be used in patients who interrupt a 15 seconds respiratory hold • May be affected by extreme levels of peep and low tidal volume • Prone for errors in measurement as the change is small
"Mini"-fluid challenge (100 mL)	6%	Requires a precise technique for measuring cardiac output
"Standard" fluid challenge (300–500 mL)	15%	Requires a direct measurement of cardiac output, induces fluid overload if repeated

(ICP: intracranial pressure; IVC: inferior vena cava)

SUMMARY

The primary hemodynamic goal in the management of critically ill patients needs the assessment and manipulation of circulatory system to provide adequate tissue delivery of oxygen and essential metabolic substrates. Newer dynamic measures, which rely on real-time measurements of certain physiological parameters have replaced earlier static measures of volume status. Ultimately, clinical judgment, proper interpretation of measurements, and appropriate therapeutic measures are the most important aspects of hemodynamic monitoring. Traditional methods continue to have a role in assessment of critically ill patients but newer technologies have expanded circulatory monitoring systems.

SUGGESTED READING

1. De Backer D, Aissaoui N, Cecconi M, Chew MS, Denault A, Hajjar L, et al. How can assessing hemodynamics help to assess volume status? Intensive Care Med. 2022;48(10):1482-94.
2. Huygh J, Peeters Y, Bernards J, Malbrain ML. Hemodynamic monitoring in the critically ill: an overview of current cardiac output monitoring methods. F1000Res. 2016;5:F1000 Faculty Rev-2855.
3. Kulkarni AP, Govil D, Samavedam S, Srinivasan S, Ramasubban S, Venkataraman R, et al. ISCCM Guidelines for hemodynamic monitoring in the critically ill. Indian J Crit Care Med. 2022;26(Suppl 2):S66-76.
4. Monnet X, Teboul JL. Passive leg raising: five rules, not a drop of fluid! Crit Care. 2015;19(1):18.
5. Pinsky MR, Cecconi M, Chew MS, De Backer D, Douglas I, Edwards M, et al. Effective hemodynamic monitoring. Crit Care. 2022;26(1):294.
6. Pinsky MR. Functional hemodynamic monitoring. Crit Care Clin. 2015;31(1):89-111.

CHAPTER

13 Acute Coronary Syndrome

Poorva Dilip Magarkar

INTRODUCTION

Acute coronary syndrome (ACS) is a medical emergency which requires prompt diagnosis and care. Patients with ACS complain of moderate-to-severe chest discomfort that lasts >20 minutes. Atypical presentations are not uncommon in women, diabetic patients, and the elderly. The ACS can be classified into:

- Unstable angina (UA)
- Non-ST-elevation myocardial infarction (NSTEMI)
- ST-elevation myocardial infarction (STEMI)

This classification of ACS is based on clinical features which includes electrocardiogram (ECG) findings and biochemical markers of myocardial necrosis.

Unstable angina: Symptoms and signs of myocardial infarction (MI) with transient or no ECG changes (ST-segment depression or T-wave inversion) without elevation of cardiac enzymes. UA is due to unstable plaque which causes aggregation of platelets but without coronary obstruction. These patients carry high risk of developing an NSTEMI or STEMI.

NSTEMI: Symptoms and signs of MI with ECG changes (ST-segment depression or T-wave inversion) with elevation of cardiac enzymes which indicates myocardial necrosis.

STEMI: Symptoms and signs of MI with ST-elevations in ECG. It is due to prolonged ischemia because of total or near total occlusion of the coronary arteries due to plaque erosion leading to rupture, or fissuring, or dissection of coronary arteries that result in an obstructing thrombus causing myocardial necrosis.

PATHOPHYSIOLOGY

Acute coronary syndromes are usually triggered by the rupture of an atheromatous plaque or fissure formation in plaque in the coronary arteries, which causes thrombotic response leading to variable obstruction to the blood flow and causes ischemic injury to the myocardium. In UA and NSTEMI, the obstruction to flow is incomplete, whereas in STEMI, it is complete.

CLINICAL PRESENTATION

Clinical signs and symptoms include chest pain, discomfort in the upper extremity, mandibular or epigastrium, shortness of breath, diaphoresis, nausea, vomiting, fatigue, or syncope. Pain radiating to the left arm, right shoulder, or both arms, and presence of diaphoresis is more likely due to ischemia. These symptoms are not specific for ACS and sometimes may not occur at all. Atypical symptoms may be seen in women, elderly, diabetics, or immunocompromised group.

INVESTIGATIONS

- *ECG:* Presence of ST-segment elevation is the hallmark sign of STEMI. UA and NSTEMI present as generalized symmetrical T-wave inversion and ST-segment depression. Changes in ECG which are suggestive of STEMI [in the absence of left ventricular hypertrophy (LVH)/left bundle branch block (LBBB)] are as follows—New ST-elevations at the J point in at least two contiguous leads ≥2 mm (0.2 mV) in men or ≥1.5 mm (0.15 mV) in women in leads V2–V3 and/or of ≥1 mm (0.1 mV) in other contiguous chest or limb leads. The specificity of ST-elevation caused by STEMI is increased in the presence of ST depression in the reciprocal leads. New LBBB is considered as STEMI equivalent. ST elevation in right precordial leads V4R for right ventricular (RV) MI. ST depression in precordial leads (V1–V3) for posterior MI. Pathological "Q" waves. Sgarbossa's criteria are used to diagnose STEMI in patients with LBBB. ST-segment elevation (concordant) of ≥1 mm in ≥1 lead, ST-segment depression (concordant) of ≥1 mm in ≥1 lead of V1–V3, excessive discordance (proportionally) of STE in ≥1 lead anywhere with ≥1 mm STE, as defined by ≥25% of the depth of the preceding S-wave.
    - NSTEMI or UA will have ST segment depression or deep T-wave inversion without Q waves or no ECG changes.
- *Echocardiography:* It localizes area and extent of myocardial ischemia/infarction by showing regional wall motion abnormality (RWMA), pick up complications of ACS such as mitral valve regurgitation, tricuspid valve regurgitation, papillary muscles rupture, ventricular septal rupture (VSR), ventricular free wall rupture, left ventricular aneurysm, and ventricular thrombosis.
- *Cardiac biomarkers:* Biochemical markers of myocardial damage and signify myocardial injury leading to myocardial-cell necrosis. The preferred cardiac biomarker is troponin, as it has high clinical sensitivity and specificity. It is essential to do serial enzyme tests to detect a rise and/or fall in cardiac biomarkers. Troponin should be measured at the time of first clinical assessment, within 6 hours of the onset of pain, and in the 6–12 hours time frame after onset of pain and levels may remain elevated for up to 2 weeks.

- *A complete blood count:* Leukocytosis may be seen in MI, prothrombin time, activated partial thromboplastin time (APTT), liver and renal function test, and electrolytes.

MANAGEMENT

Stabilize the patient, follow airway, breathing, and circulation (ABCs) approach and simultaneously monitor for hemodynamic instability.

- *Give pain relief:* Sublingual nitroglycerine (0.4 mg) may be repeated twice or thrice or as an intravenous (IV) infusion (5–200 μg/min) if patient has persistent chest pain, hypertension, or heart failure (HF). Avoid nitrates, if hypotension systolic blood pressure (BP) <90 mm Hg, bradycardia (<50 beats/min), intake of phosphodiesterase inhibitors like sildenafil, inferior wall MI, and suspected right ventricular (RV) involvement. Morphine sulfate 2–4 mg IV initially with increments of 1–2 mg IV, repeated at 5–15 minutes for persistent chest pain unresponsive to nitroglycerine.
- *Give antiplatelets*: A combination of nonenteric coated aspirin (160–325 mg orally or chewed) and clopidogrel (300–600 mg orally) given as a loading dose. For elderly (>75 year) clopidogrel loading is with 75 mg, followed by aspirin (80–325 mg/day) indefinitely and clopidogrel 75 mg/day for at least 1 year. Prasugrel (60 mg) or ticagrelor (180 mg) can be used as an alternative to clopidogrel.
- *Anticoagulants*: The choice of anticoagulant depends upon the initial management strategy in ACS and varies from case-to-case. Low-molecular-weight heparins [enoxaparin 1 mg/kg 12-hourly subcutaneously (SC) or dalteparin 120 U/kg 12-hourly SC], or fondaparinux are commonly used agents.
- *Reperfusion therapy:* Coronary angioplasty with or without stent placement for the culprit vessel is the treatment of choice for STEMI when it is performed with a door-to-balloon time (<90 minutes) by a skilled provider.

  If patient is unable to reach a percutaneous coronary intervention (PCI)-capable hospital within 120 minutes of an STEMI, then fibrinolytic therapy should be administered within 30 minutes of hospital arrival in the absence of any contraindications. Fibrinolysis is restricted to patients with STEMI, presenting early (<3 hours) and at low risk of bleeding. Fibrinolysis can be given as a definitive treatment at centers without PCI facility, or as a bridging therapy prior to shifting for PCI. The recommended dosage regimen for tissue plasminogen activator (t-PA) is a 15 mg IV bolus followed by an infusion of 0.75 mg/kg (maximum 50 mg) over 30 minutes, followed by an infusion of 0.5 mg/kg (maximum 35 mg) over 60 minutes **(Table 1)**.

TABLE 1: Reperfusion therapy.

Agents	*Dose and administration*
Alteplase (tPA)	*90 minutes infusion:* 15 mg intravenous (IV) bolus, followed by infusion 0.75 mg/kg for 30 minutes (maximum 50 mg), then 0.5 mg (maximum 35 mg) over the next 60 minutes; total dose not to exceed 100 mg; 60 mg administered within first hour, then 20 mg during second and third hour
Reteplase (rPA)	Two 10 unit boluses, each administered over 2 minutes, 30 minutes apart
Tenecteplase (TNK)	• Single bolus administration over 5 seconds; dose based on patient weight (maximum dose 50 mg): • <60 kg: 30 mg; 60–69 kg: 35 mg; 70–79 kg: 40 mg; 80–89 kg: 45 mg; and ≥90 kg: 50 mg
Streptokinase	150,000 units IV infusion over 30–60 minutes

- *Statins:* Start 80 mg of atorvastatin or equivalent statin as early as possible and preferably before PCI in patients not on statin. The dose can later be decreased to achieve the target lipids [low-density lipoprotein (LDL) <70–100 mg/dL].
- *β-blockers*: Oral β-blockers should be started within the first 24 hours in those without evidence of HF, low cardiac output, shock, bradyarrhythmias, or conduction blocks, and other conventional contraindication like asthma. Cardioselective agents without intrinsic sympathomimetic activity are preferred. Metoprolol (50–200 mg/day) is the most commonly used agent.
- *Angiotensin-converting enzyme (ACE) inhibitor or angiotensin receptor blocker (ARB):* It should be started within 24 hours of onset of ACS who have pulmonary congestion, HF, STEMI with anterior location, or left ventricular ejection fraction (LVEF) ≤40% in the absence of any contraindications to the therapy.
- *Aldosterone antagonists:* Spironolactone, eplerenone recommended in those patients who are on therapeutic doses of an ACE inhibitor or ARB and beta blocker with an LVEF ≤40% and either symptomatic HF or diabetes mellitus.

COMPLICATIONS

Postinfarction complication rates have fallen since the advent of early reperfusion strategies. Patients with large infarction, silent infarction, late presentation, and delayed or incomplete reperfusion, remain at high risk for complications.

- *Arrhythmia:* Accelerated idioventricular rhythm (AIVR), is often seen immediately following successful reperfusion, does not require any specific intervention. Ventricular tachycardia (VT) is often associated with increased mortality. Correct potassium (K) and magnesium (Mg) levels in the setting of an infarction ($K > 4$ mEq/L and Mg >2 mEq/L). Right coronary artery infarct is associated with proximal atrioventricular (AV) nodal conduction disease. Left anterior descending/septal infarct is associated with distal (infranodal) conduction disease.

- *Heart failure:* Clinical symptoms of left ventricular (LV) dysfunction range from mild HF (e.g., rales or S3) to cardiogenic shock.
- *Ventricular free wall rupture:* It presents with hypotension and signs of cardiac tamponade. Any clinical suspicion needs immediate echocardiography and emergent surgery is usually the only chance for survival.
- *Mitral regurgitation (MR):* Ischemic MR may be caused by mitral annular dilatation in LV dysfunction, papillary muscle dysfunction, or papillary muscle rupture. MR secondary to papillary muscle rupture may be severe, suspected in patients with a new pansystolic murmur in the setting of HF, or hemodynamic compromise. Echocardiography [transthoracic echocardiograms (TTE) and transesophageal echocardiograms (TEE)] is essential for diagnosis and determining the etiology. Immediate surgery is indicated in patients with suspected papillary muscle rupture with the use of nitroprusside or intra-aortic balloon pump (IABP) in the setting of hypotension to stabilize the patient until surgery.
- *Ventricular septal rupture (VSR):* It is suspected in patients with new pansystolic murmur or palpable thrill with signs of worsening biventricular failure. Echocardiography is needed to detect and localize the VSR. All patients with a VSR require early surgical therapy. IABP or nitroprusside can be used to bridge patients to surgery by reducing the shunt.
- *Embolism:* Patients suffering a large anterior wall MI will develop a mural thrombus. Echocardiography should be performed in all patients with an MI to determine the presence of either a mural thrombus or akinetic segments that predispose to thrombus formation. Anticoagulation along with antiplatelets will be required after PCI.
- *Pericardial effusions/pericarditis:* Pericardial effusions are rarely life-threatening. Post-MI pericarditis can present from the first days after MI up to 6 weeks following infarct. This complication is due to local pericardial irritation. This is treated with high-dose aspirin 650 mg every 8 hours plus colchicine 0.5–0.6 mg twice daily, especially in early pericarditis. Dressler syndrome is a type of postinfarction pericarditis that occurs 1–8 weeks after the infarct. It is thought to be immune mediated and is best treated with high-dose aspirin.
- *Aneurysm*: The characteristic ECG findings of LV aneurysms are Q waves with persistent ST elevations. Anteroapical aneurysms (due to left anterior descending artery occlusion) are more common than inferoposterior

aneurysms. Acute aneurysms lead to decompensated HF and cardiogenic shock. For patients with refractory symptoms, surgery may be considered to repair a chronic aneurysm.

- *Recurrent myocardial infarction:* Chest pain after an MI may represent recurrent ischemia from incomplete revascularization, infarct extension, reinfarction, or postinfarction angina. Increases in creatine kinase myocardial band CK-MB isoenzymes after downtrending may be a more useful marker of reinfarction as troponins may not be useful due to their persistent elevation beyond 1 week. Aggressive medical therapy with anti-ischemic medications (e.g., aspirin, heparin, nitrates, and beta blockers) is important. Revascularization should be considered in patients whose symptoms are refractory. Reinfarction due to stent thrombosis usually has a severe anginal pain refractory to medical therapy and evolving ST elevations on ECG. These findings require immediate revascularization efforts.

SUMMARY

Acute myocardial infarction and unstable angina are often clinically indistinguishable at first. There is a much more evidence base for the treatment of management of ACS. Clinical examination, ECG, along with echocardiography are needed to exclude alternate diagnosis and to detect complications if any. Early risk stratification and prognostication with validated scoring systems, examination, biomarkers are effective means of guiding and escalation of therapy.

SUGGESTED READING

1. Amsterdam EA, Wenger NK, Brindis RG, Casey DE Jr, Ganiats TG, Holmes DR Jr, et al. 2014 AHA/ACC guideline for the management of patients with non-ST-elevation acute coronary syndromes: executive summary: a report of the American College of Cardiology/American Heart Association Task Force on Practice Guidelines. Circulation. 2014;130(25):2354.
2. Anderson JL, Morrow DA. Acute myocardial infarction. N Engl J Med. 2017;376:2053-64.
3. Ibanez B, James S, Agewall S, Antunes MJ, Bucciarelli-Ducci C, Bueno H, et al. 2017 ESC guidelines for the management of acute myocardial infarction in patients presenting with ST-segment elevation: The Task Force for the management of acute myocardial infarction in patients presenting with ST-segment elevation of the European Society of Cardiology (ESC). Eur Heart J. 2018;39(2):119-77.
4. Libby P. Mechanisms of acute coronary syndromes and their implications for therapy. N Engl J Med. 2013;368(21):2004-13.
5. Smith SW, Dodd KW, Henry TD, Dvorak DM, Pearce LA. Diagnosis of ST-elevation myocardial infarction in the presence of left bundle branch block using the ST-elevation to S-wave ratio in a modified Sgarbossa rule. Ann Emerg Med. 2012;60(6):766-76.
6 Thygesen K, Alpert JS, Jaffe AS, Simoons ML, Chaitman BR, White HD, et al. Joint ESC/ACCF/AHA/WHF Task Force for the Universal Definition of Myocardial Infarction. Third universal definition of myocardial infarction. Circulation. 2012;126(16):2020-35.

CHAPTER

14

Postcardiac Arrest Management

Bindu Mulakavalupil

POSTCARDIAC ARREST MANAGEMENT

Postresuscitation can be considered a multiorgan illness **(Box 1 and Table 1)**.

PATHOPHYSIOLOGY

Systemic ischemia followed by reperfusion triggers a systematic inflammatory response syndrome which can cause an inappropriate vasodilation and microvascular function which alone with dysregulated coagulopathy can cause early organ dysfunction. Lung protective ventilation avoiding hyperventilation and hyperoxia should be the norm **(Boxes 2 and 3)**.

BOX 1: Early postresuscitation priorities.

- Provide adequate oxygenation and ventilation
- Reverse shock and stabilize hemodynamics
- Identify and treat reversible cause of cardiac arrest
- Apply neuroprotective therapies—therapeutic hypothermia
- Correct metabolic disturbances

TABLE 1: Early hemodynamic resuscitation goals following cardiac arrest.

Resuscitation priority	*Monitor and goal*	*Therapy*
Preload optimization	• Response to fluid challenge • CVP 8–12 mm Hg • Echo cardiac function and IVC variation • Stroke volume variation	Fluid challenge
Perfusion pressure	MAP 65–100 mm Hg	• Norepinephrine • Dopamine • Vasopressin
Perfusion optimization	• Global perfusion markers • $ScvO_2$ >70% • Lactate clearance • Clinical perfusion markers • Urine output (UOP) • >0.5 cm^3/kg/h • Peripheral skin perfusion	• Dobutamine • Milrinone • IABP • PRBC transfusion

(CVP: central venous pressure; IABP: intra-aortic balloon pump; IVC: inferior vena cava; MAP: mean arterial pressure; PRBC: packed red blood cells; $ScvO_2$: central venous oxygen saturation)

BOX 2: Acute respiratory management.

- *Lung-protective mechanical ventilation:*
  - Low tidal volume <7 cc/kg (ideal body weight)
  - Plateau airway pressure <30 cmH_2O
- *Avoid hyperventilation:*
  - Goals $PaCO_2$ 38–42 mm Hg
  - Hyperventilation ($PaCO_2$ <35 mm Hg) should not be used to compensate for metabolic acidosis unless severe (pH <7.0)
- *Avoid hyperoxia:*
  - Rapidly titrate FiO_2 to SpO_2 >95% (or PaO_2 >70 mm Hg)

(FiO_2: fraction of inspired oxygen; $PaCO_2$: partial pressure of arterial carbon dioxide; PaO_2: arterial oxygen pressure; SpO_2: oxygen saturation)

BOX 3: Therapeutic cooling guidelines.

- *Perform and document neurologic exam:*
  - *Eligible patient:* GCS <8 and/or no purposeful response to verbal commands
- *Hypothermia induction:*
  - Cooled intravenous (IV) fluids:
    - 4°C 0.9% normal saline, 20–30 mL/kg bolus over 30 minutes as tolerated
  - Surface ice packs
  - Place core body temperature monitor (i.e., esophageal or bladder probe)
- *Shivering control:*
  - Early sedation and neuromuscular blockade:
    - Midazolam 2–10 mg/h
    - Propofol 20–50 μg/kg/min
    - Fentanyl 50–150 μg/h
    - Vecuronium 0.1 mg/kg IV q45 min or as needed
    - Rocuronium 0.5 mg/kg IV q1 h as needed
    - Cisatracurium 0.15 mg/kg bolus followed by 3 μg/kg/min infusion
  - Adjuncts:
    - Magnesium sulfate 5 g IV over 5 hours
    - Extremity skin counter warming
- *Maintain goal 32–34°C for 12–24 hours:*
  - Recheck serum electrolytes and ABG on reaching goal temperature
- *Rewarming:*
  - Slow controlled rewarming
  - 0.25–0.5°C/h–37.5°C
  - Stop sedation once temperature reaches 36.5°C
  - Maintain normothermia (prevent hyperthermia) for 48 hours

(ABG: arterial blood gas; GCS: Glasgow Coma Scale)

The category of a patient can be assessed quickly on arrival to better stratify the initial probability of survival and risk of different complications. Precise research definitions of the categories use scoring systems assessed within 6 hours of return of pulses, but clinical examination can usually sort patients into categories. Neurologic examination cannot be assessed if drugs or paralytics are confounding **(Box 4)**.

In the heart, it can present as acute myocardial dysfunction which can cause myocardial stunning and acute coronary syndrome **(Flowchart 1)**.

BOX 4: Postcardiac arrest category.

Category 1—Awake (follows commands)
- 80% chance of survival; 60% chance of good functional recovery <5% chance of multiple organ failure

Category 2—Coma with preserved brainstem reflexes
- 60% chance of survival; 40% chance of good functional recovery
- 20% chance of multiple organ failure

Category 3—Coma with preserved brainstem reflexes and severe cardiopulmonary failure
- 40% chance of survival; 20% chance of good functional recovery
- 40% chance of multiple organ failure

Category 4—Coma with loss of brainstem reflexes
- 10% chance of survival; 7% chance of good functional recovery
- 35% chance of multiple organ failure

Flowchart 1: Adult immediate postcardiac arrest care.

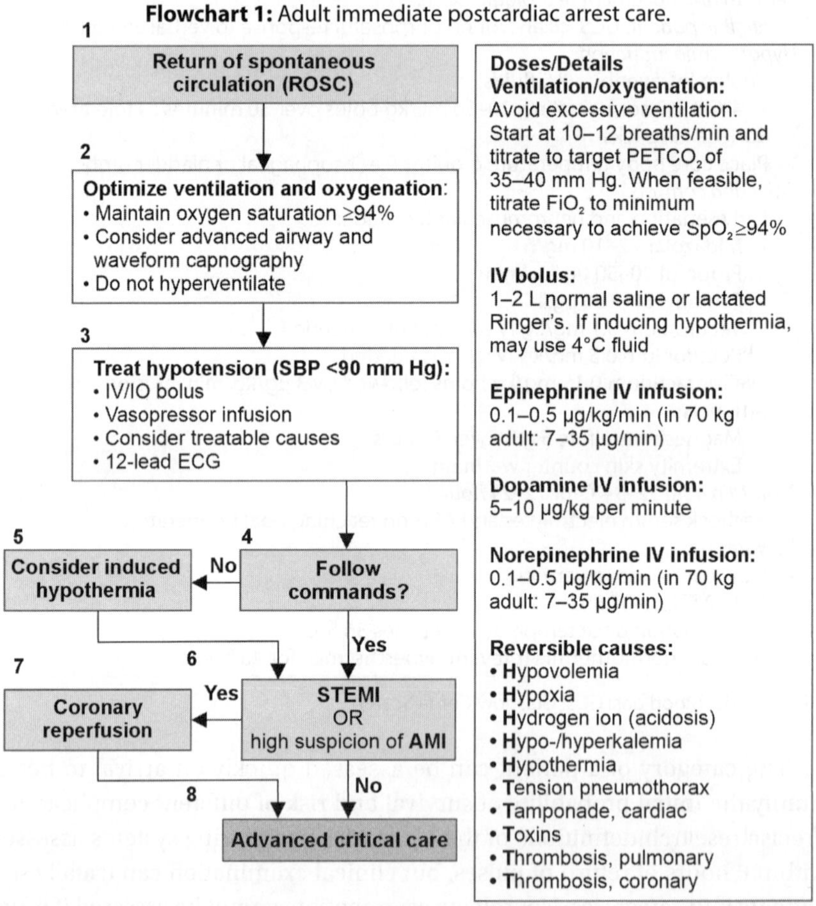

(AMI: acute myocardial infarction; ECG: electrocardiogram; FiO_2: fraction of inspired oxygen; IO: intraosseous; IV: intravenous; $PETCO_2$: partial pressure end-tidal carbon dioxide; SBP: systolic blood pressure; SpO_2: oxygen saturation; STEMI: ST-elevation myocardial infarction)

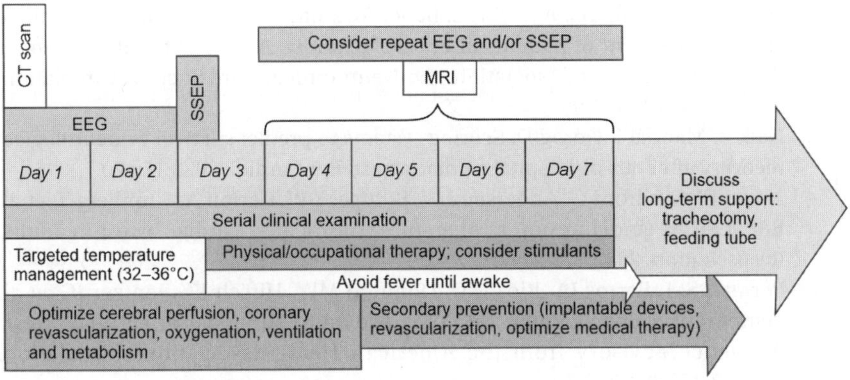

Fig. 1: Rational approach to neurologic treatment, monitoring, and testing after cardiac arrest. (CT: computed tomography; EEG: electroencephalogram; MRI: magnetic resonance imaging; SSEP: somatosensory evoked potential)

Brain can suffer from ischemic perfusion injury and impaired autoregulation.

Rational approach to neurologic treatment, monitoring, and testing after cardiac arrest is summarized in **Figure 1**.

When patients exhibit clear clinical improvement, there is no need for any tests.

For patients remaining in a coma, hypothermia treatment followed by therapy and stimulation may improve recovery.

Early electroencephalogram (EEG) monitoring can allow detection and treatment of seizures and to supplement estimations of prognosis.

Absence of cortical response on somatosensory evoked potential (SSEP) or malignant EEG patterns after hypothermia treatment help identify patients with poor prognosis. Magnetic resonance imaging (MRI) of the brain helps quantify the extent and location of injury, which in turn assists in decisions about continuing long-term support in light of patient and surrogate wishes.

SUMMARY

Postcardiac arrest management focuses on stabilizing the patient, preventing further injury, and optimizing neurological and cardiac recovery. This involves a coordinated approach encompassing hemodynamic support, neurological protection, respiratory management, and ongoing evaluation of the patient's condition, including potential reversible causes of the arrest. Early interventions, like targeted temperature management and coronary revascularization, play a critical role in improving survival and long-term outcomes.

SUGGESTED READING

1. Granfeldt A, Avis SR, Nicholson TC, Holmberg MJ, Moskowitz A, Coker A, et al. Advanced airway management during adult cardiac arrest: a systematic review. Resuscitation. 2019;139:133-43.

2. Hirsch KG, Abella BS, Amorim E, Bader MK, Barletta JF, Berg K, et al. Critical care management of patients after cardiac arrest: A scientific statement from the American Heart Association and Neurocritical Care Society. Circulation. 2024;149(2):e168-e200.
3. Naik R, Mandal I, Gorog D. Scoring systems to predict survival or neurological recovery after out-of-hospital cardiac arrest. Eur Cardiol. 2022;17:e20.
4. Nolan JP, Sandroni C, Andersen LW, Böttiger BW, Cariou A, Cronberg T, et al. ERC-ESICM guidelines on temperature control after cardiac arrest in adults. Resuscitation. 2022;172:229-36.
5. Perman SM, Bartos JA, Rios MD, Donnino MW, Hirsch KG, Jentzer JC, et al. Temperature management for comatose adult survivors of cardiac arrest: A science advisory from the American Heart Association. Circulation. 2023;48(12):982-8.
6. Sandroni C, Cariou A, Cavallaro F, Cronberg T, Friberg H, Hoedemaekers C, et al. Prognostication in comatose survivors of cardiac arrest: an advisory statement from the European Resuscitation Council and the European Society of Intensive Care Medicine. Resuscitation. 2014;85:1779-89.

CHAPTER

15 Vasopressors and Inotropes

Bindu Mulakavalupil

INTRODUCTION

When patients are hemodynamically unstable, an important and potentially lifesaving intervention is the use of vasoactive therapies to restore appropriate tissue perfusion by increasing blood flow and thereby increasing oxygenation. Vasoactive agents can be categorized by their activity and are often divided into two types: vasopressors and inotropes.

The term vasopressor refers to a class of drugs that cause vasoconstriction. Typically, increasing vasoconstriction leads to an increase in systemic vascular resistance (SVR), which leads to increase in blood pressure.

The term inotrope refers to a class of drugs that increase the strength of cardiac contraction. Increasing the strength of cardiac contractions will increase the stroke volume (SV). By increasing SV, the intent is to increase the cardiac output (CO) and therefore increase blood pressure.

Vasopressors and inotropic drugs are divided into two types based on their effects: adrenergic and nonadrenergic.

The adrenergic agonists function at adrenergic receptors (α1, α2, β1, and β2) and dopaminergic (DA) receptors. The nonadrenergic agonists exert their effect primarily via the vasopressin-specific receptor (V1 and V2) or by inhibition of phosphodiesterase 3, which potentiates the effect of cyclic adenosine monophosphate (cAMP) **(Tables 1 to 3)**.

TABLE 1: Physiologic actions of receptors stimulated by vasopressors.

Receptor	*Physiologic response*
Dopamine (DA)	Vasodilation of major vascular beds (renal, coronary, cerebral, and splanchnic) and increased renal blood flow
β1 cardiac	Inotropy and chronotropy
β2	Peripheral vasodilation and bronchial smooth muscle dilation
α1	Vasoconstriction
Vasopressin 1 (V1)	Vasoconstriction
Vasopressin 2 (V2)	Water retention

TABLE 2: Dosages of common vasopressors.

Drug	*Dose*
Dopamine	*Low dose:* <5 μg/kg/min; *Moderate dose:* 5–10 μg/kg/min *High dose:* >10 μg/kg/min
Dobutamine	2.0–20 μg/kg/min
Epinephrine	• *For refractory hypotension:* Typical dosing is 1–4 μg/min • (1:10,000 solution) • For anaphylaxis, the dose and route change, based on the presence of shock: – *Without evidence of shock:* 0.3–0.5 mg (300–500 μg) intramuscular (IM) q 5–10 min (1:1,000) – *With evidence of shock:* 0.1 mg (100 μg) intravenous (IV), which is 1.0 mL of 1:10,000 dilution IV given slowly over 3–5 minutes or infused at 5–15 μg/min
Norepinephrine	0.03–3.0 μg/kg/min
Vasopressin	• 0.04 U/min • Not titrated
Phenylephrine	• 0.5–8 μg/kg/min • 100–180 μg/min IV drip
Isoproterenol	2–10 μg/min
Milrinone	50 μg/kg bolus, and then 0.25–1 μg/kg/min

TABLE 3: Effect of vasopressors on hemodynamic variables.

Drug	*MAP*	*SVR*	*HR*	*CO*
Dopamine (moderate-high dose)	Increased	Increased	Increased	Increased
Dobutamine	Variable	Decreased		Increased
Epinephrine	Variable	Increased	Increased	Increased
Norepinephrine	Increased	Increased	0 → decreased	Increased
Vasopressin	Increased	Increased		Increased
Phenylephrine	Increased	Increased	0 → decreased*	0 → increased
Isoproterenol	Decreased	Decreased	Increased	Variable
Milrinone	Variable	Decreased		Increased

*Phenylephrine can produce reflex bradycardia as a side effect of hypertension.
(CO: cardiac output; HR: heart rate; MAP: mean arterial blood pressure; SVR: systemic vascular resistance)

Norepinephrine is a strong agonist of α receptors and moderate agonist of β receptors, with greater β1 action than β2. The effect is vasoconstriction greater than inotropy or chronotropy. This drug's effect on α receptors is increased with increasing doses. Norepinephrine increases left ventricular afterload, SV, and both systolic blood pressure (SBP) and diastolic blood pressure (DBP). The indications for norepinephrine include hypotensive states such as septic shock, neurogenic shock, and severe hypotension secondary to pulmonary embolism. Norepinephrine may not be appropriate for single agent use in cardiogenic shock secondary to the increased afterload it produces; however, it can be combined with dobutamine in this setting. The dose is 0.03–3.0 μg/kg/min. Side effects of norepinephrine include reflex bradycardia, hypertension (HTN), arrhythmias, and dyspnea. Norepinephrine is contraindicated in patients with sulfite allergies and may increase the risk of mesenteric or peripheral vascular thrombosis.

Vasopressin acts on V1 receptors, which cause vasoconstriction, and V2 receptors, which result in water retention. The primary indication for vasopressin in shock is to augment catecholamines in the treatment of septic shock, where it is used as a second pressor agent.

The typical dosing of vasopressin is 0.04 U/min for the treatment of shock. This drug is not titrated. Side effects include cardiac ischemia, arrhythmias, mesenteric ischemia, and HTN. One advantage of vasopressin is that it maintains its effects in acidic and hypoxic environments, which are typical in shock.

SUMMARY

Vasopressors and inotropes are vital medications used in critical care to stabilize patients with hemodynamic instability. "Vasopressors" increase blood pressure by constricting blood vessels, primarily through stimulating alpha-adrenergic receptors, and are used in hypotension, especially in septic shock. Common vasopressors include "norepinephrine", "epinephrine", and "vasopressin". Their side effects can include tissue ischemia and arrhythmias.

"Inotropes" enhance heart contractility, improving cardiac output in conditions like heart failure or cardiogenic shock. They act on beta-adrenergic receptors or through other pathways. Key inotropes include "dobutamine" and "milrinone", with potential side effects like tachyarrhythmias and hypotension.

In clinical practice, vasopressors and inotropes are often combined, depending on the cause of instability. Continuous monitoring and careful titration are essential to balance their benefits and minimize complications such as ischemia or arrhythmias.

SUGGESTED READING

1. Oxford Handbook of Critical Care (Oxford Medical Handbooks) 3rd edition.
2. Shoemaker WC, Grenvik A, Ayres SM, Holbrook PR. Ionotropic therapy. In: Shoemaker WC, Grenvik A, Ayres SM, Holbrook PR (Eds). Textbook of critical care, 4th edition; 2024.

CHAPTER 16

Shock

Mehul Shah, Charudatt Vaity

INTRODUCTION

Shock is a medical emergency that occurs when the body's vital organs do not receive enough oxygen and nutrients. It is a life-threatening condition that requires immediate attention in critical care medicine. The management of shock involves a systematic approach to quickly identify and treat the underlying cause. In this article, we will simplify the approach to shock in critical care, focusing on the key steps involved in its assessment and management.

DEFINITION

Acute circulatory failure associated with inadequate oxygen utilization by the cells.

Oxygen delivery (DO_2) is the product of cardiac output (CO) and the oxygen content of arterial blood.

DO_2 (mL/min) can be summarized by the following equation:

$$DO_2 = CO \times [(1.34 \times Hb \times SaO_2) + (PaO_2 \times 0.003)]$$

Where, Hb is the hemoglobin concentration (g/L), SaO_2 is the arterial hemoglobin (Hb) oxygen saturation, and PaO_2 is the arterial oxygen partial pressure.

$$CO = HR \times SV \text{ (preload, afterload, and contractility)}$$

Where, CO = cardiac output, HR = heart rate, and SV = stroke volume.

DO_2 in adults at rest is approximately 1,000 mL/min, while oxygen consumption (VO_2) is about 250 mL/min.

CLASSIFICATION

Shock is categorized based on its etiology, with the four primary types being hypovolemic, cardiogenic, distributive, and obstructive shock **(Fig. 1)**. Each type has distinct hemodynamic and clinical features, necessitating specific management strategies. Accurately identifying the type of shock is crucial for initiating appropriate treatment:

1. *Hypovolemic shock:* Characterized by a decrease in blood volume eventually leading to reduced blood flow and tissue perfusion.

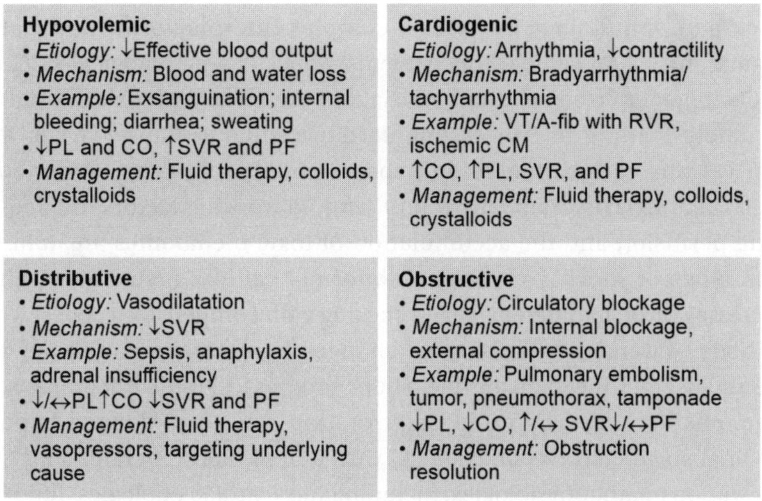

Fig. 1: Different shock types and their characteristics. (A-fib: atrial fibrillation; CM: cardiomyopathy; CO: cardiac output; PF: pressure filling; PL: preload; RVR: rapid ventricular response; SVR: systemic vascular resistance; VT: ventricular tachycardia)
Source: Adapted from Kashani K, Omer T, Shaw AD. The intensivist's perspective of shock, volume management, and hemodynamic monitoring. Clin J Am Soc Nephrol. 2022;17(5):706-16.

2. *Cardiogenic shock:* Cardiogenic shock (CS) is a multifactorial, hemodynamically complex syndrome, characterized by profound and refractory circulatory collapse due to impaired myocardial contractility, resulting in systemic hypoperfusion, metabolic acidosis, and refractory multiorgan system dysfunction. The two most commonly recognized etiologies of CS are acute myocardial (AMI-CS) and heart failure associated (HF-CS) cardiogenic shock).
3. *Distributive shock:* It is characterized by peripheral vasodilatation, leading to a reduction in blood pressure and tissue perfusion. Distributive shock is often seen in sepsis, anaphylaxis, or neurogenic factors leading to systemic vasodilation and altered microcirculatory flow.
4. *Obstructive shock:* In obstructive shock, there is a tangible obstruction of blood flow, such as pulmonary embolism, cardiac tamponade, or tension pneumothorax.

Shock may present with different clinical manifestations depending on the type and stage. Usual symptoms include hypotension, tachycardia, tachypnea, obtundation or abnormal mental status, cold, clammy extremities, mottled skin, oliguria, metabolic acidosis, and hyperlactatemia. Accurately identifying the type of shock is crucial for initiating appropriate treatment and improving patient outcomes.

PATHOPHYSIOLOGICAL PRINCIPLES

Shock pathophysiology includes a complex interplay of hemodynamic, inflammatory, and cellular mechanisms. Shock is a pathological state that results in generalized cellular hypoxia and the release of toxic substances, ultimately leading to irreversible cardiovascular collapse. It can arise from various causes, including hypovolemia, cardiogenic dysfunction, sepsis, anaphylaxis, traumatic injury, and neurogenic factors. Inadequate tissue perfusion and the accumulation of toxic metabolites are common in all types of shock, resulting in abnormal cellular metabolism. Shock progresses through different stages, starting with compensated shock, where the body undergoes physiological changes to maintain oxygen delivery. If compensatory mechanisms fail, shock progresses to the uncompensated stage, characterized by rapid deterioration due to prolonged hypoxia. The final stage is irreversible shock, with a high mortality rate. Shock can have various pathophysiologies, including intracardiac etiologies, fluid loss, obstruction, and activation of the inflammatory cascade. Understanding the pathophysiology of shock is crucial for timely and specific management to prevent complications and improve patient outcomes.

THERAPEUTIC PRINCIPLES

Shock management in the intensive care unit (ICU) is multifaceted and targets reinstating tissue perfusion, optimizing oxygen delivery, and addressing the underlying cause. Hemodynamic support, fluid resuscitation, vasoactive medications, and inotropic agents are commonly utilized to stabilize patients in shock. Additionally, source control, antimicrobial therapy, and mechanical circulatory support may be indicated based on the specific etiology. Therapeutic principles in shock involve timely recognition, classification, and management of the underlying cause to prevent complications and stabilize the patient's condition. The administration of endogenous catecholamines (epinephrine, norepinephrine, and dopamine) and vasopressor agents is a common approach to increase CO and treat shock. Other therapeutic options being explored include newer agents such as vasopressin, selepressin, calcium-sensitizing agents, cardiac-specific myosin activators, and natriuretic peptides, although their clinical outcomes are yet to be proven. Effective management also involves addressing microvascular flow alterations and inflammatory activation in shock patients, with potential interventions including histone deacetylase inhibition, nuclear factor kappa B (NF-κB) inhibition, and targeted delivery of dexamethasone. Additionally, early monitoring of clotting, and treatment of acidosis and hypothermia can help reduce bleeding complications in hemorrhagic shock.

CHALLENGES AND CONSIDERATIONS

The diagnosis and management of shock in the ICU present various challenges, including the need for rapid assessment, tailored interventions, and vigilant monitoring. The dynamic nature of shock requires ongoing reassessment and adjustment of therapeutic measures to optimize patient outcomes. The use of advanced hemodynamic monitoring techniques, such as echocardiography and pulmonary artery catheterization, may aid in the management of complex cases. Optimal management of patients with shock in the ICU requires a systematic assessment of all organ systems, considering the underlying cardiac disease, severity of shock, involvement of other organ systems, patient age, and comorbidities. The mainstay of management is supportive care, including the use of acute mechanical circulatory support devices. However, the management of shock in the ICU can be challenging due to the heterogeneity of the patient population, and the need for specialized knowledge and skills in cardiac intensive care. In addition, the identification and management of rare causes of shock, such as idiopathic capillary leak syndrome, hemophagocytic lymphohistiocytosis, systemic mastocytosis, and toxic shock syndrome, require prompt recognition and appropriate treatment. Early diagnosis and treatment are crucial in improving outcomes for patients in shock, and a multidisciplinary approach involving intensive care specialists, cardiologists, and other healthcare professionals is essential.

MANAGEMENT OF SHOCK IN ICU

Initial Assessment and Recognition

Clinicians should always be on the lookout for signs and symptoms of shock, including hypotension, tachycardia, altered mental status, oliguria, and cool extremities. Rapid evaluation of the vital signs, tissue perfusion, and end-organ function, such as mental status, urine output, and peripheral perfusion, is invaluable for identifying and categorizing the type of shock.

Hemodynamic Stabilization and Supportive Measures

Early resuscitation with saline or balanced electrolytes is usually the primary step in dealing with hypovolemic and distributive shock. In incidences of failure to fluid resuscitation or persistent hypotension, the initiation of vasopressor agents such as norepinephrine can be included to sustain blood pressure and restore tissue perfusion. For patients with CS, the use of inotropic agents such as dobutamine, and mechanical circulatory support devices such as intra-aortic balloon pumps or ventricular assist devices, may be essential to supplement cardiac function and boost perfusion.

Targeted Diagnostics

Acquiring blood samples for comprehensive laboratory testing, including complete blood count, electrolyte panel, coagulation studies, arterial blood gas analysis, and lactate levels, facilitates the evaluation of organ dysfunction and metabolic derangements associated with shock. Depending on the suspicion, imaging modalities such as bedside ultrasound, chest X-ray, computed tomography (CT) scans, or echocardiography may be indicated to identify underlying causes, such as cardiac dysfunction, pulmonary embolism, or obstructive pathologies.

Identification and Treatment of Underlying Cause

In case of distributive shock, notably septic shock, identification and curbing of the infectious source through blood cultures, imaging studies, and potential surgical intervention are crucial to optimizing patient outcomes. In patients with CS secondary to acute coronary syndromes, immediate consideration of revascularization procedures, such as percutaneous coronary intervention (PCI) or coronary artery bypass grafting (CABG) might be imperative to restore coronary blood flow and preserve cardiac function. Rapid recognition and intervention to address conditions such as tension pneumothorax, cardiac tamponade, or aortic dissection through emergent procedures such as needle decompression, pericardiocentesis, or surgical repair is necessitated in obstructive shock.

ONGOING MONITORING AND ADJUSTMENT

Constant assessment of hemodynamic parameters, such as mean arterial pressure, central venous pressure, CO, and mixed venous oxygen saturation, is instrumental in guiding the titration of fluids, vasopressors, and inotropes to achieve targeted hemodynamic goals. Consecutive monitoring of renal function, hepatic enzymes, and arterial blood gas parameters informs the assessment of end-organ perfusion and guides the intensity of supportive measures and interventions.

MULTIDISCIPLINARY COLLABORATION AND SPECIALIZED INTERVENTIONS

Collaboration with critical care pharmacists, respiratory therapists, nutrition support teams, and consultants in cardiology, surgery, infectious diseases, and interventional radiology is needed in robust management of complex shock cases.

For refractory shock cases, consideration of advanced therapies such as extracorporeal membrane oxygenation (ECMO) for severe cardiopulmonary failure or continuous renal replacement therapy for renal dysfunction may be necessary to support organ function and survival.

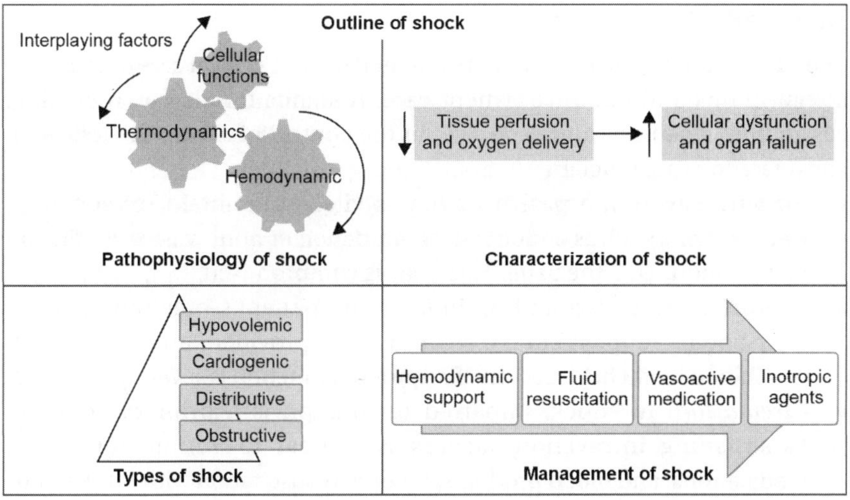

Fig. 2: Outline of shock in ICU.
Source: Adapted from references 2, 4, 5, 6, and 9.

CONTINUOUS REASSESSMENT AND DE-ESCALATION

Frequent reassessment of the patient's clinical status, intervention response, and evolving needs ensures that management strategies are adjusted dynamically to align with the patient's changing condition. As shock resolves and hemodynamic stability improves, a stepwise de-escalation of supportive measures, including gradually tapering vasopressors and reassessing the need for invasive monitoring, is essential to facilitate the transition to post-shock care and eventual ICU discharge. This algorithmic approach provides a structured and comprehensive framework for managing shock in the ICU, emphasizing the significance of rapid recognition, targeted diagnostics, and multidisciplinary collaboration in delivering optimal care to critically ill patients experiencing this life-threatening condition. Shock management's dynamic and iterative nature necessitates ongoing assessment, adjustment, and tailored interventions to address the underlying pathophysiology and optimize patient outcomes in the ICU setting **(Fig. 2)**.

APPROACH TO SHOCK

Step 1: Recognition and Initial Assessment

The first step in managing shock is to recognize its presence. Common signs of shock include low blood pressure, rapid heart rate, altered mental status, cold and clammy skin, and decreased urine output. Once identified, the healthcare team initiates an initial assessment, which involves evaluating the patient's vital signs, oxygen levels, and overall clinical status. This helps determine the severity of shock and guides subsequent interventions.

Step 2: ABCDE Approach

The ABCDE approach is a systematic method used in critical care to prioritize interventions and optimize patient care. It stands for airway, breathing, circulation, disability, and exposure. In the context of shock, the following considerations are crucial:

- *Airway:* Ensuring a patent airway is vital to maintain oxygenation. Interventions such as endotracheal intubation or noninvasive ventilation may be required if the patient's airway is compromised.
- *Breathing:* Assessing and optimizing the patient's breathing pattern is essential. Supplemental oxygen may be provided, and mechanical ventilation might be necessary if respiratory function is severely impaired.
- *Circulation:* In shock, impaired circulation is a primary concern. Establishing intravenous access is critical to administer fluids, medications, and blood products. Volume resuscitation with intravenous fluids, such as crystalloids or colloids, is often initiated to restore blood flow and improve organ perfusion.
- *Disability:* Evaluating the patient's neurological status helps identify any potential brain injury or impaired cerebral perfusion. It involves assessing the patient's level of consciousness, pupillary reactions, and motor responses.
- *Exposure:* The patient should be undressed to facilitate a thorough physical examination. This step allows the healthcare team to identify any potential sources of infection or external bleeding that could contribute to shock.

Step 3: Identification of the Underlying Cause

Once the ABCDE approach is initiated and stabilization measures are underway, the healthcare team focuses on identifying the specific cause of shock. There are various types of shock, including hypovolemic shock (due to blood loss), CS (due to heart failure), septic shock (due to severe infection), and anaphylactic shock (due to allergic reactions). Diagnostic tests, such as blood tests, imaging, and invasive monitoring, may be utilized to determine the underlying cause accurately.

Step 4: Tailored Treatment

Once the cause of shock is determined, treatment strategies are tailored to address the specific condition. These may include:

- *Fluid resuscitation:* In cases of hypovolemic shock, replenishing the lost blood volume with appropriate fluids is crucial. However, in other types of shock, excessive fluid administration may be detrimental. Individualized fluid management based on the patient's condition is essential.

- *Medications:* Specific medications, such as vasopressors (e.g., norepinephrine) or inotropes (e.g., dobutamine), may be administered to improve blood pressure and cardiac function.
- *Source control:* In cases of septic shock, identifying and treating the underlying infection is vital. This may involve administering antibiotics, draining abscesses, or performing surgical interventions.
- *Supportive care:* Patients in shock require close monitoring, including continuous vital sign monitoring, frequent laboratory tests, and hemodynamic monitoring.

SUMMARY

Shock is a life-threatening condition that is broadly classified based on its etiology as hypovolemic, cardiogenic, distributive, and obstructive. As each type of shock has distinct hemodynamic and clinical features, accurately identifying the type and implementing targeted management strategies is crucial. Effective management of shock in critical care medicine requires a systemic and dynamic approach to identify and treat the underlying cause. Its management strategy can be summarized in four crucial steps: (1) Recognition and identification of the type of shock; (2) Hemodynamic stabilization through interventions, such as fluid resuscitation, vasopressor or inotrope support, and device support, as required; (3) Identification and treatment of the underlying cause, which may require targeted diagnostics and collaborative efforts across medical specialties; (4) Continuous monitoring and assessment of patient condition to ensure appropriate intensity of supportive measures and interventions that continually evolve during the treatment course depending on patient response. This operational framework highlights the need for ongoing reassessment and tailored interventions to address the intricate pathophysiological aspects of shock and enhance patient outcomes. Once the shock subsides, meticulous stepwise de-escalation of supportive measures ensures a smooth transition to postshock care, underlining the significance of adaptability in the ever-evolving landscape of critical care medicine.

SUGGESTED READING

1. Bonanno FG. Physiopathology of shock. J Emerg Trauma and Shock. 2011;4(2):222-32.
2. Doerschug KC, Schmidt GA. Shock: diagnosis and management. In: Oropello JM, Pastores SM, Kvetan V (Eds). Critical Care, 2nd edition. New York, NY: McGraw-Hill; 2017.
3. Forsythe RM, Peitzman AB. Chapter 13. Management of shock. In: Feliciano DV, Mattox KL, Moore EE (Eds). Trauma, 6th edition. New York, NY: McGraw Hill; 2008.
4. Jones PM. Shock. In: Fuller J, Granton J, McConachie (Eds). Handbook of ICU Therapy, 3rd edition. London: Cambridge University Press; 2014. pp. 13-9.
5. Kashani K, Omer T, Shaw AD. The intensivist's perspective of shock, volume management, and hemodynamic monitoring. Clin J Am Soc Nephrol. 2022;17(5):706-16.

6. Kislitsina ON, Rich JD, Wilcox JE, Pham DT, Churyla A, Vorovich EB, et al. Shock-classification and pathophysiological principles of therapeutics. Curr Cardiol Rev. 2019;15(2):102-13.
7. Martin ND, Codner P, Greene W, Brasel K, Michetti C; AAST Critical Care Committee. Contemporary hemodynamic monitoring, fluid responsiveness, volume optimization, and endpoints of resuscitation: an AAST critical care committee report. Trauma Surg Acute Care Open. 2020;5(1):e000411.
8. McLean B. Chapter 7. Diagnosis and management of shock. In: McLean B (Ed). Fundamental Critical Care Support, 4th edition. Mount Prospect, IL: Society of Critical Care Medicine; 2007. pp. 1-16.
9. Standl T, Annecke T, Cascorbi I, Heller AR, Sabashnikov A, Teske W. The nomenclature, definition and distinction of types of shock. Dtsch Arztebl Int. 2018;115(45):757-68.
10. Vincent JL, De Backer D. Circulatory shock. N Engl J Med. 2013;369(18):1726-34.
11. Wheeler DS, Carcillo JA. Shock. In: Wheeler D, Wong H, Shanley T (Eds). Pediatric Critical Care Medicine, 2nd edition. London: Springer; 2014.

SECTION

5 Abdominal Disorders

CHAPTER 17

Acute Kidney Injury

Harsh Parikh

INTRODUCTION

Acute kidney injury (AKI) occurs in 1–7% of all hospitalized patients and in 30–50% of patients in the intensive care unit (ICU), indicating its substantial impact on hospital patient populations. Despite advancements in therapeutic techniques, morbidity and mortality associated with AKI remain substantial, with rates between 20 and 60%.

By definition, AKI is an acute deterioration of renal function in critically ill patients. AKI is characterized by a rapid decline in renal function, typically identified by an increase in serum creatinine levels or a decrease in urine output. It is a critical condition that requires prompt diagnosis and management to prevent further renal damage.

Acute kidney injury may contribute to the initiation or progression of cardiovascular diseases, proteinuria, and chronic kidney disease (CKD). Preventive strategies, including the avoidance of nephrotoxic agents and the optimization of hemodynamic status, represent the most effective interventions for AKI. Renal replacement therapy (RRT) remains the fundamental approach for managing severe AKI in the ICU.

The Kidney Disease: Improving Global Outcomes (KDIGO) definition of AKI: A clinical syndrome characterized by a rapid decline in kidney function, typically identified by an increase in serum creatinine levels or a decrease in urine output. This condition can result from various etiologies and requires prompt recognition and management to prevent further renal impairment **(Table 1)**.

RISK STRATIFICATION FOR ACUTE KIDNEY INJURY

All patients admitted to the ICU must be categorized according to their risk of developing AKI, the likelihood of progression to more severe stages of AKI, and the necessity for RRT. Early identification of kidney injury allows for the implementation of interventions, including the removal of the injury's cause, avoidance of nephrotoxic agents, and optimization of hydration and hemodynamics, to mitigate the progression of AKI.

TABLE 1: Kidney Disease: Improving Global Outcomes (KDIGO) (2012) criteria for acute kidney injury (AKI) staging based on serum creatinine and urine output.

Stage	*Serum creatinine (SCr) criteria*	*Urine output criteria*
1.	Increase ≥26 µmol/L within 48 hours or increase ≥1.5–1.9 × baseline SCr	<0.5 mL/kg/h for 6–12 hours
2.	Increase 2–2.9 × baseline SCr	<0.5 mL/kg/h for ≥12 hours
3.	Increase ≥3 × baseline SCr or increase 354 µmol/L or commenced on renal replacement therapy, irrespective of stage	<0.3 mL/kg/h for ≥24 hours or anuria for ≥12 hours

Source: KDIGO (2012).

The susceptibility to AKI is influenced by several risk factors, including advanced age, hypertension, diabetes mellitus, preexisting CKD, burns, cardiac surgery, trauma leading to rhabdomyolysis, volume depletion, fluid overload, nephrotoxic medications, sepsis, cardiac failure, persistent shock, and the administration of vasopressors.

Clinical findings include reduced urine output, volume depletion, a large cumulative positive fluid balance, hypotension, cold extremities, and prolonged capillary refill time.

Laboratory parameters include a progressive increase in serum creatinine, and hypoalbuminemia.

PREVENTION AND EARLY MANAGEMENT OF ACUTE KIDNEY INJURY

All ICU patients necessitate vigilant monitoring for the prompt detection of subclinical AKI. Ongoing and adaptive monitoring using defined clinical criteria and/or biomarkers is crucial for detecting subclinical AKI in high-risk groups.

APPLICATION OF ACUTE KIDNEY INJURY CARE BUNDLES

The AKI care bundle encompasses the optimization of hemodynamic and volume status, management of hyperglycemia, and nephrotoxins stewardship.

Blood pressure targets in critically ill patients are essential for preventing AKI and its progression.

- Mean arterial pressure (MAP) should exceed 70–75 mm Hg.
- Diastolic blood pressure (DBP) exceeding 55 mm Hg.
- Mean perfusion pressure (MPP) exceeds 60 mm Hg.
- Mean arterial pressure should exceed 80–85 mm Hg in individuals with chronic hypertension.

Volume optimization using crystalloids, preferably balanced salt solutions, is recommended. The administration of isotonic 0.9% saline [normal saline (NS)] for large-volume resuscitation is associated with a significant incidence of hyperchloremic acidosis, which may adversely affect renal function.

Nephrotoxin stewardship entails the meticulous oversight of pharmaceuticals that have the potential to induce renal impairment, particularly in patients with critical illnesses. The objective is to evaluate and mitigate the risk associated with nephrotoxin exposure while not requiring the cessation of all nephrotoxic medications. Essential strategies encompass:

- *Assessment of nephrotoxin utilization:* It is essential to evaluate the necessity and appropriateness of nephrotoxic medications, confirming that their application is warranted and that alternative options are explored.
- Utilize medications that are non-nephrotoxic or exhibit reduced nephrotoxicity whenever possible.
- Monitor blood levels of nephrotoxic drugs such as vancomycin and aminoglycosides to prevent excessive concentrations, if available.
- Adjust drug dosages or administration intervals to reduce nephrotoxicity when discontinuation of the medication is not feasible.
- Contrast-induced nephropathy (CIN) refers to kidney damage that occurs following the administration of contrast agents during imaging procedures. To avoid that utilization of low or iso-osmolar contrast agents while minimizing the volume of contrast can be done. Administering isotonic fluids, specifically normal saline, can enhance hydration and mitigate the risk of CIN.

DIAGNOSIS OF ACUTE KIDNEY INJURY IN LABORATORY SETTINGS

Serum creatinine is the most widely used endogenous biomarker for assessing kidney function and diagnosing AKI. The primary limitations of serum creatinine are its exclusive assessment of renal excretory function, its elevation only following a substantial decrease in glomerular filtration rate (GFR), and its susceptibility to various nonrenal factors such as volume status, muscle mass, medications, and dietary habits. In the evaluation of GFR in patients with AKI, measuring urine creatinine clearance over a minimum duration of 8 hours is preferable to shorter intervals.

The "Kinetic GFR" concept, which considers the dynamic fluctuations in GFR among critically ill patients, is currently gaining attraction. The primary site of injury in most types of AKI is the renal tubular epithelium, rather than the glomeruli. Urinary indicators are considered more sensitive than blood markers for the early detection of AKI due to the initial damage occurring in renal tubular cells. Early diagnosis of AKI can be achieved by assessing the levels of L-type fatty acid-binding protein (L-FABP) and neutrophil gelatinase-associated lipocalin (NGAL) in urine. Urine NGAL levels serve as a predictor for the severity and mortality associated with AKI. Combining biomarkers with clinical characteristics may provide a more effective approach to scheduling RRT.

DRUG DOSING

Multiple factors influence drug dosage in AKI, such as volume status, administration method (bolus versus infusion), and type of RRT. Patients with AKI often exhibit complex medical conditions and are usually treated with a range of medications. This can result in adverse drug interactions, inappropriate prescribing, omissions, and either under- or overdosing. Aminoglycosides must be avoided in patients with AKI when less nephrotoxic alternatives are available. The combination of vancomycin and an aminoglycoside increases the risk of nephrotoxicity.

NUTRITION

Nutritional requirements in patients with AKI vary significantly and should be customized based on the individual's preexisting nutritional status, catabolic rate, severity of AKI, underlying conditions, comorbidities, and the type and intensity of RRT. Patients in the ICU experiencing AKI receive energy provisions of 25–30 kcal/kg/day, equating to 100–130% of their resting energy expenditure. Protein consumption in individuals with AKI during critical illness is outlined as follows:

- *Not on RRT:* 1.3–1.7 g/kg/day.
- *Intermittent RRT:* 1 g/kg/day, with a maximum limit of 1.5 g/kg/day.
- In continuous renal replacement therapy (CRRT), the maximum dosage is 1.7 g/kg/day.

INDICATIONS FOR RENAL REPLACEMENT THERAPY IN ACUTE KIDNEY INJURY

Indications can be absolute or relative.

Absolute includes:

- Refractory hyperkalemia ($K > 6.5$ mEq/L)
- Refractory acidemia is defined by metabolic or mixed acidosis, indicated by a pH level lower than 7.15.
- Clinical manifestations of uremia encompass bleeding diathesis, pericarditis, and encephalopathy.
- Persistent volume overload associated with organ edema
- Dialysable toxins

Relative indications include specific circumstances or conditions that suggest the appropriateness of a particular intervention or treatment.

- The presence of progressive oliguria or anuria (urine output <200 mL/24 hours) unresponsive to medical intervention.
- Progressive azotemia; blood urea nitrogen (BUN) levels exceed 100 mg/dL and do not respond to medical intervention.
- Life-threatening electrolyte imbalances, including hypermagnesemia and hypercalcemia, arise in the setting of AKI.
- Hyperthermia resistant to conventional cooling techniques.
- Anticipating the worsening of electrolyte imbalances linked to AKI, including tumor lysis syndrome and rhabdomyolysis.

Timing of Renal Replacement Therapy

A universal consensus regarding the initiation and cessation of RRT remains absent. The decision is ultimately clinical in nature.

Modality of Renal Replacement Therapy in Acute Kidney Injury

Several modalities of RRT for critically ill patients with AKI are available, broadly classified into continuous and intermittent therapies.

ONGOING TREATMENTS

- Continuous renal replacement therapy is a dialysis modality utilized for patients with AKI, providing renal support through a continuous process. This therapy is particularly beneficial in critically ill patients who require hemodynamic stability and fluid management.
- Continuous venovenous hemofiltration (CVVH) is a renal replacement therapy utilized in critically ill patients to manage AKI. This technique involves the continuous removal of solutes and excess fluid from the blood, thereby maintaining electrolyte balance and acid–base homeostasis.
- Continuous venovenous hemodialysis (CVVHD) is a RRT utilized for patients with AKI. It operates by continuously filtering blood through a dialysis membrane, allowing for the removal of waste products and excess fluid. This method is particularly beneficial for hemodynamically unstable patients, as it provides a gentler approach compared to intermittent dialysis.
- Continuous venovenous hemodiafiltration (CVVHDF) is a RRT that combines both diffusion and convection to remove solutes and excess fluid from the blood in critically ill patients.
- Peritoneal dialysis (PD) is a medical procedure used to remove waste products and excess fluid from the body when the kidneys are unable to perform these functions adequately.

Intermittent therapies refer to treatment regimens that are administered in cycles, alternating between periods of treatment and periods of rest or no treatment. This approach is often utilized to enhance therapeutic efficacy while minimizing side effects. Intermittent hemodialysis (IHD) is a medical procedure utilized for the treatment of renal failure, involving the periodic removal of waste products and excess fluids from the blood through an artificial kidney. This method is characterized by its scheduled sessions, typically occurring several times a week, to maintain electrolyte balance and overall health in patients with compromised renal function.

Hybrid therapies or prolonged intermittent renal replacement therapy (PIRRT) include sustained low-efficiency hemodialysis (SLED) and sustained low-efficiency hemodiafiltration (SLED-f). Sustained low-efficiency hemodialysis (SLED) refers to a dialysis modality characterized by prolonged treatment sessions at reduced blood flow rates, aiming to optimize solute clearance while minimizing hemodynamic instability.

Sustained low-efficiency hemodiafiltration (SLED-f) is an RRT technique characterized by its prolonged duration and lower efficiency compared to traditional methods.

Surveillance During Renal Replacement Therapy

See **Table 2.**

Anticoagulation in Renal Replacement Therapy

Anticoagulation is generally required for acute RRT. Anticoagulation reduces filter clotting and improves the efficacy of RRT as well as prolongs the filter life. Replacing the hemofilter due to clotting of the circuit may reduce the time on CRRT from 24 to 16 hours a day, thereby reducing the delivery of an adequate CRRT dose.

Anticoagulant Options During Continuous Renal Replacement Therapy (Box 1)

Unfractionated or standard heparin (UFH) is the anticoagulant agent most commonly used in CRRT to prolong the life of the extracorporeal circuit. Regional citrate anticoagulation (RCA) is a procedure that prevents blood clotting during CRRT by infusing citrate into the circuit during renal replacement therapy to chelate ionized Ca^{2+} forming calcium-citrate complexes, thus preventing coagulation of blood. This technique is characterized by its ability to maintain anticoagulation locally while minimizing systemic effects. Blood gas analysis and ionized calcium should be conducted every 4 hours initially, transitioning to every 8 hours once stable acid-base status and ionized calcium levels are achieved.

TABLE 2: The parameters that should be assessed when a patient is on renal replacement therapy (RRT).

Neurological status		
Look for dialysis disequilibrium syndrome	Patients who had CKD and currently initiated on renal replacement therapy	
GCS	Daily	
Hemodynamic parameters		
Clinical parameters	Edema, daily weight, JVP, heart and lung auscultation	Need hourly monitoring depending on clinical status
Static/dynamic parameters	CVP, PCWP/SVV, PPV, aortic flow velocity	As per availability and based on clinical status
Fluid status		
Cumulative balance		Daily
Continuous intake and output chart		Hourly for those on CRRT
Acid–base status		
Blood gas analysis	Every 6th hourly at initial presentation	Once daily after hemodynamic stabilization
Electrolytes		
Potassium	8th hourly initially	Once daily after achieving stable levels
Sodium, magnesium, phosphorus, and calcium		Daily, S Na monitored at least 6-hourly while on CRRT
Anticoagulation		
Unfractionated heparin	APTT, activated clotting time	4th hourly
Regional citrate anticoagulation	Blood gas analysis and ionized calcium	4th hourly initially and 8th hourly after achieving stable acid–base status and ionized calcium level
Blood parameters		
Hemoglobin, WBC count, platelet count		Daily
Solute clearance		
Blood urea, serum creatinine urea		Daily
Kt/V, URR; prescribed dose in CRRT; delivered dose		Daily

Contd…

Contd...

Sieving coefficient	Effluent urea/blood urea	Daily
Clearance	Sieving coefficient × effluent dose	Daily
Nutrition		
Total energy intake; protein intake		Daily
Liver parameters		
Serum albumin; liver enzymes; serum ammonia; and serum bilirubin levels		To be verified on initiation of RRT and for every 72 hours after clinical stabilization
Vascular access		
Exit site; blood flow through access; tunnel infection		Daily

(APTT: activated partial thromboplastin time; CKD: chronic kidney disease; CRRT: continuous renal replacement therapy; CVP: central venous pressure; GCS: Glasgow Coma Scale; JVP: jugular venous pressure; Kt/V: 'K' stands for clearance—the amount of urea your dialyzer can remove (L/min), 't' stands for time—the duration of treatment (minutes), and 'V' stands for volume—the amount of body fluid (liters); PCWP: pulmonary capillary wedge pressure; PPV: pulse pressure variation; SVV: stroke volume variation; URR: urea reduction ratio)

BOX 1: Anticoagulant options during continuous renal replacement therapy.

- Unfractionated heparin
- LMWH
- Citrate
- No anticoagulation
- Saline flushes
- Prostacyclin
- Direct thrombin inhibitors
- Hirudin and argatroban
- Serine protease inhibitors
- Nafamostat

(LMWH: low-molecular-weight heparin)

WEANING FROM RENAL REPLACEMENT THERAPY

- There is no universal consensus about weaning from RRT. Spontaneous improvement in urine output (UO) from oliguric to nonoliguric state (UO >400 mL/day) or urine creatinine clearance of >15–20 mL/min may be considered as the reliable clinical parameters to consider weaning from RRT. A progressive UO of >400 mL/day without diuretics showed the highest sensitivity and specificity.

SUMMARY

In the ICU, renal replacement therapy is critical for managing patients with acute kidney injury or severe fluid overload. Commonly used modalities include continuous renal replacement therapy and intermittent hemodialysis. CRRT is often preferred in unstable, critically ill patients due to its slower, continuous process, allowing better fluid and solute removal without causing hemodynamic instability. RRT in the ICU helps control electrolyte imbalances, remove toxins, and manage acid–base disturbances. It is essential in multi-organ failure or sepsis management, providing crucial support while allowing time for renal recovery or serving as long-term therapy.

SUGGESTED READING

1. Bellomo R, Ronco C, Kellum JA, Mehta RL, Palevsky P. Acute renal failure: definition, outcome measures, animal models, fluid therapy and information technology needs: the second international consensus conference of the Acute Dialysis Quality Initiative group. Crit Care. 2004;8(4):R204-12.
2. Kidney disease: Improving Global Outcomes (KDIGO) acute kidney injury workgroup. KIDGO clinical practice guideline for acute kidney injury. Kidney Int Suppl. 2012;2(Suppl. 1):1-138.
3. Levey AS, Eckardt KU, Dorman NM, Cheung M, Jadoul M, Winkelmayer WC, et al. Nomenclature for kidney function and disease: report of a Kidney Disease: Improving Global Outcomes (KDIGO) Consensus Conference. Kidney Int. 2020;97(6):1117-29.
4. Mehta RL, Kellum JA, Shah SV, Molitoris BA, Ronco C, Warnock DG, et al. Acute Kidney Injury Network: report of an initiative to improve outcomes in acute kidney injury. Crit Care. 2007;11(2):R31.
5. Mishra RC, Sodhi K, Prakash KC, Tyagi N, Chanchalani G, Annigeri RA, et al. ISCCM Guidelines on Acute Kidney Injury and Renal Replacement Therapy. Indian J Crit Care Med. 2022;26(Suppl 2):S13-S42.

CHAPTER 18

Acute Liver Failure

Apurva Kakatkar

ACUTE LIVER FAILURE

Acute onset liver dysfunction in individuals without underlying chronic liver disease associated with deranged liver function tests (LFTs), liver related coagulopathy, and hepatic encephalopathy (HE). Many of the times, this terminology is incorrectly used for acute deterioration of chronic liver disease.

Depending upon the interval from onset of symptoms to development of encephalopathy, acute liver failure (ALF) is divided in hyperacute, acute, and subacute liver failure. Disease duration of >28 weeks from onset of symptoms to encephalopathy is labeled as chronic liver disease **(Figs. 1A to C)**.

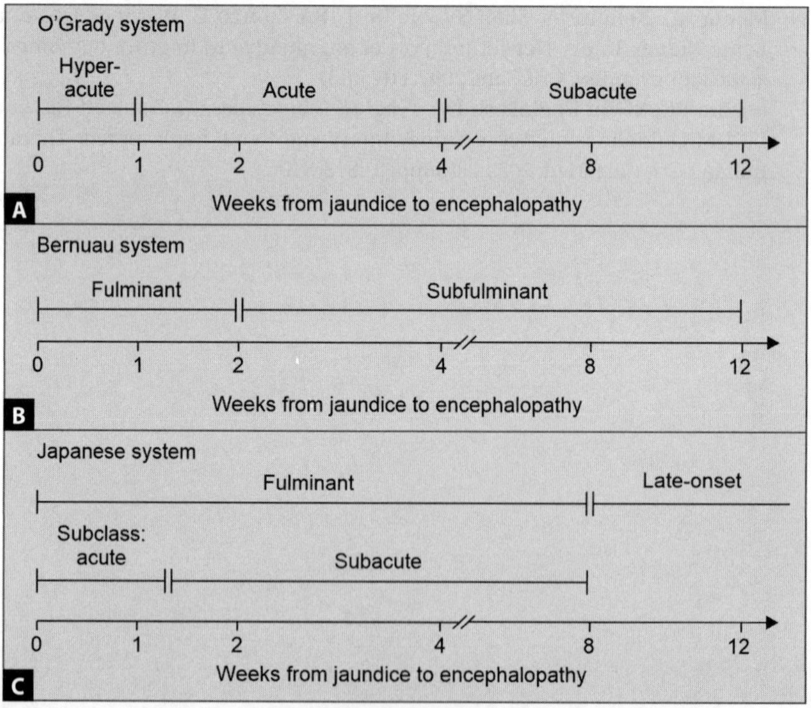

Figs. 1A to C: ALF presentations.

HYPER ACUTE LIVER FAILURE

- Jaundice to encephalopathy duration <7 days.
- Severe coagulopathy
- Marked increase in enzymes but low-to-moderate rise in bilirubin.
- Raised intracranial pressure (ICP)
- Multiorgan dysfunction
- More chances of spontaneous recovery hence better prognosis.
- Most commonly secondary to paracetamol or hepatitis A or B.

ACUTE LIVER FAILURE

- Jaundice to encephalopathy duration is 8–28 days.
- Gradual onset of symptoms.
- Commonly due to idiosyncratic drug overdose or viral infection.

SUBACUTE LIVER FAILURE

- Jaundice to encephalopathy duration 5–12 weeks.
- Marked increase in bilirubin, mild-to-moderate coagulopathy, mild increase in enzymes.
- Splenomegaly, ascites, and shrunken liver.
- Chances of spontaneous recovery are poor.
- Once the encephalopathy develops then transplant is the only treatment for survival.

ETIOLOGY

Drug Induced

- Paracetamol
- Phosphorus
- Alcohol
- *Amanita phalloids* mushrooms
- Cocaine
- Kava-Kava
- Methylenedioxymethamphetamine (MDMA)
- Antituberculous drugs
- Flucloxacillin
- Statins

Infection

- Viral hepatitis A, B, C, and E
- Cytomegalovirus
- Herpes simplex
- Varicella
- Dengue

Congenital

Wilson's disease

Vascular

- Right heart failure
- Ischemia of hepatic artery
- Budd–Chiari

Autoimmune

- Hemophagocytic syndrome
- Vasculitis

Malignancy

- Hepatocellular carcinoma
- Lymphoma
- Carcinoma colon

Pregnancy

- HELLP (hemolysis, elevated liver enzymes, and low platelets)
- Acute fatty liver of pregnancy (AFLP)
- Preeclamptic acute liver rupture.

Traumatic

- Capsular hematoma
- Crush injury
- Hyperthermia induced liver injury

Idiosyncratic Drug Reaction

- Nonsteroidal anti-inflammatory drug (NSAID)
- Anticonvulsants
- Aspirin (in children)

APPROACH TO THE DIAGNOSIS CAUSE OF ACUTE LIVER FAILURE

Drug-induced ALF

Paracetamol

Suicidal intention or accidental ingestion of excessive dose or staggered dose over a period of time.

Toxicology screening to detect circulating levels.

Very high aminotransferase levels usually >10,000, normal bilirubin, metabolic acidosis, high lactates, and kidney injury are strongly suspicious of paracetamol overdose.

- Paracetamol level
- LFTs—high aminotransferase levels usually >10,000, normal bilirubin, and high international normalized ratio (INR).
- Arterial blood gas (ABG)—metabolic acidosis, high lactates.
- Renal function test (RFT)—acute kidney injury (AKI), low urea level is suggestive of severe liver failure.

Non-paracetamol

Proper history—prescribed/nonprescribed drugs taken in last 6 months. History of ingestion of supplements or herbal medicines should be obtained. 10% of drug-induced liver injury patient progress to ALF, but once progressed to ALF will die or require emergency liver transplant (LT).

The MDMA (ecstasy) induced liver injury presents with severe hyperthermia, multiorgan involvement, and severe rhabdomyolysis profound coagulopathy mimicking like severe heat stroke.

Some of the drugs such as anticonvulsant, sulfa group, and antibiotics present like DRESS (drug reaction with eosinophilia and systemic symptoms). Presents such as fever, eosinophilia, rash, and lymphadenopathy.

Viral Hepatitis

Immunoglobulin M (IgM) antibodies for hepatitis A and E, hepatitis B surface antigen, and core antibody, hepatitis B virus (HBV) deoxyribonucleic acid (DNA), Epstein-Barr virus (EBV), herpes simplex virus (HSV), cytomegalovirus (CMV), varicella serology in immunocompromised person, and dengue serology.

Autoimmune Hepatitis

- History of other autoimmune syndromes.
- Significantly positive autoantibody levels—antinuclear antibodies (ANA), antismooth muscle antibodies (ASMA), antisoluble liver antigen, antineutrophil cytoplasmic antibody (ANCA), and human leukocyte antigen (HLA) typing.
- High globulin level
- Need coformation by liver biopsy.

Uncommon Etiology for Acute Liver Failure

- Budd-Chiari syndrome—typically presents with abdominal pain, ascites, and hepatomegaly.
- Diagnosed on liver Doppler.
- Wilson's disease—young age, Coombs negative hemolytic anemia, and high bilirubin to alkaline phosphatase ratio. Kayser-Fleischer ring in 50% patients, low ceruloplasmin levels, low uric acid levels, and renal dysfunction.

- Mushroom poisoning—history of ingestion of mushroom, presents with severe vomiting and diarrhea, hypovolemic shock, renal failure, and liver failure.
- ALF in pregnancy—in third trimester of pregnancy, hemolysis, elevated liver enzymes, low platelet (HELLP) syndrome, and AFLP. In a known case of preeclampsia need to rule out rupture liver.
- Heat stroke—drug induced or after exercise in high temperature.
- Secondary ALF—The cause of ALF is not hepatic. Raised liver enzymes and coagulopathy secondary to sepsis, malaria, leptospirosis, rickettsia, and hemophagocytic syndrome.

INVESTIGATIONS

- CBC—look for low hemoglobin (Hb) (hemolytic anemia), white cell count increased or decreased in infection, malignancy, eosinophilia (in drug reactions), and thrombocytopenia in HELLP.
- LFTs and RFTs
- Lactate dehydrogenase (LDH)—high in malignancy
- Paracetamol levels
- Two-dimensional echocardiography (2D Echo)—to rule out right heart failure.
- Computed tomography (CT) abdomen—to look for malignancy, splenomegaly, liver rupture in pregnancy, and lymphadenopathy.
- Liver biopsy to rule out autoimmune hepatitis or malignancy, acute pancreatitis, and vascular patency.
- Coagulation profile—prothrombin time (PT)/INR, activated partial thromboplastin time (APTT), fibrinogen, factor V cultures
- Electrocardiogram (ECG), X-ray chest.

CLINICAL FEATURES

- *Hepatic encephalopathy:* Intracranial hypertension (ICH) and HE of various grades is the most common finding in ALF. Manifestations of HE are agitation, headache, vomiting, asterixis, hyperreflexia, and clonus. Usually, diagnosis of exclusion after excluding other causes of drowsiness such as hypoglycemia, hypercapnia, stroke, seizure, hyponatremia, and effect of sedatives. Depending upon neuropsychiatry evaluation graded from I to IV, I being the mildest form and IV severe HE.
- *West Haven criteria:*
    - Lack of awareness, short attention span, and difficulty with addition.
    - Lethargy, inappropriate behavior, mild disorientation, and difficulty with subtraction.
    - Somnolence, respond to verbal stimuli, disoriented, and confused
    - Coma

Patients with encephalopathy grade >3 needs to be intubated and ventilated, should be monitored for seizure, and treated appropriately with antiepileptic drugs.

Patient with shorter duration of jaundice to encephalopathy may progress to ICH and manifest as hypertension, bradycardia, and mydriasis. Persistent hyperammonemia (levels 150–200) after initial resuscitation indicates high chances of ICH. ICP monitoring is used to monitor ICP.

- *Systemic inflammatory response syndrome (SIRS):* Altered balance between pro and anti-inflammatory immune response. Reduced complement levels. This leads to severe immunosuppression, presents with hyperdynamic circulation with severe hypotension due to hypovolemia with severe vasodilation. Sepsis needs to be ruled out from SIRS.
- *Metabolic acidosis with lactic acidosis:* High lactates are because of poor lactate clearance due to liver cell failure.
- *Hypoxia and acute respiratory distress syndrome (ARDS):* Hypoxia can be because of aspiration due to poor airway protection due to low Glasgow Coma Scale (GCS), hepatic hydrothorax, hepatopulmonary syndrome, or poor ventilation due to large ascites.
- *Hypoglycemia:* Due to impaired glycogenolysis, impaired gluconeogenesis, and poor glycogen stores.
- *Coagulopathy:* Reduced circulatory procoagulant as well as anticoagulant. Increased coagulation tendency due to protein C and protein S deficiency. Deranged coagulation in the form of increased INR reduced all cell line. In spite of all of this, usually the thromboelastogram (TEG) is normal and actual chances of bleeding are less.
- Thrombocytopenia
- Heart—high output failure
- Bone marrow suppression
- Pancreatitis
- Acute kidney injury and hepatorenal syndrome
- Glucocorticoid deficiency causing hypotension

Sepsis: Impaired leukocyte function increases chances of infection, bacterial, fungal, or viral. Patient should be watched for any new onset fever, worsening neurological status, hemodynamic instability after initial improvement, elevating biomarkers for infection like C-reactive protein or procalcitonin. Patient on long-term antibiotics should be observed for fungal infection and fungal infection biomarkers to be checked.

MANAGEMENT

Very little in specific management, more role of supportive care.

- Withdrawal of hepatotoxic drug in drug-induced liver injury.
- N-acetylcysteine (NAC) in paracetamol overdose.
- Copper chelating agent in Wilson's disease.

- Hemoperfusion in *Amanita phalloides* toxicity
- L-carnitine and hemodialysis in valproate overdose
- Transjugular intrahepatic portosystemic shunt (TIPS), thrombus removal in portal vein thrombosis
- Steroids in autoimmune hepatitis and sometimes in alcoholic hepatitis.

SUPPORTIVE CARE

- *Airway:* Consider intubation and mechanical ventilation when encephalopathy progresses to grade 3 encephalopathy. Lung protective ventilation is preferred. Target normocapnia, avoid hypercapnia or hypocapnia.
- *Treat hypovolemia:* Fluid boluses and maintenance fluid to keep normovolemia, avoid overresuscitation and hypervolemia, crystalloid is preferred fluid of choice. Start vasopressors in case of persistent hypotension, norepinephrine is the preferred drug of choice. Volume overload is as detrimental as hypotension.
- Hypoglycemia is very common, needs frequent monitoring of blood glucose, large rapid boluses cause osmotic shift and should be avoided. Hyperglycemia can worsen rise in ICP and should be avoided. Strict normoglycemia should be targeted.
- Hyponatremia should be avoided and should maintain sodium concentration between 140 and 150 mmol/L, rapid change of s. sodium levels should be avoided.
- Watch for high lactates and metabolic acidosis. High lactates is poor prognostic marker.
- Renal replacement therapy (RRT)—apart from routine indications of RRTV such as acidosis, hyperkalemia, and uremia, early RRT is considered in ALF in hyperammonemia, worsening encephalopathy. RRT also helps in temperature and sodium management. Continuous mode of RRT is preferred over intermittent as it prevents large hemodynamic or metabolic fluctuation and eventually prevents rise in ICP.
- *Blood and blood product transfusion:* Trigger for blood transfusion is Hb 7 or <7. Routine correction of PT/INR or other coagulation abnormality is not indicated unless there is bleeding or for ICP insertion. Venous thromboprophylaxis should be considered unless contraindicated.
- *Infection:* Keep close eye for worsening encephalopathy, signs of infection, or SIRS. Care bundles should be followed strictly. Surveillance culture should be sent periodically. Consider antifungals in case of prolonged antibiotic therapy or positive biomarkers for fungal infection.
- *Hepatic encephalopathy:* Lactulose and rifaximin has no role in reducing ammonia. In patients with grade 3 encephalopathy, intubate ventilate to protect airway. Evaluation for signs of raised ICP should be done. For evaluation of raised ICP transcranial Doppler is noninvasive alternative to invasive ICP monitoring.

- *Indications for invasive ICP monitoring:* Grade 3 or 4 coma, intubated and ventilated, presence of >1 of the following: (1) Young patient with hyperacute or acute presentation, (2) ammonia level >150–200 µmol/L, not responding to IV fluids and RRT, (3) renal impairment, and (4) requirement of vasopressor >0.1 µg/kg/min.
- *Treatment for raised ICP*: Mannitol or 3% sodium chloride is administered in acute surge in ICP. Hyperventilation (for short duration), hypothermia, and indomethacin can be used in uncontrolled ICH.

- *Role of plasma exchange:* Plasma exchange undertaken in first 3 days of admission to ICU shown to have benefit in decreasing raised ICP and demonstrate mortality benefit in patients who did not receive transplantation.
- *Artificial liver devices:* Liver assist devices supposedly provide bridge to transplant or recovery, unfortunately, no such device is yet proven its benefit.
  - *Molecular absorbent and recirculating system (MARS):* MARS utilizes a hollow fiber, double-sided, albumin impregnated, dialysis membrane designed to extract protein-bound toxin into albumin dialysate. These devices improve HE, but no mortality benefit. Extracorporeal liver assist device (EALD) did not show any mortality benefit.

Liver transplant: Patients who do not respond to medical management and heading toward LT need to be identified early. Liver transplantation should be considered in those who are fulfilling King's college or Clichy criteria **(Box 1)**.

BOX 1: King's college criteria.

Acute liver failure (ALF) due to paracetamol:
- Arterial pH <7.3 after resuscitation and >24 hours since ingestion
- Lactate >3 mmol/L
- The following three criteria:
  1. Hepatic encephalopathy >grade 3
  2. Serum creatinine >300 µmol/L
  3. International normalized ratio (INR) >6.5

ALF not due to paracetamol:
- INR >6.5
- Three out of five of the following criteria:
  1. *Etiology:* Indeterminate etiology hepatitis, drug-induced hepatitis
  2. Age <10 years or >40 years
  3. Interval jaundice-encephalopathy >7 days
  4. Bilirubin >300 µmol/L
  5. INR >3.5

Beaujon–Paul Brousse criteria (Clichy)
- Confusion or coma (hepatic encephalopathy stage 3 or 4)
- Factor V <20% of normal if age <30 years
- Factor V <30% if age >30 years

PROGNOSIS

Prognostic models are available that help to select patients who will die without transplant.

SUMMARY

"Acute liver failure" is a rapid loss of liver function, occurring within days or weeks, in individuals without preexisting liver disease. It results in severe liver dysfunction, coagulopathy (impaired blood clotting), and encephalopathy (brain dysfunction due to liver toxins). Common causes include "viral hepatitis (hepatitis A, B, E)", drug-induced liver injury (most notably "acetaminophen overdose"), autoimmune liver disease, and toxins.

Symptoms of ALF include jaundice, confusion, altered consciousness, and abnormal bleeding. The condition progresses quickly and can lead to multiorgan failure, making early diagnosis and treatment crucial.

Management focuses on supportive care in an intensive care unit, addressing complications such as cerebral edema, infections, and coagulopathy. In some cases, liver transplantation may be necessary if the liver fails to regenerate. Without timely intervention, ALF can be fatal, underscoring the need for urgent medical attention.

SUGGESTED READING

1. Bernal W, Wendon J, Lee WM, Larsen FS, Williams R. Acute liver failure. J Hepatol. 2015;62(1 Suppl):S112-20.
2. McPhail Mark JW, Wendon JA, Bernal W. Meta-analysis of performance of Kings's College Hospital Criteria in prediction of outcome in non-paracetamol-induced acute liver failure. J Hepatol. 2010;53(3):492-9.
3. O'Grady JG, Alexander GJ, Hayllar KM, Williams R. Early indicators of prognosis in fulminant hepatic failure. Gastroenterology. 1989;97(2):439-45.
4. Wiesner R, Edwards E, Freeman R, Harper A, Kim R, Kamath P, et al. United Network for Organ Sharing Liver Disease Severity Score Committee. Model for end-stage liver disease (MELD) and allocation of donor livers. Gastroenterology. 2003;124(1):91-6.

CHAPTER

19 Acute on Chronic Liver Failure

Vikas Gupta

ACUTE ON CHRONIC LIVER FAILURE MANAGEMENT IN INTENSIVE CARE UNIT

Acutely decompensated cirrhosis refers to the development of ascites, encephalopathy, gastrointestinal hemorrhage, or any combination of these disorders in patients with cirrhosis. Acute on chronic liver failure (ACLF) reflects the development of extrahepatic and/or intrahepatic organ failure(s) **(Fig. 1)** in a patient with cirrhosis and is associated with high short-term mortality.

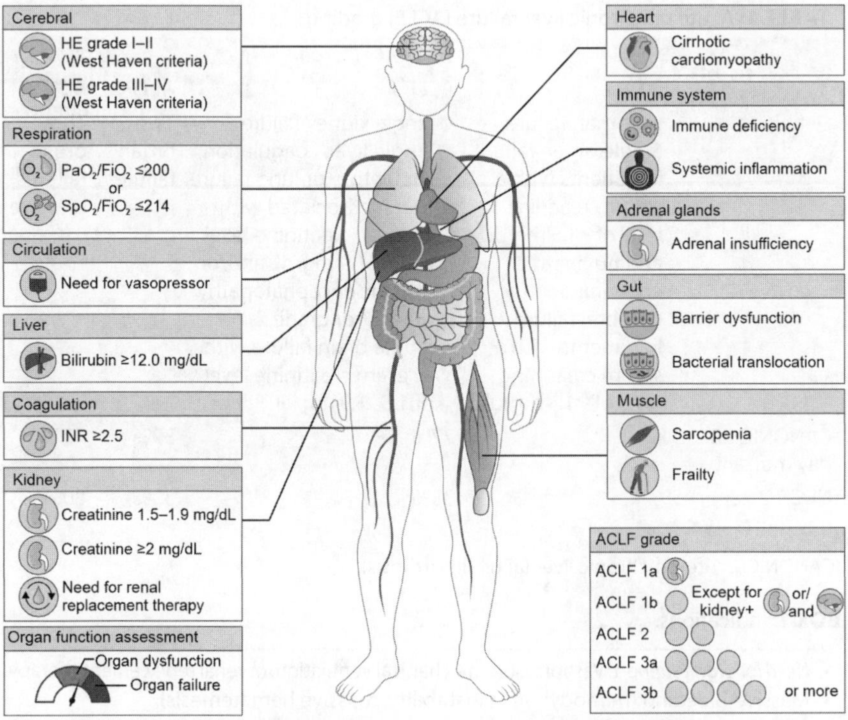

Fig. 1: Various organ systems involved in acute on chronic liver failure (ACLF). (FiO_2: fraction of inspired oxygen; HE: hepatic encephalopathy; INR: international normalized ratio; PaO_2: arterial oxygen pressure; SpO_2: oxygen saturation)

The goals of intensive care management of patients suffering ACLF are to rapidly recognize and treat inciting events (e.g., infection, severe alcoholic hepatitis, and severe bleeding) and to aggressively support failing organ systems to ensure that patients may successfully undergo liver transplantation.

ACUTE ON CHRONIC LIVER FAILURE GRADING

Broadly, ACLF is classified into 0, 1, 2, and 3 grades depending on the number of organ failures **(Table 1)**.

VARIOUS ORGAN SYSTEMS INVOLVED IN ACUTE ON CHRONIC LIVER FAILURE

There is various organ systems involved in acute on chronic liver failure **(Fig. 1)**.

PROPOSED CRITERIA FOR ADMISSION TO INTENSIVE CARE UNIT IN PATIENTS WITH ACUTE ON CHRONIC LIVER FAILURE

Diagnostic Workup for Acute on Chronic Liver Failure (Box 1)

While approaching ACLF patient, first we have to identify the precipitant cause and grading the severity of ACLF.

TABLE 1: Acute on chronic liver failure (ACLF) grading.

	ACLF grade			
	ACLF 0	*ACLF 1*	*ACLF 2*	*ACLF 3*
Definition	• No organ failure • Single organ failure in patients with a serum creatinine level of <1.5 mg/dL and no hepatic encephalopathy • Cerebral failure in patients with a serum creatinine level of <1.5 mg/dL	• Single kidney failure • Single liver, coagulation, circulatory or lung failure that is associated with a serum creatinine level of 1.5–1.9 mg/dL and/or hepatic encephalopathy grade 1 or grade 2 • Single brain failure with a serum creatinine level of 1.5–1.9 mg/dL	Two organ failures	Three organ failures or more
CANONIC 28-day mortality	5%	22%	32%	77%
HEGITO 28-day mortality	5%	33%	33%	80%

(CANONIC: acute-on-chronic liver failure in cirrhosis)

BOX 1: Indications.

- *Need for organ support:* Vasopressors, mechanical ventilation, or renal replacement therapy
- Massive bleeding (hemodynamic instability, massive hematemesis)
- Severe (grade III or IV) hepatic encephalopathy (airway protection)
- Septic shock requiring vasopressors or sepsis with elevated lactate (>4 mmol/L) or organ dysfunction

APPROACH TO PATIENT WITH ACUTE ON CHRONIC LIVER FAILURE (FLOWCHART 1)

All patients should be prognosticated at admission using either the Chronic Liver Failure Consortium (CLIF-C) ACLF or ACLF grading.

Precipitating Events should be Identified and Treated

Box 2 shows the identification of precipitants.

Flowchart 1: Approach to patient with acute on chronic liver failure (ACLF).

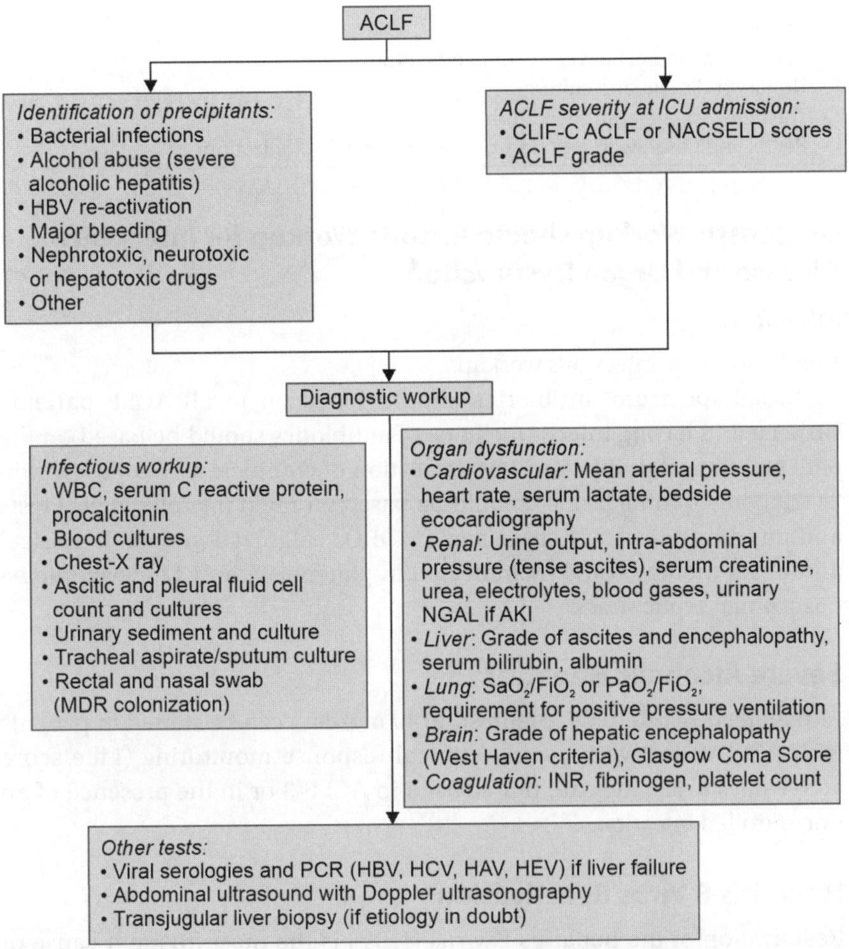

(AKI: acute kidney injury; CLIF-C: Chronic Liver Failure Consortium; FiO_2: fraction of inspired oxygen; HAV: hepatitis A virus; HBV: hepatitis B virus; HCV: hepatitis C virus; HEV: hepatitis E virus; ICU: intensive care unit; INR: international normalized ratio; MDR: multidrug-resistant; NACSELD: North American Consortium for the Study of End Stage Liver Disease; NGAL: neutrophil gelatinase-associated lipocalin; PaO_2: arterial oxygen pressure; PCR: polymerase chain reaction; SaO_2: oxygen saturation; WBC: white blood cell)

BOX 2: Identification of precipitants.

- Bacterial infections
- Alcohol abuse (severe alcoholic hepatitis)
- Hepatitis B virus (HBV) reactivation
- Major bleeding
- Nephrotoxic, neurotoxic, or hepatotoxic drugs
- Other

BOX 3: Infectious workup.

- White blood cell (WBC), serum C reactive protein, and procalcitonin
- Blood cultures
- Chest X-ray
- Ascitic and pleural fluid cell count and cultures
- Urinary sediment and culture
- Tracheal aspirate/sputum culture
- Rectal and nasal swab [multidrug-resistant (MDR) colonization]

Diagnostic Workup should Include Workup for Infectious Disease and Organ Dysfunction

Infections

Box 3 shows the infectious workup.

Broad-spectrum antibiotics should be given in all ACLF patients suspected of having infection choice of antibiotics should be based on the patients' clinical profile. Early de-escalation of empirical antibiotics (within 24–72 hours of time frame) should be based on rapid microbiological tests and multidrug-resistant organisms (MDRO) colonization data. Empirical antifungal therapy could be indicated in patients with ACLF developing a nosocomial septic shock.

Severe Alcoholic Hepatitis

Although corticosteroids (prednisone 40 mg/day) can be started in patients with ACLF-1 or 2 with careful clinical response monitoring (Lille score at 4–7 days 0.45), they are not advised in ACLF-3 or in the presence of an uncontrolled infection.

Hepatitis B Virus Reactivation

Reactivation of the hepatitis B virus (HBV) is the most frequent cause of ACLF. In this situation, early implementation of effective antiviral medication (tenofovir 245 mg/day or entecavir 0.5 mg/day) increases short-term survival.

In patients with HBV-related ACLF, liver transplantation should be considered in those with a severe presentation [e.g., model for end-stage liver disease (MELD) score >30; ACLF-2 or 94% –3].

Variceal Bleeding

A serious side effect of portal hypertension is acute variceal hemorrhage from esophageal/gastric varices, which can result in severe bleeding and shock.

Management

- Consider early intubation is advised in cirrhotic/ACLF patients with concurrent hepatic encephalopathy (HE), respiratory distress, or high volume hematemesis (>500 mL blood)
- Massive blood transfusion protocol as appropriate
- Thromboelastography (TEG)-based correction of coagulopathy
- Terlipressin [(0.5–2.0 mg intravenous (IV) q 6 h]
- Balloon tamponade device like the Sengstaken–Blakemore or Minnesota tube may be used.
- TIPS

INTENSIVE CARE UNIT MANAGEMENT OF ACUTE ON CHRONIC LIVER FAILURE

Suggested criteria for ICU admission in patients with ACLF **(Box 4)**.

Box 5 shows the intensive care unit management of acute on chronic liver failure.

BOX 4: Indications of ICU admission.

- *Need for organ support:* Vasopressors, mechanical ventilation, or renal replacement therapy
- Massive bleeding (hemodynamic instability, massive hematemesis)
- Severe (grade III or IV) hepatic encephalopathy (airway protection)
- Septic shock requiring vasopressors or sepsis with elevated lactate (>4 mmol/L) or organ dysfunction

BOX 5: Intensive care unit management of acute on chronic liver failure (ACLF).

Management of septic shock:
- Consider balanced crystalloid solutions as first-line resuscitation fluid for hypotensive ACLF patients. Human albumin is recommended in patients requiring substantial amounts of fluids and vasopressors
- Administration of fluids should be guided by dynamic parameters (bedside echocardiography, stroke volume/pulse pressure variation, and passive leg raises)
- *Goals of resuscitation:* Maintain a mean arterial pressure (MAP) >65 mm Hg [if no acute kidney injury (AKI)]
- Normalize serum lactate levels
- Norepinephrine as the vasopressor of choice
- Continuous infusion of terlipressin or vasopressin when MAP is inadequate despite moderate doses of norepinephrine

Contd...

Contd...

- *Transfusion policy:* Threshold for red blood cell transfusion is Hb <70 g/L. Less restrictive approaches (Hb <80 g/L) if microcirculation is altered, especially in Child–Pugh C patients

Fluid therapy for conditions other than septic shock:

- Balanced crystalloid solutions as first-line therapy
- *Threshold for red blood cell transfusion:* Hb <70 g/L
- Transfusion of blood products/factor concentrates guided by viscoelastic tests in bleeding patients
- 20% albumin is the fluid of choice in patients with ACLF and spontaneous bacterial peritonitis, HRS-AKI, and in those requiring large volume paracentesis

Respiratory support:

- *Noninvasive systems:* High flow nasal cannula in moderate hypoxemic respiratory failure and non-invasive mechanical ventilation in patients with hypercapnia (if patient protecting airway)
- *Invasive mechanical ventilation:* Apply protective strategies with low tidal volumes (≤6 mL/kg), and low plateau (<30 cmH_2O), and driving pressures (<15 cmH_2O)
- Highly selected ACLF patients with refractory hypoxemia ($PaFiO_2$ <150) could benefit from prone position. It should be indicated early and maintained for at least 16–24 hours
- Early extracorporeal membrane oxygenation (ECMO) is contraindicated in the majority of ACLF patients (futile intervention)
- Tracheostomy is only recommended in highly selected patients on prolonged invasive mechanical ventilation (10–14 days)

Management of kidney failure:

- Patients with HRS-AKI should be treated with vasopressors (i.e., terlipressin, norepinephrine second line) plus albumin
- Continuous RRT should be started at standard doses (25–30 mL/kg/h) in patients with AKI and one of the following criteria: persistent hyperkalemia (>6.5 mmol/L), persistent metabolic acidosis (pH <7.2), therapy-resistant fluid overload, and oliguria

Management of kidney failure:

- Patients with HRS-AKI should be treated with vasopressors (i.e., terlipressin, norepinephrine second line) plus albumin
- Continuous RRT should be started at standard doses (25–30 mL/kg/h) in patients with AKI and one of the following criteria: persistent hyperkalemia (>6.5 mmol/L), persistent metabolic acidosis (pH <7.2), therapy-resistant fluid overload, and oliguria

Prevention of second infections: Measures to prevent catheter-related infections[a] and ventilator-associated pneumonia[b] are recommended

[a]Hand hygiene, use of alcohol/chlorhexidine-containing skin antiseptics with sterile dressing, sterile barrier precautions, catheter insertion site selection (subclavian >jugular >femoral), and timely central line removal

[b]Elevation of the head of bed (>30°), chlorhexidine mouthwash, and subglottic suctioning

(Hb: hemoglobin; HRS: hepatorenal syndrome; RRT: renal replacement therapy)

MANAGEMENT OF ORGAN FAILURE(S)

Neurological Failure

The therapy of an ACLF patient with altered mental status should focus on protecting the airway, confirming the diagnosis of HE, or other etiologies, treating any potential precipitating causes, and assessing the effectiveness of ammonia-lowering treatments.

Blood ammonia levels should not be routinely measured in critically sick cirrhotic patients.

Sedation-short-acting drugs like dexmedetomidine or propofol are preferred. Benzodiazepines should be avoided.

Lactulose is the cornerstone of therapy for HE. Typical dosing strategies include 20 g orally every hour until the first bowel movement and then titrated to maintain 2–3 soft bowel movements daily. Lactulose may be administered by nasogastric tube or as a retention enema of 200 g/300 mL of solution. Careful monitoring of electrolytes to prevent dehydration and hypernatremia is desirable.

Rifaximin, a minimally absorbed antibiotic, has demonstrated efficacy in prevention of HE-related events.

No role for continuous renal replacement therapy (CRRT) to improve neurologic outcomes in ACLF (only in ALF).

Respiratory Failure

Management of respiratory failure depends on the cause.

- Pulmonary complications like acute respiratory failure (pneumonia, acute lung injury, or hepatic hydrothorax)
- Respiratory complications either as the result of cirrhosis such as portopulmonary hypertension and hepatopulmonary syndrome or indirect results of cirrhosis chest wall edema, hepatic hydrothorax, and tense abdominal ascites.

Diagnostic tests such as echocardiography and pulmonary artery catheterization should be done in patients with unexplained hypoxia.

Circulatory Failure

It can be due to decompensated cirrhosis or cirrhotic cardiomyopathy.

Crystalloids should be utilized for first fluid treatment in patients with ACLF and hypotension and patients who need a lot of fluids and vasopressors, human albumin is recommended. Norepinephrine is the first-line vasopressor for patients with ACLF and hypotension resistant to fluid treatment. Potential second-line treatments for people who do not respond well to norepinephrine include terlipressin or vasopressin continuous infusion. Target a mean arterial pressure (MAP) of >65 mm Hg. Stress dose steroids to be added as per septic shock regimen. If patients are on nonselective β-blockers (NSBB) it should be stopped. Somatostatin administration may be advised in these patients until β-blockers may be restarted.

Renal Failure/Acute Kidney Injury

Acute kidney injury (AKI) is the most common extrahepatic organ failure in ACLF. AKI can be caused by structural or functional causes of AKI.

The hepatorenal syndrome (HRS)-AKI is defined as an increase in serum creatinine ≥0.3 mg/dL within 48 hours or ≥50% from baseline value **(Tables 2 and 3)**. Besides HRS-AKI and hypovolemia/prerenal azotemia, intrinsic renal/parenchymal causes of AKI in ACLF include acute tubular

TABLE 2: Classification of hepatorenal syndrome (HRS).

Classification diagnostic criteria	
HRS-AKI	• Increase in serum creatinine by ≥0.3 mg/dL (26.5 µmol/L) within 48 hours • Urine output ≤0.5 mL/kg body weight for ≥6 hours • ≥50% increase in serum creatinine from baseline (last available outpatient serum creatinine within 3 months)
HRS-NAKI	HRS-AKD: • eGFR <60 mL/min/1.73 m^2 for <3 months in the absence of structural causes • <50% increase in serum creatinine from baseline (last available outpatient serum creatinine within 3 months) HRS-CKD: eGFR <60 mL/min/1.73 m^2 for ≥3 months in the absence of structural causes

(AKI: acute kidney injury; AKD: acute kidney disease; CKD: chronic kidney disease; NAKI: non-acute kidney injury; eGFR: estimated glomerular filtration rate)

TABLE 3: Hepatorenal syndrome (HRS).

HRS-AKI	• ↑ in serum creatinine (sCr) ≥0.3 mg/dL (≥26.5 µmol/L) in 48 hours; or ↑ ≥50% in 3 months • No response after volume expansion with albumin 1 g/kg/day × 48 hours • Cirrhosis with ascites • Absence of shock • No current or recent use of nephrotoxic drugs (diuretics, NSAIDs) • *Absence of parenchymal kidney disease:* – No proteinuria (>500 mg/day) – No hematuria (>50 RBC/HPF) – Normal kidney ultrasonography	
New	*Criteria*	
	HRS-AKD	*HRS-CKD*
HRS-NAKI	• ↑ in SCr <50% in 3 months • eGFR <60 mL/min/1.73 m^2 • No other cause of kidney disease • Cirrhosis with ascites	• eGFR <60 mL/min/1.73 m^2 • No other cause of kidney disease • Cirrhosis with ascites

(AKI: acute kidney injury; AKD: acute kidney disease; CKD: chronic kidney disease; eGFR: estimated glomerular filtration rate; HPF: high power field; NAKI: non-acute kidney injury; NSAIDs: nonsteroidal anti-inflammatory drugs; RBC: red blood cells)

Flowchart 2: Causes of AKI in ACLF.

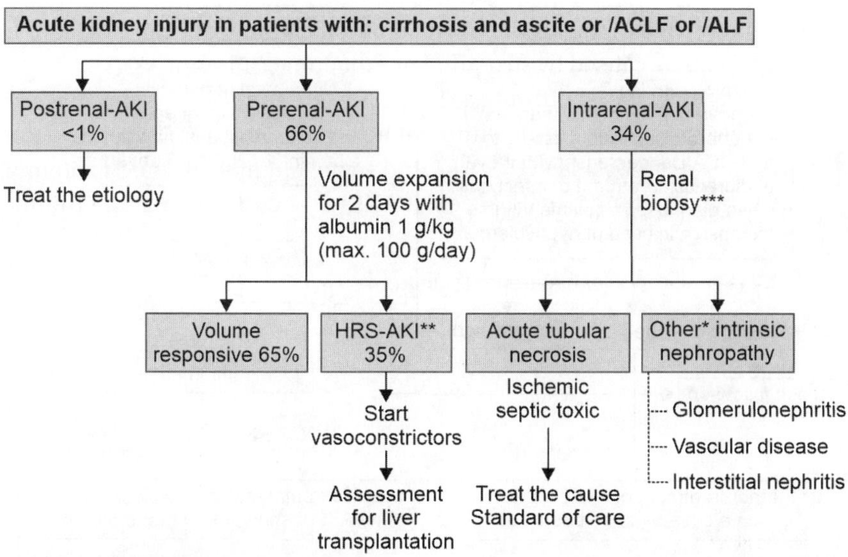

* The list is not exhaustive
** According to the ICA definition
*** If high suspicion of glomerular etiology

(ACLF: acute on chronic liver failure; AKI: acute kidney injury; ALF: acute liver failure; HRS: hepatorenal syndrome)

necrosis (ATN), nephrotoxicity, interstitial nephritis, and glomerulonephritis **(Flowchart 2)**. Urinalysis and urine examination may differentiate functional versus structural causes of AKI. Clinically, HRS-AKI primarily occurs in patients with ascites, advanced liver disease (i.e., jaundice/cholestasis) and hypotension due to splanchnic/systemic vasodilation. To date, therapies for HRS-AKI in ACLF include vasoconstrictor therapy which includes norepinephrine/terlipressin and albumin. Albumin dose is 1 g/kg/day on presentation (max 100 g daily) and then 20–60 g daily as required **(Flowchart 3)**. Norepinephrine is preferred over terlipressin in patients with history of ischemic cardiopathy. Prerenal azotemia (i.e., diuretics, diarrhea) is usually reversible following discontinuation of the precipitating cause. The severity of AKI associated with bacterial infection depends on the resolution of the infection.

The role of intermittent or CRRT in renal failure (HRS-AKI or ATN-AKI) is primarily as bridges to liver transplant (LT). In patients who are LT candidates, RRT can serve as a bridge to LT to improve pre-LT metabolic profile and metabolic status. Current guidelines recommend starting CRRT at standard doses (25–30 mL/kg/h) in the presence of one or more of the following criteria: persistent hyperkalemia (>6.5 mmol/L), persistent metabolic acidosis (pH <7.2), therapy-resistant fluid overload, and anuria (<50 m/L 12 hours).

Flowchart 3: Therapies for AKI in ACLF.

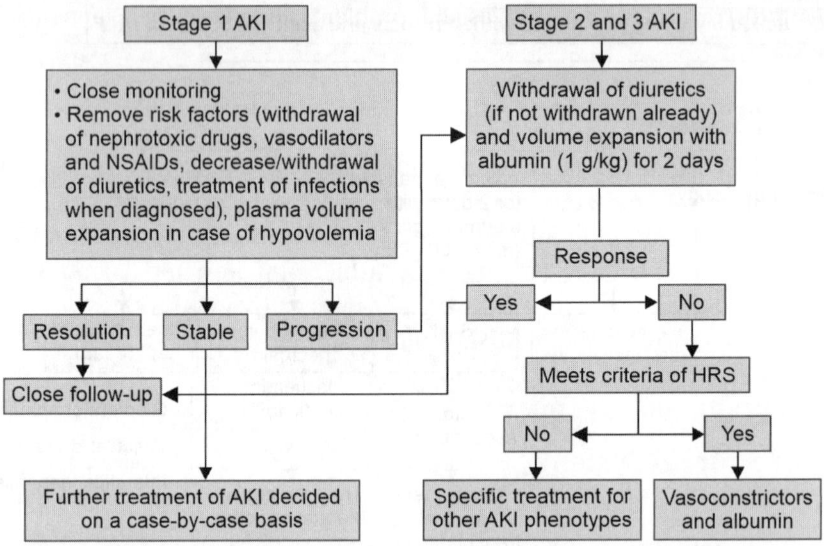

(ACLF: acute on chronic liver failure; AKI: acute kidney injury; HRS: hepatorenal syndrome; NSAIDs: nonsteroidal anti-inflammatory drugs)

Prerenal azotemia (i.e., diuretics, diarrhea) is usually reversible following discontinuation of the precipitating cause. The severity of AKI associated with bacterial infection depends on the resolution of the infection.

Coagulation Failure and Hemostatic Disorders

Traditional coagulation assays, such as the INR, and bleeding risk in ACLF do not correlate well. While measuring platelet function, fibrinolysis, and premature clot dissolution in real time, viscoelastic testing [i.e., TEG and rotational thromboelastometry (ROTEM)] provides a functional evaluation of changed pro- and anticoagulant pathways.

Due to the low risk of bleeding during paracentesis (0–3.3%) and thoracentesis (2%), standard preprocedural coagulation testing is not necessary in cases of decompensated cirrhosis or ACLF. 140 patients with platelets ≤50–60 × 10^9/L have increased reported bleeding rates during liver biopsies. Transjugular liver biopsy, especially in individuals with low platelet counts or extended INR, has been demonstrated to be generally safe. In spite of the uncertainty around the ideal fibrinogen level in surgical and bleeding patients, fibrinogen levels >1.5 g/L are advised in the absence of viscoelastic tests.

Low-volume cryoprecipitate or human fibrinogen concentrate transfusions are preferred to high-volume fresh frozen plasma that also includes anticoagulants when correction is required. Despite the fact that there are serious worries about bleeding in cirrhotic patients, a conservative transfusion target (7 mg/dL) was not worse than a liberal strategy (9 mg/dL) regardless of age or vascular problems and may even be beneficial for survival.

Liver Failure

Liver and coagulation failures are clinical signs of advanced liver disease. Liver failure is the most relevant organ failure in terms of prognosis in patients with ACLF. LT is the only currently available treatment capable to definitively correcting these failures. Patients with ACLF 2 or 3 after initial supportive therapy show very poor prognosis at short-term with mortality rates >50% at 1 month. These patients should be evaluated for salvage LT.

SPECIFIC TREATMENTS

Liver Support Systems

In ACLF 2–3 patients, supportive therapy [therapeutic plasma exchange (TPE) or albumin dialysis systems] may be considered as a bridge for LT, even though it is not the standard of care, particularly in the case of high bilirubin levels with vasoplegia, bile cast nephropathy, renal failure, coagulopathy, and/or severe HE.

Early Liver Transplantation

An early assessment for liver transplantation should be proposed for all patients with severe ACLF (ACLF-2 or -3). Given high waitlist mortality, the window for LT in patients with severe ACLF 2–3 is extremely narrow. Patient with ACLF-3 should be prioritized on a MELD-NA [Model for End-Stage Liver Disease (NOT appropriate for patients under the age of 12)] driven waiting list to reduce the excess of mortality. Delaying liver transplantation for patients with severe ACLF (ACLF-2 or -3) increase the risk of waitlist and posttransplant mortality.

Futility of Liver Transplantation

Several scores have been developed to predict 1-year post-LT mortality in patients with ACLF-3, trying to identify the "too sick population" for transplantation. A TAM (Transplantation for ACLF-3 patients Model) score higher than 2 [three of the following: age ≥53 years, pre-LT arterial lactate ≥4 mmol/L, mechanical ventilation with PaO_2/FiO_2 ≤200, and pre-LT white blood cell (WBC) ≤10 g/L] is associated with very low 1-year post-LT survival 8–10%. Severe frailty, ongoing sepsis, infection by multidrug-resistant bacteria, PaO_2/FiO_2 ratio <150, circulatory failure requiring a dose of norepinephrine >1 µg/kg/min and arterial lactate >9 mmol/L have also been suggested as clinical criteria to deny or postpone LT in these critically-ill patients.

TABLE 4: The CLIF—organ failure score system.

Organ/system	*Subscore = 1*	*Subscore = 2*	*Subscore = 3*
Liver	Bilirubin <6 mg/dL	Bilirubin ≥6 mg/dL and <12 mg/dL	Bilirubin ≥12 mg/dL
Kidney	Creatinine <2 mg/dL	Creatinine ≥2 mg/dL and <3.5 mg/dL	Creatinine ≥3.5 mg/dL or renal replacement
Brain (West-Haven grade for HE)	Grade 0	Grade 1–2	Grade 3–4
Coagulation	INR <2.0	INR ≥2.0 and <2.5	INR ≥2.5
Circulatory	MAP ≥70 mm Hg	MAP <70 mm Hg	Use of vasopressors
Respiratory			
PaO_2/FiO_2	>300	≤300 and >200	≤200
or	or	or	or
SpO_2/FiO_2	>357	>214 and ≤357	≤214

(FiO_2: fraction of inspired oxygen; INR: international normalized ratio; HE: hepatic encephalopathy; MAP: mean arterial pressure; PaO_2: arterial oxygen pressure; SpO_2: oxygen saturation)

PROGNOSTIC SCORES

The CLIF-C ACLF, NACSELD (the North American Consortium for the Study of End Stage Liver Disease), and AARC scores each have their own prognosis score for each of the three primary definitions of ACLF. Due to the fact that Child–Pugh and MELD scores do not take extrahepatic organ failures into account, they perform poorly in ACLF. Whatever the score, evaluations made after a few days of complete organ support (3–7 days) rather than at diagnosis have a considerably higher accuracy in predicting mortality. It has been suggested that CLIF-C ACLF score should take the role of MELD-NA as the measure for prioritizing patients with ACLF in the waiting list for LT due to its greater predictive accuracy. An anticipated mortality of >90% at 28 days is associated with a CLIF-C ACLF score of ≥70 or the existence of four or more organ failures at days 3–7.

THE CLIF—organ failure score system is summarized in **Table 4**.

SUMMARY

Rapid identification and treatment of precipitating events as well as systematic control of organ failures are the objectives of intensive care management of ACLF. In patients with ACLF, early, adequate antibiotic therapy improves outcomes. Dynamic tools like bedside echocardiography are advised for patients with circulatory failure, and balanced crystalloid should be the first choice of resuscitation fluid. Vasoconstricting drugs, like terlipressin, are linked to the reversal of HRS-AKI, with better immediate results for ACLF responders. When evaluating prognosis, take into account organ failure prognostic ratings (such as CLIF-C ACLF) **(Table 4)**. However, there are still certain LT contraindications that need to be identified. Early liver transplantation increases survival in individuals with severe ACLF.

SUGGESTED READING

1. Artzner T, Michard B, Weiss E, Barbier L, Noorah Z, Merle JC, et al. Liver transplantation for critically ill cirrhotic patients: stratifying utility based on pretransplant factors. Am J Transplant. 2020;20(9):2437-8.
2. Bernal W, Karvellas C, Saliba F, Saner FH, Meersseman P. Intensive care management of acute-on-chronic liver failure. J Hepatol. 2021;75(Suppl 1): S163-77.
3. European Association for the Study of the Liver. EASL Clinical Practice Guidelines on acute-on-chronic liver failure. J Hepatol. 2023;79(2):461-91.
4. Karvellas CJ, Gustot T, Fernandez J. Management of the acute on chronic liver failure in the intensive care unit. Liver Int. 2023;00:1-14.

CHAPTER

20 Pancreatitis

Apurva Kakatkar

SEVERE ACUTE PANCREATITIS

Pancreatitis is inflammation of pancreas caused by premature activation of pancreatic enzymes, leading to autodigestion of pancreas and peripancreatic tissue. Alcohol and bile stones are the two leading causes of acute pancreatitis. Pancreatitis associated with organ dysfunction, local or systemic complication is called severe acute pancreatitis (SAP). The criteria to diagnose pancreatitis are: (1) Abdominal pain consistent with pancreatitis, (2) Serum amylase or lipase >3 times normal, and (3) Imaging suggestive of pancreatitis.

CAUSES

- *Mechanical:* Gallstone, biliary sludge, ampullary or periampullary carcinoma, duodenal stricture/obstruction
- *Toxic:* Ethanol, methanol
- *Metabolic:* Hyperlipidemia, hypercalcemia
- *Drugs:*
    - *Antibiotics:* Isoniazid, tetracycline, pentamidine
    - *Diuretics:* Frusemide, thiazide
    - *Immunosuppressants:* Azathioprine, steroids
    - *Anti-inflammatory:* Salicylates
    - Antiretroviral
    - *Antipsychotics:* Valproates
- *Infection:*
    - *Bacterial: Mycoplasma, Legionella*
    - *Viral:* Coxsackie, mumps, hepatitis B
    - Fungal
    - Parasitic
- *Trauma:* Iatrogenic, blunt trauma abdomen, endoscopic retrograde cholangiopancreatography (ERCP)
- *Congenital:* Anatomical defect
- *Vascular:* Ischemia, vasculitis
- *Miscellaneous:* Hypothermia, pregnancy, postrenal transplant.

SEVERITY

Multiple scoring systems such as Ranson's criteria **(Box 1)** which involves monitoring multiple laboratory parameters and calculated over 48 hours; Imrie which also takes 48 hours parameters of bedside index of severity of acute pancreatitis (BISAP) score, and involves blood urea nitrogen (BUN), age, mental status, systemic inflammatory response syndrome (SIRS), and pleural effusion; and APACHE II >8 is suggestive severe pancreatitis **(Table 1)**.

LOCAL COMPLICATIONS

Pancreatic pseudocyst: Approximately 5% patients have pancreatic pseudocyst caused due to leakage of pancreatic duct. Mostly asymptomatic, but can present with pain, bleeding, infection, or rupture. Pseudocyst can rarely cause gastric outlet obstruction or biliary obstruction, or portal or splenic vein thrombosis.

Pancreatic necrosis: Patients with pancreatic necrosis on computed tomography (CT) should be closely monitored for infection. In case of suspected infection, image guided aspiration is recommended. Proven infection will need antibiotics and debridement or drainage.

BOX 1: Ranson's criteria.

Ranson's criteria on admission:
- Age >55 years
- A white blood cell count >16,000 cells/μL
- Blood glucose >11 mmol/L (>200 mg/dL)
- Serum LDH >350 IU/L
- Serum AST >250 IU/L

Ranson's criteria after 48 hours of admission:
- Fall in hematocrit by >10%
- Fluid sequestration of >6 L
- Hypocalcemia (serum calcium <2.0 mmol/L) (<8.0 mg/dL)
- Hypoxemia (PO_2 <60 mm Hg)
- Increase in BUN to >1.98 mmol/L (>5 mg/dL) after intravenous (IV) fluid hydration
- Base deficit of >4 mmol/L

The prognostic implications of Ranson's criteria are as follows:
- Score 0–2: 2% mortality
- Score 3–4: 15% mortality
- Score 5–6: 40% mortality
- Score 7–8: 100% mortality

(AST: aspartate aminotransferase; BUN: blood urea nitrogen; LDH: lactate dehydrogenase; PO_2: partial pressure of arterial oxygen)

Source: Adapted from Ranson JH, Rifkind KM, Roses DF, Fink SD, Eng K, Spencer FC. Prognostic signs and the role of operative management in acute pancreatitis. Surg Gynecol Obstet. 1974:139(1):69-81.

TABLE 1: APACHE II: A severity of disease classification system.[a]

Physiologic variable[b]	*Point score*								
	+4	+3	+2	+ 1	0	+ 1	+2	+3	+4
1. Temperature	≥41°	39–40.9°	–	38.5–38.9°	36–38.4°	34–35.9°	32–33.9°	30–31.9°	≤29.9°
2. Mean arterial pressure (mm Hg)	≥160	130–159	110–129	–	70–109	–	50–69	–	≤49
3. Heart rate	≥180	140–179	110–139	–	70–109	–	55–69	40–54	≤39
4. Respiratory rate (nonventilated or ventilated)	≥50	35–49	–	25–34	12–24	10–11	6–9	–	≤5
5. *Oxygenation:* i. FiO_2 ≥0.5: Use $A\text{-}aDO_2$	≥500	350–499	200–349	–	<200	–	–	–	–
ii. FiO_2 <0.5: Use PaO_2 (mm Hg)	–	–	–	–	>70	61–70	–	55–60	<55
6. Arterial pH	≥7.7	7.6–7.69	–	7.5–7.59	7.33–7.49	–	7.25–7.32	7.15–7.24	<7.15
7. Serum sodium (Na) (mmol/L)	≥180	160–179	155–159	150–154	130–149	–	120–129	111–119	≤110
8. Serum potassium (K) (mmol/L)	≥7	6–6.9	–	5.5–5.9	3.5–5.4	3–3.4	2.5–2.9	–	<2.5
9. *Serum creatinine (mg/dL):* Double point score for acute renal failure	+3.5	2–3.4	15–1.9	–	0.6–1.4	–	<0.6	–	–
10. Hematocrit (Hct) (%)	≥60	-	50–59.9	46–49.9	30–45.9	–	20–29.9	–	<20
11. White blood cell (WBC) (in 1,000s)	≥40	–	20–39.9	15–19.9	3–14.9	–	1–2.9	–	<1

Contd...

Contd...

Physiologic variable[b]	***Point score***								
12. Glasgow Coma Score (GCS)	Score = 15 minus actual GCS								
• Acute physiology score is the sum of the 12 individual variable points. • Add 0 points for the age <44. 2 points: 45–54 years; 3 points: 55–64 years; 5 points: 65–74 years; 6 points: ≥75 years. • Add chronic health status points: two points if elective postoperative patient with immunocompromise or history of severe organ insufficiency: five points for nonoperative patient or emergency postoperative patient with immunocompromise or severe organ insufficiency.[c]									
13.[d] Serum HCO_3 (venous-mmol/L) use only if no ABGs	52 ≥ 52	41–51.9	–	32–40.9	22–31.9	–	18–21	15–17.9	<15

nterpretation of APACHE II scores (predicted mortality rate).

0–4 = ~4% death rate, 10–14 = ~15% death rate, 20–24 = ~40% death rate, 30–34 = ~75% death rate.

5–9 = ~8% death rate, 15–19 = ~25% death rate, 25–29 = ~55% death rate, over 34 = ~85% death rate.

[a]APACHE II score = acute physiology score + age points + chronic health points. Minimum score = 0; maximum score = 71. Increasing score is associated with increasing risk of hospital death.

[b]Choose worst value in the past 24 hours.

[c]Chronic health status: Organ sufficiency (e.g., hepatic, cardiovascular, renal, and pulmonary) or immunocompromised state must have preceded current admission.

[d]Optional variable: Use only if no arterial blood gases (ABGs).

Source: Adapted from Knaus WA, Draper EA, Wagner DP, Zimmerman JB. APACHE II: A severity of disease classification system. Crit Care Med. 1985;13(10): 818-29.

INDICATIONS OF INTENSIVE CARE UNIT ADMISSIONS

- Pancreatitis associated with organ dysfunction such as hypotension, hypoxia, tachypnoea, and acute kidney injury (AKI).
- Age >70
- Obesity
- Presence of pleural effusion
- Necrosis >30%
- APACHE II >8
- High C-reactive protein (CRP).

IMAGING IN SEVERE ACUTE PANCREATITIS

- *Ultrasound abdomen:* It is preferred choice of investigation in early stage of pancreatitis, to look for gallstone as cause of pancreatitis, size of bile duct.
- *X-ray chest:* To look for pleural effusion, also can detect gas under diaphragm in acute abdomen cases where diagnosis is not sure.
- *Contrast-enhanced computed tomography (CECT):* In pancreatitis, CT scan is the choice of imaging for diagnosis, severity staging, and detection of complication. CECT abdomen should not be done before 72 hours as early CT may not show necrosis or collection and will not change the management in first week, however, if uncertain about diagnosis, then CT should be done to rule out other causes of acute abdomen such as perforation, obstruction, perforation, or mesenteric ischemia. In severe acute pancreatitis, follow-up CT is recommended after 7–10 days. Additional CT is indicated in case of clinical deterioration or failure to show continuous improvement or when some invasive intervention is required.
- *Endoscopic ultrasonography (EUS):* Microlithiasis, drainage of peripancreatic collection.
- *Endoscopic retrograde cholangiopancreatography:* In case of ascending cholangitis, acute gallstone pancreatitis, gallstone pancreatitis with common bile duct (CBD) obstruction.
- *Magnetic resonance imaging (MRI) abdomen or magnetic resonance cholangiopancreatography (MRCP):* To replace CECT in case of allergy to contrast or kidney injury. MRCP to rule out occult CBD stones.

Balthazar CT severity index is the scoring system based on CT findings and graded on the basis of percentage pancreatic necrosis or collection around pancreas along with severity and mortality associated with them **(Table 2)**.

LAB PARAMETERS TO DIAGNOSE CAUSE AND SEVERITY OF ACUTE PANCREATITIS

Complete hemogram with hematocrit.

- *Renal function test (RFT):* To look for AKI, high BUN on admission is suggestive of severe pancreatitis.

TABLE 2: Balthazar score: CT diagnosis and staging of acute pancreatitis.

CT grade	*CT finding*		*Points*
A	Normal pancreas		0
B	Pancreatic enlargement		1
C	Pancreatic inflammation and/or peripancreatic fat		2
D	Single peripancreatic fluid collection		3
E	Two or more fluid collections and/or retroperitoneal air		4
Necrosis			***Points***
None			0
<30%			2
30–50%			4
>50%			6
CT severity index (CT grade + necrosis score)		***Complications***	***Mortality***
0–3		8%	3%
4–6		35%	6%
7–10		92%	17%

Source: Balthazar EJ. CT diagnosis and staging of acute pancreatitis. Radiol Clin North Am. 1989;27(1):19-37.

- *Liver function test (LFT):* Do rule out gallstone as a cause of pancreatitis-elevated bilirubin and alkaline phosphatase is suggestive of obstruction, need to rule out cholangitis serum amylase, serum lipase, serum and ionized calcium levels.
- *Serum triglycerides levels:* Levels should be >1,000 mg/dL to diagnose hypertriglyceridemia as cause of pancreatitis.
- *Arterial blood gas (ABG):* To look for hypoxia (sign of organ damage), acidosis, ionized calcium, and lactates.
- Lactate dehydrogenase (LDH) levels
- C-reactive protein
- Procalcitonin to detect infection. Low procalcitonin is strong negative predictor of infection.

MANAGEMENT

The patient should be assessed in detail and look for organ dysfunction and hemodynamic compromise. Pancreatitis should be treated like any other vasodilatory shock with SIRS.

The initial approach is to assess and manage airway, breathing, and circulation (ABC).

- *Resuscitation:* The preferred choice is balanced crystalloid solution, 5–10 mL/kg to meet the resuscitation goals like urine output of 0.5 mL/kg/h, hematocrit around 35–44%, mean arterial pressure (MAP) >65 mm Hg. Avoid fluid overload. Consider early use of vasopressors if required to maintain MAP target. Monitor the hemodynamics and resuscitative goals frequently.
- *Pain management:* Intravenous analgesia in the form of opioid or nonopioid analgesia. If this is not sufficient then thoracic epidural analgesia. Patient-controlled analgesia is preferred.
- *Organ support:* In case of hypoxia use high-flow nasal cannula or noninvasive or invasive ventilator as per oxygen requirement and ability of secretion clearance.
- *Treat the cause:* Gallstone, hyperlipidemia, and hypercalcemia should be treated appropriately.
- *Nutrition:* Early enteral nutrition is advocated to prevent translocation of bacteria. Low fat diet, oral if tolerated, or nasogastric if no gastric outlet obstruction and adequate gastric emptying. Nasojejunal feeding in case of impaired gastric emptying. Partial or total parenteral nutrition when patient is not able to tolerate feeds at all. In hypertriglyceridemic pancreatitis zero fat diet.
- *Antibiotics:* Avoid use of antibiotics in first week. No role of prophylactic antibiotics. Antibiotics are indicated in subgroup of patients with cholangitis or infected wall of collections or sepsis or any other infection such as pneumonia and urinary tract infection (UTI). Broad-spectrum antibiotic in case of clinical deterioration and possible or proven infection.
- General supportive care in intensive care unit (ICU) such as deep venous thrombosis (DVT) prophylaxis, ventilator-associated pneumonia (VAP) bundle, and physiotherapy.
- *Pancreatic pseudocyst:* Encapsulated collection is usually sterile. In case of suspected infection fine needle aspiration under image guidance should be done and in proven infection or if causing gastric outlet, biliary or intestinal obstruction due to large pseudocyst. It can be drained endoscopically or percutaneously or surgically or ongoing pain or discomfort after 8 weeks.
- *Pancreatic necrosis:* Contains heterogenous material. High risk of mortality and morbidity is associated with infected necrosis. Usually, the infection peaks around end of second week. New onset or worsening sepsis, diagnosis is radiological (CECT), or by image guided fine needle aspiration to diagnose infection. Empirical antibiotics should be started and can be adjusted as per culture sensitivity. Infected necrosis need to be drained percutaneously or endoscopically or surgically.

- *Surgery in pancreatitis:* Indication of surgery in pancreatitis are: (1) As a step up approach to percutaneous or endoscopic drain. Infected pancreatic necrosis needs aspiration or necrosectomy. The preferred duration for surgical intervention is after 4 weeks when clear demarcation of infected tissue is there; (2) Abdominal compartment syndrome, the initial approach should be conservative only if fails then decompression by laparotomy; (3) Bowel ischemia or necrotizing cholecystitis with acute pancreatitis; (4) Ongoing bleeding with failed endovascular embolization; (5) Bowel fistula extending to peripancreatic collection. Whenever possible minimal invasive like transgastric endoscopic necrosectomy or video-assisted retroperitoneal debridement (VARD).
- *Role of ERCP:* ERCP should be considered when signs of ascending cholangitis like dilatation of CBD with significantly elevated/rising bilirubin or in patients with evidence of persistent choledocholithiasis like elevated bilirubin or impacted stone. MRCP or EUS are other alternatives for ERCP.
- *Abdominal compartment syndrome:* Avoid large volume resuscitation, adequate sedation and paralysis are rare surgical intervention to reduce intra-abdominal pressure.
- *Hemorrhagic pancreatitis:* Caused of erosion of splenic or gastroduodenal artery near pancreas. Diagnosis is by CT angiography to detect bleeding vessel, and active bleeding is treated by embolization of bleeding vessel.
- *Acute respiratory distress syndrome (ARDS):* Patients of pancreatitis with ARDS are treated with standard ARDS protocol—lung protective ventilation, optimum positive end-expiratory pressure (PEEP), plateau pressures <30 cmH_2O, prone ventilation if PaO_2/FiO_2 (P/F) ratio <150 mm Hg.

SUMMARY

Alcohol and gallstone is most common cause. The diagnostic criteria is abdominal pain, elevated amylase and lipase 3 times normal and imaging suggestive of pancreatitis. Severe acute pancreatitis is association of organ dysfunction with local or systemic complications. Contrast enhanced CT scan is the investigation of choice. ERCP and MRCP are the modalities used in case of gallstone pancreatitis with common bile duct obstruction for diagnosis of and therapeutic intervention. Balthazar CT scoring is widely used scoring system based on CT finding and percentage of necrosis. The treatment of severe acute pancreatitis is: (1) Fluid resuscitation; (2) pain management; (3) organ support; (4) treat the cause; (5) nutrition; (6) treatment of complications for drainage of collection indications are infection or gastric outlet obstruction, can be done percutaneously or EUS guided. Surgery in pancreatitis: The ideal time to intervene is around 4th week when clear demarcation is there. (7) General supportive care like DVT prophylaxis, VAP bundle, physiotherapy.

SUGGESTED READING

1. Gliem N, Ammer-Herrmenau C, Ellenrieder V, Neesse A. Management of severe acute pancreatitis: An Update. Digestion. 2021;102(4):503-7.
2. Leppäniem A, Tolonen M, Tarascon A, Segovia-Lohse H, Gamberini E, Kirkpatrick AW, et al. 2019 WSES guidelines for the management of severe acute pancreatitis. World J Emerg Surg. 2019;14:27.
3. Mederos MA, Reber HA, Girgis MD. Acute pancreatitis: A review. JAMA. 2021;325(4):382-90.
4. Tenner S, Baillie J, DeWitt J, Vege SS; American College of Gastroenterology. Guideline: Management of acute pancreatitis. Am J Gastroenterol. 2013;108(9):1400-15.

CHAPTER 21

Abdominal Compartment Syndrome

Charudatt Vaity

ABDOMINAL COMPARTMENT SYNDROME

Normal intra-abdominal pressure (IAP) is 5–7 mm Hg.

Abdominal perfusion pressure (APP) is calculated using the following formula:

$$APP = MAP - IAP$$

Where, MAP is mean arterial pressure.

The following are definitions from the World Society for Abdominal Compartment Syndrome (WSACS):

- *Intra-abdominal hypertension (IAH)* is defined as sustained or repeated pathological elevations in IAP >12 mm Hg.
- *Abdominal compartment syndrome* is a sustained IAP >20 mm Hg (with or without an APP <60 mm Hg) that is associated with new organ dysfunction or failure.

Intra-abdominal hypertension may be graded according to severity as follows:

- *Grade 1:* 12–15 mm Hg
- *Grade 2:* 16–20 mm Hg
- *Grade 3:* 21–25 mm Hg
- *Grade 4:* ≥26 mm Hg

Abdominal compartment syndrome may be primary (due to abdominal pathology) or secondary to one or more extra-abdominal processes.

Risk factors associated with the development of IAH and abdominal compartment syndrome are as follows:

- *Diminished abdominal wall compliance:*
  - Abdominal surgery with tight primary closure
  - Trauma, burns, and obesity
  - Prone positioning
- *Increased abdominal contents:*
  - *Intraluminal:* Ileus, gastroparesis, and pseudo-obstruction
  - *Extraluminal:* Ascites, hemoperitoneum, and pneumoperitoneum

- *Capillary leak:*
    - Severe sepsis, trauma, pancreatitis, and burns
    - Hypothermia
    - Acidosis
    - Massive transfusion
    - Fluid resuscitation, positive fluid balance
- *Other/Miscellaneous:*
    - Mechanical ventilation
    - Positive end-expiratory pressure (PEEP) >10 cmH_2O
    - Increased head of bed angle
    - Shock or hypotension

HOW TO MEASURE INTRA-ABDOMINAL PRESSURE?

Clinical examination has a low sensitivity for diagnosing IAH.

The IAP can be measured directly or indirectly **(Fig. 1)** as given in the following text.

- *Directly:* Via the introduction of a needle into the abdomen (e.g., during laparoscopy).
- *Indirectly:*
    - Transduction of pressure via an intra-abdominal viscus can be used to measure IAP using a noninvasive technique (bladder, stomach, colon, and uterus).

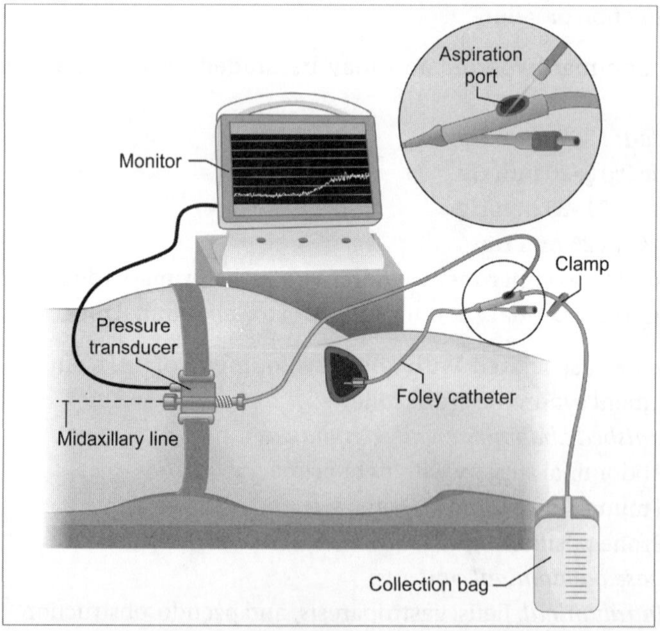

Fig. 1: Measurement of intra-abdominal pressure.

- Intravesical pressure is the most commonly used method and is performed via a urinary bladder catheter.
- 25 mL of sterile saline is introduced into the bladder and the drainage bag is reconnected and cross-clamped.
- A 16 G needle is connected to a pressure transducer and introduced via the culture port site of the catheter.

PATHOPHYSIOLOGICAL EFFECTS OF IAH ON OTHER ORGAN SYSTEMS

Respiratory

- Raised IAP causes basal atelectasis and collapse due to diaphragmatic splinting and reduced chest wall and lung compliance.
- There is increased ventilation/perfusion (V/Q) mismatch, hypoxemia, and hypercapnia.
- The application of PEEP and use of positive pressure ventilation (PPV) will worsen venous return and cardiac output (CO).

Cardiovascular

- The raised IAP is transmitted directly to the abdominal vasculature.
- There is a reduction in CO secondary to reduced venous return to the right ventricle (due to venous compression) and increased afterload (due to arterial compression).
- The reduction in CO will further reduce the APP.
- Increased intrathoracic pressure due to diaphragmatic splinting may further compromise CO.

Neurological

- Increased intracranial pressure (ICP) can occur secondary to the impedance of cerebral venous return due to raised intrathoracic pressure.
- The ICP may be increased further due to cerebral vasodilatation caused by concomitant hypoxemia and hypercapnia.

Renal

- There is direct transmission of the raised IAP to the renal vasculature, which in combination with a reduction in CO reduces renal blood flow.
- The raised IAP is also transmitted to the renal outflow tract, causing increased pressure within the tubules and reducing the filtration gradient.
- Compensatory activation of the renin-angiotensin-aldosterone (RAA) system further worsens the renal insult.

Gastrointestinal and Hepatic

- The hypoperfusion caused by critical illness is exacerbated by venous hypertension, which results in bowel wall edema.
- This may cause bowel ischemia and bacterial translocation, increasing the risk of developing sepsis.
- There is reduced flow in the hepatic artery, vein, and portal system, which contributes to liver dysfunction.
- Biliary stasis resulting from increased pressure within the biliary tree.

PRINCIPLES OF MANAGING ABDOMINAL COMPARTMENT SYNDROME (FLOWCHART 1)

Untreated abdominal compartment syndrome is associated with a mortality approaching 100%. Multiorgan failure will result and is a consequence of the severity and duration of IAH. It is important to think about "opening the abdomen" and of which patient and when. The open abdomen has become a proactive strategy against last resort methods as it was in the past. Specific indications for open abdomen:

- Severe necrotizing pancreatitis
- Abdominal sepsis

Flowchart 1: Principles of managing abdominal compartment syndrome.

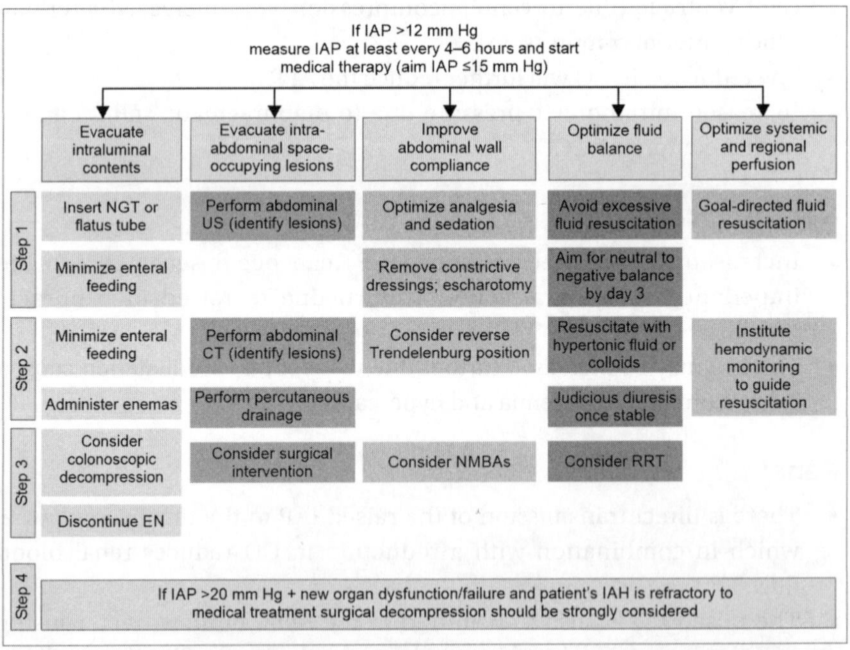

(CT: computed tomography; EN: enteral nutrition; IAP: intra-abdominal pressure; NGT: nasogastric tube; NMBAs: neuromuscular blocking agents; RRT: renal replacement therapy; US: ultrasound)

- Damage control surgery post-trauma
- Emergent vascular surgery

ISSUES AND COMPLICATIONS ASSOCIATED WITH OPEN ABDOMEN

Patients with open abdomen present a number of specific management issues and complications which are listed below.

- *Nursing issues:*
  - Skin care; skin around the wound is often moist and prone to damage.
  - Patient turning and positioning
  - Pain control
- *Significant fluid loss:*
  - Postoperative fluid losses can be as high as several liters per day.
  - Unreliable fluid balance
- *Malnutrition:* The open abdomen is a significant source of protein/nitrogen loss.
- *Infection risk:* Gauze changes and wound care make safeguarding sterility almost impossible.
- Visceral injury and adhesions
- Ileus
- *Abdominal wall-related:*
  - Large ventral abdominal wall hernias following definitive closure
  - Inability to definitively close
- Significant risk of enterocutaneous fistulation

Management of Patients with Open Abdomen

- Correction of hypothermia, coagulopathy, and acidosis.
- Lung protective ventilatory strategy
- Adequate sedation, analgesia, and neuromuscular blockade.
  - Target Richmond Agitation-Sedation Score (RASS)—4 during the acute resuscitation phase
  - Paralysis
- *Nutritional support and fluid resuscitation:*
  - Enteral feeding is safe in a patient with an intact gastrointestinal (GI) tract.
  - Supplement protein—an estimate of 2 g of nitrogen per liter of abdominal fluid output should be included in the nitrogen balance calculations of any patient with an open abdomen.
- Antibiotics tailored to the clinical situation
- Monitoring for abdominal compartment syndrome
- Adequate source control with bedside washouts as necessary

  The aim is for definitive closure within 8 days of initial laparostomy.

SUMMARY

The abdominal compartment syndrome is a potentially life-threatening condition caused by increased intra-abdominal pressure. It can lead to severe consequences for multiple organ systems. The diagnosis of ACS relies on measuring IAP, with values above 15 mm Hg indicating intra-abdominal hypertension, a risk factor for ACS. The management of ACS involves improving abdominal compliance, evacuating intra-abdominal contents, optimizing fluid balance, and supporting organ function. Prevention includes identifying and treating underlying causes, monitoring IAP in high-risk patients, and avoiding excessive fluid administration. The World Society for Abdominal Compartment Syndrome has published guidelines for the management of IAH and ACS, which can improve patient outcomes and reduce mortality.

SUGGESTED READING

1. Berry N, Fletcher S. Abdominal compartment syndrome. Contin Educ Anaesth Crit Care Pain. 2012;12(3):110-17.
2. Dutton WD, Diaz JJ, Miller RS. Critical care issues in managing complex open abdominal wound. J Intensive Care Med. 2012;27(3):161-71.
3. Kirkpatrick AW, Roberts DJ, De Waele J, Jaeschke R, Malbrain ML, De Keulenaer B, et al. Intra-abdominal hypertension and the abdominal compartment syndrome: updated consensus definitions and clinical practice guidelines from the World Society for Abdominal Compartment Syndrome. Intensive Care Med. 2013;39(7):1190-206.

SECTION

6 Neurological Disorders

CHAPTER

22 Acute Ischemic Stroke

Vivek Jain

INTRODUCTION

It is defined as sudden loss of blood circulation to an area of brain, typically in a vascular territory, resulting in a corresponding loss of neurological function.

KEY CONCEPT IN MANAGEMENT OF STROKE

A key concept in stroke management is the presence of a central area of tissue ischemia. This core is surrounded by a hypoperfused but potentially salvageable penumbral zone. The blood flow to the ischemic core is insufficient to maintain electrophysiological activity and cellular integrity. However, the surrounding penumbra has the potential for complete functional recovery if blood flow is restored promptly and adequately.

PREHOSPITAL MANAGEMENT

To detect potential stroke patients in prehospital settings, the Cincinnati prehospital stroke scale, an adaptation of the National Institutes of Health Stroke Scale (NIHSS), is employed. Dysarthria, facial drooping, and arm drift for 10 seconds are required. A score of 1 denotes a 75% likelihood of having a stroke, whereas a score of 3 denotes an 85% or higher chance.

Face Arm Speech Test (FAST) prehospital stroke scale/Cincinnati prehospital stroke scale is shown in **Table 1**.

Clinical features of stroke according to territory is shown in **Table 2**.

Bamford classification of stroke is shown in **Table 3**.

TABLE 1: Face Arm Speech Test (FAST) prehospital stroke scale.

	Yes	*No*
Facial droop?		
Arm drift?		
Speech abnormal?		
Positive screen if response to any question is positive		

TABLE 2: Clinical features of stroke according to territory.

Site of ischemia/infarction	*Clinical features*
Anterior cerebral artery (ACA)	Weakness of contralateral leg behavior changes
Middle cerebral artery (MCA)	• Weakness of contralateral face and arm • Aphasia, dysarthria • Hemianopia • Inattention to stimuli • Sensory deficit
Posterior cerebral artery (PoCA)	• Visual field deficits • Sensory deficits
Vertebrobasilar system	• Dizziness, ataxia, impaired balance • Pupil and eye movement abnormalities • Changes in voice and swallowing • Weakness and sensory changes • Decreased consciousness
Cerebral vein and sinuses	• Decreased consciousness • Headache • Vomiting

TABLE 3: Bamford classification of stroke.

	Features	*Anatomy*
Total anterior circulation syndrome (TACS)	All three criteria has to be present to diagnose total anterior circulation syndrome: 1. Unilateral motor, sensory deficit or both affecting at least two of face, arm, or leg 2. Higher cerebral dysfunction (e.g., dysphasia, dyspraxia) 3. Homonymous hemianopia	Occlusion of MCA
Partial anterior circulation syndrome (PACS)	Two of the three components of TACS	Occlusion of MCA/ branch of ACA
Lacunar syndrome (LACS)	1. Pure motor or sensory deficit affecting at least two of face, arm, or leg 2. Sensorimotor deficit not meeting TACS/PACS criteria 3. Ataxic hemiparesis 4. Dysarthria and clumsy hand	Occlusion of small, deep penetrating artery causing subcortical stroke
Posterior circulation syndrome (POCS)	1. Isolated homonymous hemianopia or cortical blindness 2. Brainstem or cerebellar syndromes/ cranial nerve palsy 3. Loss of consciousness	Brainstem/ cerebellum/ occipital lobe

(ACA: anterior cerebral artery; MCA: middle cerebral artery)

Determine the time when the patient's neurological condition last appeared to be normal. Inform the receiving emergency department (ED) of the patient's arrival, so that staff members there can get equipped and quickly start the patient's treatment.

EMERGENCY DEPARTMENT CARE

Within 20 minutes of the ED's arrival, conduct a quick neurological evaluation and activate the stroke team.

Condiitions that mimic stroke:

- Brain mass/hemorrhage/contusion
- Epilepsy-post ictal state, Todd's palsy
- Hypoglycemia/hyponatremia
- Intoxication/infection
- Migraine

Assess the patient with a neurological screening test, such as the NIHSS. The NIHSS is a method for determining the degree of stroke-related disability. It is made up of 11 components, including best gaze, visual loss, facial palsy, motor arm, motor leg, limb ataxia, sensory, best language, dysarthria, extinction, and inattention. A score of 0 denotes normal function, while a score of 42 or higher indicates impairment.

INVESTIGATIONS

- *Imaging:* A plain computed tomography (CT) scan of the brain should be obtained to exclude hemorrhagic stroke. The recommended door-to-CT scan completion time is 25 minutes, and the CT scan must be read by the neurologist in 45 minutes. In the case of an ischemic stroke, the CT brain plain may show signs, including the hyperdense vascular sign, hypodensity, loss of gray-white distinction, sulcal effacement, and the insular ribbon sign. Calculate the ASPECTS (Alberta Stroke Program Early CT Score) using CT imaging, where 10 points represent a normal CT scan. A score of 0 indicates widespread involvement across the middle cerebral artery (MCA) territory. For intravenous thrombolysis, the ASPECTS should be 6 or higher.
- *Blood tests:* Full blood count, urine routine, creatinine, C-reactive protein (CRP), erythrocyte sedimentation rate (ESR), thyroid function tests (TFTs), and lipid profile.
- Electrocardiogram (ECG)
- Transthoracic echocardiogram (TTE), transesophageal echocardiogram (TOE) +/– bubble-contrast echocardiogram.

ICU MANAGEMENT

ICU Admission Indications

The following are some potential indications for admission to ICU:

- Seizures
- Deteriorating neurological status and airway compromise
- Mass effect secondary to large space occupying infarcts
- Respiratory failure (secondary to neurogenic pulmonary edema, depressed central respiratory drive, aspiration, etc.)
- To facilitate interventions.

General Management of Stroke (Table 4)

The general management of stroke involves several key components to ensure comprehensive care for the patient. Each aspect targets a specific area of patient care to promote recovery and prevent complications.

Seizure Management

Aggressive treatment: Seizures should be treated immediately and effectively to prevent further neurological damage.

Prophylactic anticonvulsants: There is not enough evidence to support the routine use of anticonvulsants to prevent primary or secondary seizures

TABLE 4: Management of systemic physiological variables after acute ischemic stroke.

Oxygenation and ventilation	• Routine administration of oxygen is not recommended • Administer supplemental oxygen only if SpO_2 <95% • Intubation and mechanical ventilation may be required in patients with decreased conscious level, severe bulbar palsy, and risk factors for intracranial hypertension
Blood pressure	• Routine blood pressure (BP) lowering is not recommended • Cautious BP lowering in patients not receiving thrombolysis if • BP >220/120 mm Hg • Lower BP to <185/110 mm Hg before thrombolysis and maintain for 24 hours afterwards • Treat significant hypotension (systolic BP <90 mm Hg) with volume expansion and vasopressors
Glucose	• Maintain blood glucose between 7 and 11 mmol/L [with intravenous (IV) insulin as required] • Treat hypoglycemia (blood glucose <2.8 mmol/L) with 10% dextrose
Temperature	• Symptomatic treatment with paracetamol if temperature >37.5°C • Exclude or treat infective cause of pyrexia

in stroke patients. They should only be used if the patient has a history of seizures or if seizures occur.

Thromboprophylaxis

Anticoagulant therapy: Use of anticoagulants, such as heparin or low-molecular-weight heparin, to prevent the formation of blood clots. This is essential to reduce the risk of deep vein thrombosis (DVT) or pulmonary embolism, particularly in immobile patients.

Physiotherapy

Rehabilitation exercises: Engage patients in tailored physiotherapy sessions to strengthen weak or immobile limbs. This includes range-of-motion exercises, strength training, and mobility exercises to improve function and independence.

Early mobilization: Encourage early mobilization as soon as the patient is medically stable to prevent complications associated with immobility.

Nutritional Support

Dietary assessment: Conduct a thorough dietary assessment to determine the nutritional needs of the patient.

Feeding assistance: Provide assistance with feeding if the patient has difficulty swallowing (dysphagia) or is unable to eat independently. This may include the use of feeding tubes if necessary.

Nutritional supplements: Offer nutritional supplements to ensure the patient receives adequate vitamins, minerals, and calories for recovery.

Pressure Area Care

Regular position changes: Frequently reposition immobile patients to prevent pressure ulcers. Ideally, patients should be repositioned at least every 2 hours.

Pressure-relieving devices: Use specialized mattresses, cushions, and other pressure-relieving devices to reduce the risk of pressure sores.

Skin care: Maintain good skin hygiene and inspect the skin regularly for any signs of pressure sores or breakdown.

Specific management involves the following:

- The National Institute of Neurological Disorders and Stroke (NINDS) advises employing tissue plasminogen activator for thrombolysis within 60 minutes (door-to-needle time). Thrombolysis should be administered if the following criteria are met, and contraindications excluded.

- Intravenous (IV) alteplase [recombinant tissue plasminogen activator (rTPA)] should be given as soon as possible. The IST-3 trial (The third International Stroke Trial) (Lancet, 2012) demonstrated a clear time-dependent benefit when rTPA was administered within 4.5 hours of onset of symptoms. Dose: 0.9 mg/kg (90 mg maximum dose) of alteplase should be infused over 60 minutes with 10% of the dose administered as a bolus over 1 minute. Post-thrombolysis patient should be shifted to stroke unit or ICU within 3 hours of admission.

INTERVENTIONAL RADIOLOGY

Recanalization therapy with clot retrieval +/– intra-arterial rTPA may be considered in patients who present 6–8 hours after onset of symptoms. Additionally, it may be useful in the subset of patients with carotid or MCA occlusion who does badly with IV rTPA alone.

Criteria for mechanical thrombectomy includes:

- Age ≥18 years
- NIHSS score ≥6
- ASPECT score ≥6
- Modified Rankin scale ≤1
- Patient presenting with 24 hours of symptoms.

Consider decompressive craniectomy (DC) in patients at high risk of malignant MCA syndrome, i.e.

- >50% MCA territory stroke on CT
- >82 mL infarct volume at 6 hours on magnetic resonance imaging (MRI)
- >145 mL infarct volume at 14 hours on MRI

Decompressive craniectomy should be considered in patients who have sustained an MCA infarct (malignant MCA infarction) and meet the following criteria:

- <60 years of age
- Clinical neurological deficits in keeping with MCA infarct
- NIHSS of >15
- CT demonstrating evidence of an infarct of at least 50% of the MCA territory.

Adjuvant Therapy

Aspirin should be given within 24–48 hours of stroke. If IV thrombolysis was done then only after 24 hours. Dual antiplatelet therapy is contraindicated at present and is associated with increased risk of bleeding.

SUMMARY

The management of acute ischemic stroke encompasses a comprehensive approach that begins with prehospital care and extends through to specific medical and surgical interventions. The primary goal is to restore and maintain cerebral blood flow to prevent further neurological damage thereby reducing morbidity and mortality associated with this condition.

SUGGESTED READING

1. Adams HP, Davis PH, Leira EC, Chang KC, Bendixen BH, Clarke WR, et al. Baseline NIH Stroke Scale score strongly predicts outcome after stroke: a report of the Trial of Org 10172 in Acute Stroke Treatment (TOAST). Neurology. 1999;53(1):126-31.
2. Hofmeijer J, Kappelle LJ, Algra A, Amelink GJ, van Gijn J, van der Worp HB. Surgical decompression for space-occupying cerebral infarction [the Hemicraniectomy After Middle Cerebral Artery infarction with Life-threatening Edema Trial (HAMLET)]: a multicentre, open, randomised trial. Lancet Neurol. 2009;8(4):326-33.
3. Jüttler E, Schwab S, Schmiedek P, Unterberg A, Hennerici M, Woitzik J, et al. Decompressive surgery for the treatment of malignant infarction of the middle cerebral artery (DESTINY) a randomized, controlled trial. Stroke. 2007;38(9):2518-25.
4. Jüttler E, Bösel J, Amiri H, Schiller P, Limprecht R, Hacke W, et al. DESTINY II: Decompressive Surgery for the Treatment of malignant Infarction of the middle cerebral artery II. Int J Stroke. 2011;6(1):79-86.
5. Khurana D, Padma MV, Bhatia R, Kaul S, Pandian J, Suri V, et al. Recommendations for the early management of acute ischemic stroke: a consensus statement for healthcare professionals from the Indian Stroke Association. J Stroke Med. 2018;1(2):79-113.
6. Kothari RU, Pancioli A, Liu T, Brott T, Broderick J. Cincinnati Prehospital Stroke Scale: reproducibility and validity. Ann Emerg Med. 1999;33(4):373-8.
7. Mohr JP, Grotta JC, Wolf PA, Moskowitz MA, Mayberg MR, Von Kummer R. Stroke: Pathophysiology, Diagnosis, and Management, 5th edition. Philadelphia: Elsevier Saunders; 2011. pp. 45-59.
8. Mokin M, Ansari SA, McTaggart RA, Bulsara KR, Goyal M, Chen M, et al. Society of NeuroInterventional Surgery. Indications for thrombectomy in acute ischemic stroke from emergency large vessel occlusion (ELVO): report of the SNIS standards and guidelines committee. J Neurolnterv Surg. 2019;11(3):215-20.
9. Pexman JH, Barber PA, Hill MD, Sevick RJ, Demchuk AM, Hudon ME, et al. Use of the Albert Stroke Program Early CT score (ASPECTS) for assessing CT scan in patients with acute stroke Am J. Neuroradiol. 2001;22(8):1534-42.
10. Powers WJ, Rabinstein AA, Ackerson T, Adeoye OM, Bambakidis NC, Becker K, et al. American Heart Association Stroke Council. 2018 Guidelines for EARLY management of patients with acute Ischemic stroke: A guideline for healthcare professionals from the American Heart Association/American Stroke Association. Stroke. 2018;49(3):e46-99.

11. Powers WJ, Rabinstein AA, Ackerson T, Adeoye OM, Bambakidis NC, Becker K, et al. Guidelines for the early management of patients with acute ischemic stroke: 2019 update to the 2018 guidelines for the early management of acute ischemic stroke: a guideline for healthcare professionals from the American Heart Association/American Stroke Association. Stroke. 2019;50(12): e344-e418.
12. The National Institute of Neurological Disorders and Stroke rt-PA Stroke Study Group. Tissue plasminogen activator for acute ischemic stroke. N Engl J Med. 1995;333(24):1581-7.
13. Vahedi K, Hofmeijer J, Juettler E, Vicaut E, George B, Algra A, et al. Early decompressive surgery in malignant infarction of the middle cerebral artery: a pooled analysis of three randomised controlled trials. Lancet Neurol. 2007;6(3):215-22.
14. Vahedi K, Vicaut E, Mateo J, Kurtz A, Orabi M, Guichard JP, et al. Sequential-design, multicenter, randomized, controlled trial of early decompressive craniectomy in malignant middle cerebral artery infarction (DECIMAL Trial). Stroke. 2007;38(9):2506-17.

CHAPTER

23 Intracerebral Hemorrhage

Vivek Jain

INTRODUCTION

Intracerebral hemorrhage (ICH) refers to the spontaneous rupture of a blood vessel within the brain parenchyma, leading to the accumulation of blood in the surrounding tissues. This condition is distinct from subarachnoid hemorrhage, which involves bleeding into the space surrounding the brain. The 30-day mortality rate from ICH varies from 35 to 52%.

The causes of ICH are as follows:

- Hypertension
- Cerebral amyloid angiopathy (CAA)
- Vascular malformations
- Anticoagulant and antiplatelet medications
- Traumatic brain injury.

PATHOPHYSIOLOGY

The ICH begins with weakened vessel walls due to factors like hypertension. Ruptured vessels release blood, forming a hematoma that creates mass effect and inflammation. Disrupted neuronal function and secondary injury follow, potentially leading to herniation. Clot formation, resolution, and long-term deficits complete the pathophysiological sequence.

History

- Time of symptom initiation
- Medications-anticoagulants and antihypertensive—last dose when.

AIRWAY, BREATHING, AND CIRCULATION (ABC) MANAGEMENT

Airway: Ensure a patent airway, especially if consciousness is impaired. Position the patient to prevent airway obstruction and consider intubation if necessary for airway protection and adequate oxygenation.

Breathing: Monitor respiratory rate, oxygen saturation, and provide supplemental oxygen, if needed. Address any respiratory distress promptly.

Maintain proper ventilation to prevent hypercapnia, which can elevate intracranial pressure (ICP).

Circulation: Control blood pressure cautiously, balancing the need to maintain cerebral perfusion while avoiding excessive pressure that may worsen bleeding. Intravenous (IV) access should be established for fluid resuscitation and medication administration.

Intracerebral hemorrhage demands vigilant ABC management to optimize oxygenation, maintain stable circulation, and prevent secondary brain injury.

The target blood pressure management in ICH has evolved over time, with consideration given to individual patient characteristics and the specific situation. Generally, the following guidelines are often considered:

Hypertension control: In the acute phase of ICH, blood pressure control is important to prevent further bleeding and reduce the risk of hematoma expansion. However, aggressive lowering of blood pressure can lead to reduced cerebral perfusion.

Blood pressure goals: A common target is to reduce systolic blood pressure (SBP) to around 140–160 mm Hg. Some guidelines suggest gradually lowering blood pressure within the first hours to avoid sudden drops that could compromise cerebral perfusion.

If the initial BP is 150–220 mm Hg, then target SBP is 130–150 mm Hg never below.

If the initial BP >220 mm Hg, then target is 140–180 mm Hg SBP.

Individualization: Blood pressure targets may vary based on factors such as the patient's age, comorbidities, preexisting blood pressure levels, and the size and location of the hemorrhage.

Drugs: Intravenous labetalol is the drug of choice, preferably by IV infusion. Initial bolus dose of 10 mg IV followed by infusion of 2–8 mg/min, or intermittent boluses of 10 mg every half an hour. Maximum daily dose of IV labetalol is 300 mg/day.

It is important to monitor heart rate, and hold infusion if it is <60 beats/min. Other agents that are recommended for treating hypertension in hemorrhagic stroke are nicardipine, angiotensin-converting enzyme inhibitor, and hydralazine. Nitrates should be avoided because they tend to increase ICP.

NEUROIMAGING

Neuroimaging plays a crucial role in the diagnosis and management of ICH. Given here is a brief overview of its role:

- *Diagnosis:* Neuroimaging, typically with a noncontrast computed tomography (CT) scan of the head, is the primary tool for diagnosing ICH.

It provides immediate and clear visualization of the hemorrhage, allowing for rapid intervention and treatment decisions.

- *Hematoma assessment:* Imaging helps determine the size, location, and shape of the hematoma. This information guides treatment decisions, including whether surgical intervention is necessary.
- *Identifying underlying causes:* Neuroimaging can reveal underlying causes of ICH, such as vascular abnormalities, tumors, or structural lesions. Identifying these causes is crucial for appropriate management and preventing recurrence.
- *Monitoring hematoma evolution:* Repeat imaging, such as follow-up CT scans, can monitor the progression or resolution of the hematoma. This helps in assessing treatment efficacy and making necessary adjustments.
- *Identifying complications:* Neuroimaging can detect complications of ICH, such as hydrocephalus or herniation, which require timely intervention.
- *Guiding rehabilitation:* For survivors of ICH, imaging can provide insights into the extent of brain injury, aiding in the development of personalized rehabilitation plans.

Role of cerebral angiography: Cerebral angiography is used in ICH to:

- Identify underlying vascular issues like aneurysms.
- Map the vascular anatomy for surgery.
- Confirm vascular abnormalities.
- Guide endovascular treatments.
- Assess vessel patency after treatment.

Its use depends on the specific case and clinical need, given the procedure's invasiveness and potential risks.

In summary, neuroimaging, particularly CT scanning, is essential for diagnosing, characterizing, and managing intracerebral hemorrhage. It not only guides acute treatment decisions but also contributes to long-term care and recovery planning for patients.

MANAGEMENT OF RAISED INTRACRANIAL PRESSURE

Managing raised ICP in ICH is crucial to prevent further brain injury and improve patient outcomes. Given here is an overview of the management strategies:

- *Elevate the head of the bed:* Keep the patient's head elevated at 30° to promote venous drainage from the brain. This can help reduce ICP.
- *Control blood pressure:* Maintain blood pressure within target ranges. Hypertension can worsen bleeding, while hypotension can compromise cerebral perfusion. Medications may be necessary to achieve and maintain the desired blood pressure.

- *Osmotic agents:* Hyperosmolar agents such as mannitol or hypertonic saline can be used to reduce cerebral edema and lower ICP.
- *Mechanical ventilation:* If the patient's respiratory status is compromised, mechanical ventilation may be required to ensure adequate oxygenation and ventilation while preventing increases in CO_2, which can raise ICP.
- *Sedation and neuromuscular blockade:* These interventions can reduce agitation, pain, and the metabolic demands of the brain, helping to control ICP. They should be used judiciously to avoid oversedation.
- *Cerebral perfusion pressure (CPP):* Ensure that CPP (the pressure gradient driving blood to the brain) is maintained within a therapeutic range. This typically involves keeping the mean arterial pressure (MAP) above 70 mm Hg while controlling ICP.
- *Surgical intervention:* In cases of refractory ICP elevation or if there is an accessible hematoma causing mass effect, surgical evacuation of the hematoma may be necessary to relieve pressure.
- *Cerebral perfusion monitoring:* Invasive monitoring, such as ICP monitoring and CPP, can help guide therapy and assess treatment effectiveness.
- *Prevent secondary insults:* Avoid factors that can exacerbate elevated ICP, such as fever, seizures, or hypoxia. Proactively manage these issues.
- *Rehabilitation:* As ICP stabilizes, focus on rehabilitation to help patients recover and regain lost functions.

Management of raised ICP in ICH requires a multidisciplinary approach involving neurologists, neurosurgeons, intensivists, and nurses. Individualized care plans tailored to the patient's condition and response to treatment are essential for optimizing outcomes.

ROLE OF SURGERY

The following are the current indications for surgery based on the STICH (surgical treatment for ischemic heart failure) trial.

- A cerebellar hemorrhage with a diameter larger than 3 cm.
- High risk of hydrocephalus and brain stem compression without evacuation is anticipated.
- A lobar clot with a volume >30 mL that is <1 cm below the cortical surface.
- In some patients who are young and rapidly deteriorating, decompressive craniectomy may also be taken into consideration.
- When there is hydrocephalus and intraventricular bleeding that causes a rise in ICP and neurological impairment, external ventricular drainage is done.

BASIC CRITICAL CARE

General critical care for patients with ICH is crucial to optimize their neurological outcomes and overall well-being.

- *Frequent neurological assessment:* Continuous monitoring of the patient's neurological status is essential. Assess level of consciousness, pupillary size and reactivity, motor function, and vital signs regularly.
- *Temperature control:* Maintain normothermia as fever can exacerbate ICP. Use cooling measures or medications to control temperature when necessary.
- *Seizure prophylaxis:* Consider prophylactic antiepileptic medications in high-risk patients to prevent seizures, which can worsen ICP.
- *Fluid and electrolyte balance:* Maintain euvolemia and monitor electrolyte levels. Avoid excessive fluid administration, which can increase ICP.
- *Glucose control:* Keep blood glucose levels within a range of 140–180 mg/dL, as hyperglycemia can exacerbate brain injury.
- *Thromboprophylaxis:* Administer prophylactic anticoagulation or compression devices to prevent deep vein thrombosis and pulmonary embolism.
- *Prevention of complications:* Prevent secondary complications such as infections, pressure ulcers, and deep vein thrombosis through appropriate hygiene, turning, and pharmacological measures. Proper care for eyes should be given.
- *Nutrition:* Ensure adequate nutrition, considering the patient's caloric and protein needs, to support recovery. Precautions for aspiration should be taken. Only after a thorough swallow assessment should oral feeding be initiated.
- *Family support:* Offer emotional support to the patient's family, explaining the situation, providing updates, and involving them in decision-making when appropriate.
- *Rehabilitation planning:* Begin rehabilitation assessments and planning early to optimize functional recovery once the acute phase has stabilized.
- *Multidisciplinary team:* Collaborate with neurologists, neurosurgeons, intensivists, nurses, and rehabilitation specialists for comprehensive care.

Individualized care is essential, as the management of ICH varies based on the location, size, and underlying cause of the hemorrhage, as well as the patient's overall health and clinical response. Close monitoring, timely interventions, and a patient-centered approach are key to achieving the best outcomes for ICH patients in critical care.

SUMMARY

The management of intracerebral hemorrhage from a critical care perspective involves a multifaceted approach that requires timely and coordinated interventions to optimize patient outcomes. Key elements include rigorous neurological assessments, meticulous control of intracranial pressure and blood pressure, and proactive measures to prevent complications. The use of osmotic agents, careful monitoring of fluid and electrolyte balance, and the maintenance of normothermia are vital strategies. Additionally, seizure prophylaxis, appropriate nutritional support, and early rehabilitation planning are essential components of comprehensive care.

A multidisciplinary team comprising neurologists, neurosurgeons, intensivists, nurses, and rehabilitation specialists is indispensable for providing holistic and patient-centered care. Continuous monitoring, individualized treatment plans, and supportive care for both patients and their families are critical to enhancing recovery and long-term outcomes.

Through diligent application of these principles, the critical care management of ICH can significantly mitigate the immediate threats posed by the hemorrhage and lay the groundwork for meaningful recovery and improved quality of life for survivors.

SUGGESTED READING

1. Hemphill JC 3rd, Greenberg SM, Anderson CS, Becker K, Bedok BR, Cushman M, et al. American Heart Association Stroke Council, Council on Cardiovascular and Stroke Nursing, and Council on Clinical Cardiology. Guidelines for the management of spontaneous intracerebral hemorrhage: A guideline for healthcare professionals from the American Heart Association/American Stroke Association. Stroke. 2015;46(7):2032-60.
2. Mendelow A, Gregson B. Surgery for intracerebral hemorrhage. In: Mohr J, Wolf P, Grotta JC, Moskowitz M, Mayberg M, von Kummer R (Eds). Stroke: pathophysiology, diagnosis and management, 5th edition. WB Saunders; Philadelphia: 2011.
3. Mendelow AD, Gregson BA, Rowan EN, Murray GD, Gholkar A, Mitchell PM; STICH II Investigators. Early surgery versus initial conservative treatment in patients with spontaneous supratentorial lobar intracerebral haematomas (STICH II): a randomised trial. Lancet. 2013;382:397-408.
4. Whelton PK, Carey RM, Aronow WS, Casey DE, Kollins KJ, Himmelfarb CD, et al. ACC/AHA/AAPA/ABC/ACPM/AGS/APhA/ASH/ASPC/NMA/PCNA Guideline for the prevention, detection, evaluation, and management of high blood pressure in adults: A report of the American College of Cardiology/American Heart Association Task Force on clinical practice guidelines. Circulation. 2017;138(17):e484.

CHAPTER

24 Traumatic Brain Injury

Vivek Jain

INTRODUCTION

Traumatic brain injury (TBI) results from a sudden and often violent impact to the head **(Flowchart 1)**.

PATHOPHYSIOLOGY

Pathophysiology of Secondary Brain Injury (Flowchart 1 and Fig. 1)

Hypotension [systolic blood pressure (SBP) <90 mm Hg] and hypoxemia (SpO_2 <90%) are independent risk factors for mortality following severe head injury and should be treated aggressively.

PATHOANATOMIC CLASSIFICATION

The pathoanatomic classification of TBI categorizes injuries based on the specific anatomical locations and patterns of damage within the brain. This classification helps clinicians and researchers understand the extent

Flowchart 1: The pathophysiology of primary brain injury.

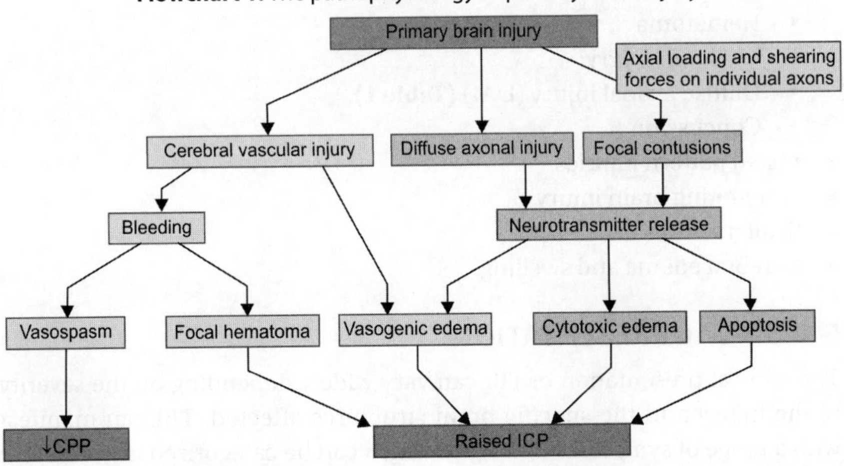

(CPP: cerebral perfusion pressure; ICP: intracranial pressure)

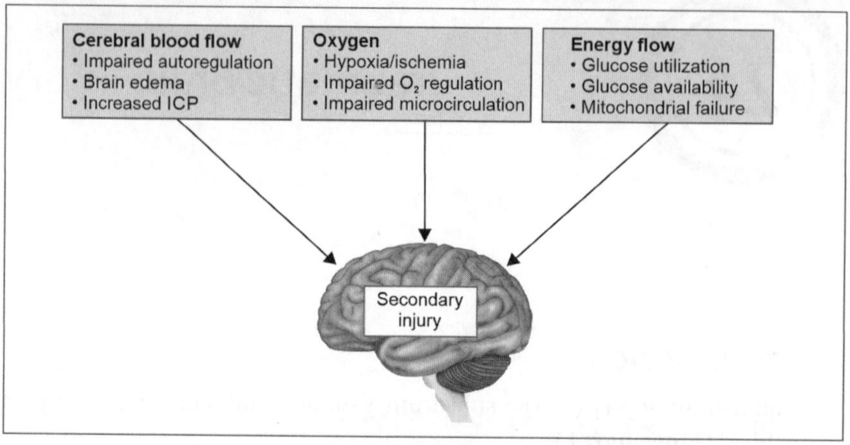

Fig. 1: Pathophysiology of secondary brain injury. (ICP: intracranial pressure)

TABLE 1: Marshall grading system for diffuse axonal injury.

Grade	*CT findings*	*Mortality*
I	No visible intracranial injury	10%
II	• Cisterns present • Midline shift <5 mm • Small, high- or mixed-density lesions <25 cc	14%
III	Cisterns compressed or absent	34%
IV	Midline shift >5 mm	56%

and severity of brain injuries. There are several common pathoanatomic classifications of TBI, including:

- *Focal (localized) brain injury:*
  - Contusion
  - Hematoma
- *Diffuse brain injury:*
  - Diffuse axonal injury (DAI) **(Table 1)**.
  - Concussion
- Mixed pattern injuries
- Penetrating brain injury
- Skull fractures
- Cerebral edema and swelling.

CLINICAL PRESENTATION

The clinical presentation of TBI can vary widely depending on the severity of the injury and the specific brain structures affected. TBI can manifest with a range of symptoms and signs, which can be categorized into different levels of severity—mild, moderate, and severe. It is important to note that

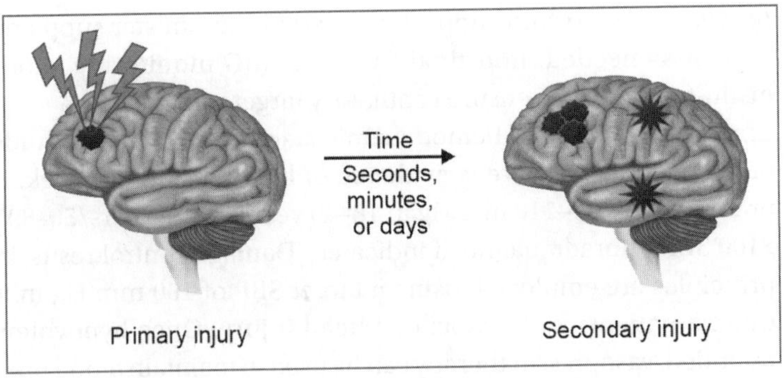

Fig. 2: Progression of primary to secondary injury.

TBI symptoms can evolve over time, and some symptoms may not become apparent until hours or days after the initial injury as shown in **Figure 2**.

SEVERITY SCORING SYSTEMS

The Glasgow Coma Scale (GCS), Full Outline of UnResponsiveness (FOUR) score, and the Marshall CT classification, are tools commonly used in the assessment and classification of TBI.

- *Glasgow Coma Scale:* The most useful classification is based on the GCS after initial resuscitation: Mild GCS ≥13, moderate GCS 9–12, and severe GCS ≤8.
- *FOUR score:* It evaluates following four components:
  1. Eye response
  2. Motor response
  3. Brainstem reflexes
  4. Respiration

ROLE OF IMAGING

Computed tomography (CT) and magnetic resonance imaging (MRI) have distinct roles in the evaluation of TBI. CT is the primary imaging modality for rapid assessment and detection of acute, life-threatening injuries, while MRI provides more detailed information about brain structure and function and is valuable for assessing TBI in the subacute and chronic phases.

MANAGEMENT

The TBI management aims to prevent further damage, stabilize the patient, and promote recovery.

Key aspects of TBI management are as follows:

- *Primary assessment and stabilization:*
  - *Airway:* Ensure a patent airway and address any immediate threats to breathing. Intubation and mechanical ventilation, if indicated.

- *Breathing:* Assess and support ventilation. Administer supplemental oxygen as needed. End-tidal CO_2 and ABG monitoring should be instituted rapidly to ensure ventilatory targets are met.
- *Circulation:* Maintain hemodynamic stability. Administer fluids and blood products if there is evidence of hypotension or shock. Blood pressure targets—110 mm Hg in 18–49 years or >70 years/50–69 years >100 SBP—noradrenaline, if indicated. Damage control resuscitation principles are employed, using a target SBP of 100 mm Hg in major trauma patients with associated head injury. Once hypovolemia is excluded, vasopressor therapy can be used to maintain blood pressure.
- *Neurological assessment:* Perform a thorough neurological examination, including the GCS score, to assess the level of consciousness.
- *Coagulation optimization:* Reversal of anticoagulant/tranexamic acid if <3 hours and moderate/severe TBI.

▪ *Intracranial pressure (ICP) management:*
  - In cases of ICP crisis, identified by signs such as neuroworsening, anisocoria, or posturing, it is crucial to promptly administer empirical hypertonic saline while awaiting a CT scan.
  - Prophylactic levetiracetam in high risk patients.
  - Continuous monitoring of ICP is essential in patients at risk of elevated ICP. This is typically done using invasive techniques such as an intraventricular catheter or an intraparenchymal monitor.
  - Noninvasive methods like transcranial Doppler (TCD) ultrasound or optic nerve sheath diameter (ONSD) measurement can provide indirect information about ICP.

Elevated ICP is defined as sustained ICP values above 20–25 mm Hg. Measures to decrease ICP are:

▪ Elevate the head of the bed to 30° to facilitate venous drainage from the brain.
▪ Maintain neck in a neutral position. Discontinue cervical collar as soon as possible (ASAP).
▪ Maintain normocapnia (normal carbon dioxide levels) to avoid hypercapnia (elevated carbon dioxide levels), which can cause vasodilation and increase ICP.
▪ Ensure adequate oxygenation to prevent hypoxia, which can also raise ICP.
▪ Use osmotic agents such as mannitol or hypertonic saline to reduce cerebral edema and lower ICP.
▪ Sedation and neuromuscular blockade may be employed to minimize patient agitation, coughing, and increased ICP due to increased intrathoracic pressure.
▪ Aggressive fever management
▪ Avoid hyponatremia

ICP monitoring with intraventricular catheter: The Brain Trauma Foundation (BTF) recommends ICP monitoring. The gold standard monitoring device is a surgically placed intraventricular catheter [which also permits removal of cerebrospinal fluid (CSF)]. A cerebral perfusion pressure (CPP) of 50–70 mm Hg should be targeted.

$$CPP = MAP - ICP$$

MAP = Mean arterial pressure

- *The BTF recommends ICP monitoring in:*
  - All salvageable patients with severe TBI and an abnormal CT brain
  - Patients with severe TBI and a normal CT if the following risk factors are present (50–60% increased risk of intracranial hypertension in these patients):
    - Age >40
    - Motor posturing
    - SBP <90 mm Hg
- *Jugular bulb oxygen saturation ($SjvO_2$):* The normal range for $SjvO_2$ is 50–75% and a value <50% necessitates intervention.
- Transcranial Doppler
- Electroencephalogram (EEG)
- *Surgical intervention*

  Indications for emergency neurosurgery include:
  - Craniotomy and evacuation of intracranial hematoma
  - Insertion of an external ventricular drain (EVD) for obstructive hydrocephalus
  - Elevation of depressed skull fracture
  - Evacuation of traumatic intracranial hemorrhage (ICH)
- *Medications:*
  - Control pain and agitation with appropriate analgesics and sedatives.
  - Manage seizures with antiepileptic drugs (AEDs) in cases of post-traumatic seizures.
  - Osmotic agents such as mannitol or hypertonic saline may be used to reduce cerebral edema.

Osmotherapy causes early volume expansion and reduced viscosity, which improves microvascular blood flow and increases circulating volume and cardiac output. This is thought to improve regional blood flow, and result in vasoconstriction in areas of intact autoregulation, thus reducing ICP and vasogenic edema formation. There is a secondary osmotic effect, which moves fluid from the intracellular to intravascular and interstitial spaces, increasing cerebral blood flow (CBF) and reducing cytotoxic edema.

Agents used include:

- *Hypertonic saline (1–2 mL/kg of 5% solution):*
  - Acts predominantly via osmotic shift of fluid

    - May also improve CBF and have an immunomodulatory function
    - Can be repeated every 4–6 hours provided serum osmolality <320 mOsm/kg and Na^+ <155 mmol/L
- *Mannitol (0.25–1 g/kg of 20% solution):*
    - In addition to the beneficial effects on blood rheology and edema formation, there is an osmotic diuresis (reduces extravascular fluid volume).
    - Potential side effects include hypovolemia, hypotension, hyperkalemia, and rebound intracranial hypertension.

Can be repeated as needed, provided serum osmolality <320 mOsm/kg and patient is normovolemic.

Routine intensive care unit (ICU) measures are important in this group:
- Ventilator associated pneumonia (VAP) care bundles
- Thromboprophylaxis (pharmacological prophylaxis is usually guided by neurosurgeons).
- Early enteral feeding (within 5 days) is associated with improved outcomes
- Stress ulcer prophylaxis
- Physiotherapy
- *Nutrition and metabolic support:* Glycemic control
    - *Calorie requirements:*
        - Caloric needs in TBI patients are typically higher due to the increased metabolic demands associated with injury and recovery.
        - A commonly used estimation is to provide 25–30 kilocalories per kilogram of body weight per day (kcal/kg/day) for patients with moderate-to-severe TBI.
    - *Protein requirements:* A typical recommendation is to provide 1.2–2.0 grams of protein per kilogram of body weight per day (g/kg/day) for TBI patients.
- *Rehabilitation:* Early rehabilitation, including physical therapy, occupational therapy, and speech therapy will optimize functional recovery.

Predictors of Poor Prognosis

- Extremes of age
- Reduced GCS motor score
- Bilateral unreactive pupils
- Absent oculocephalic reflex
- Low GCS eye and verbal score
- Untreatable raised ICP with DAI (vs. surgically amenable discrete intracranial lesion)
- Presence of extracranial complications.

SUMMARY

Traumatic brain injury remains a complex public health issue requiring multidisciplinary care. Advances in diagnostics and treatment have improved outcomes, but individual variability in injury response highlights the need for ongoing research and tailored care strategies. Continued efforts in prevention, early intervention, and rehabilitation are essential to enhance recovery and quality of life for those affected.

SUGGESTED READING

1. Adams JH, Doyle D, Ford I, Gennarelli TA, Graham DI, McLellan DR. Diffuse axonal injury in head injury: definition, diagnosis and grading. Histopathology. 1989;15(1):49-59.
2. Brain Trauma Foundation, American Association of Neurological Surgeons, Congress of Neurological Surgeons. Guidelines for the management of severe traumatic brain injury. J Neurotrauma. 2007;24(Suppl 1):S1-106.
3. Bullock R, Chestnut RM, Clifton G, Ghajar J, Marion DW, Narayan RK, et al. Guidelines for the management of severe head injury: Brain Trauma Foundation. Eur J Emerg Med. 1996;3(2):109-27.
4. Mayer AR, Yang Z, Yeo RA, Pena A, Ling JM, Mannell MV, et al. A functional MRI study of multimodal selective attention following mild traumatic brain injury. Brain Imaging Behav. 2012;6(2):343-54.
5. Raghupathi R. Cell death mechanisms following traumatic brain injury. Brain Pathol. 2004;14(2):215-22.
6. Teasdale G, Jennett B. Assessment of coma and impaired consciousness: A practical scale. Lancet. 1974;2(7872):81-4.
7. Wijdicks EF, Bamlet WR, Maramattom BV, Manno EM, McClelland RL. Validation of a new coma scale: The FOUR Score. Ann Neurol. 2005;58(4):585-93.

CHAPTER

25 Subarachnoid Hemorrhage

Vivek Jain

INTRODUCTION

Subarachnoid hemorrhage (SAH) is a critical neurological emergency characterized by bleeding into the subarachnoid space, the area between the arachnoid and pia mater membranes that cover the brain.

ETIOLOGY

85% is due to aneurysmal rupture.

Causes of SAH are listed in **Table 1**.

CLINICAL FEATURES

- Sudden severe headache (referred to as a "thunderclap" headache)
- Neck stiffness
- *Altered mental status:* The change in mental status is a critical indicator of the severity of the condition.
- Nausea and vomiting
- Photophobia
- Neurological deficits
- Seizures
- Focal neurological signs
- Loss of consciousness
- Look for Cushing's triad—hypertension, bradycardia, and irregular respiration.

SEVERITY-BASED CLASSIFICATION

Hunt and Hess classification is based on clinical grounds **(Table 2)**.

TABLE 1: Causes of subarachnoid hemorrhage.

Vascular	*Nonvascular*
Cerebral aneurysm	Head trauma
Arteriovenous malformation	Medications—anticoagulants, thrombolytics
Vasculitis	Illicit—cocaine, amphetamines
	Infections—mycotic aneurysms

TABLE 2: Hunt and Hess classification of subarachnoid hemorrhage.

Grade 1	No neurological deficits, minimal headache
Grade 2	Moderate-to-severe headache, with or without motor deficit
Grade 3	Drowsiness, confusion, or mild deficits
Grade 4	Stupor, moderate-to-severe weakness
Grade 5	Coma or extensor posturing

TABLE 3: Fisher classification of subarachnoid hemorrhage (SAH).

Grade 1	No blood on the computed tomography (CT) scan
Grade 2	Thin or <1 mm of diffuse blood
Grade 3	Localized clot in the subarachnoid space or layers of blood >1 mm thick
Grade 4	Intraventricular and intracerebral blood present in the absence of significant SAH

The Fisher classification categorizes SAH based on computed tomography (CT) scan findings as listed in **Table 3**.

ROLE OF IMAGING

Several imaging modalities are used in the evaluation of SAH:

- *Noncontrast CT scan:* It is highly sensitive in detecting acute hemorrhage.
- *CT angiography (CTA):*
  - *Vascular imaging:* CTA is used to visualize the intracranial blood vessels, helping to identify aneurysms or other vascular abnormalities that may have caused the SAH.
  - *Aneurysm characterization:* CTA provides detailed information about the size, location, and morphology of aneurysms.
- Digital subtraction angiography (DSA) is the gold standard for aneurysm detection.
- Magnetic resonance imaging (MRI) can be used to assess the age of the hemorrhage and identification of complications such as vasospasm or cerebral infarctions.

Role of lumbar puncture: Xanthochromia confirms the diagnosis of SAH when CT of the head is equivocal or negative.

MANAGEMENT

The SAH is a medical emergency. Immediate management includes the following steps:

- Airway control and ventilatory support

- Optimization of cardiovascular physiology:
    - A systolic blood pressure (SBP) <160 mm Hg or mean arterial pressure (MAP) <110 mm Hg should be targeted using intravenous (IV) antihypertensive therapy, e.g., labetalol, nitrates, hydralazine, or sodium nitroprusside (SNP).
    - An SBP <100 mm Hg should be supported with appropriate fluid resuscitation and vasopressors or inotropes.
- Neurological assessment with Glasgow Coma Scale (GCS) and Full Outline of UnResponsiveness (FOUR) score. Monitor pupils closely following sedation and ventilation.
- Prompt CT imaging
- Neuroprotective measures should be instituted.
- Liaison with neurosurgical team for definitive treatment.

Treatment of aneurysmal SAH is threefold:

1. Securing the ruptured aneurysm by surgical clipping or endovascular Coiling. Hunt and Hess grade 1, 2, and 3 require early repair. For grades 4 and 5, before repair, it is better to wait for neurological improvement.
2. Minimizing secondary brain injury and delayed neurological deficit.
3. Preventing and treating non-neurological complications.

COMPLICATIONS

- Specific complication of SAH—cerebral vasospasm and delayed cerebral ischemia (DCI)-vasospasm occurs 3–4 days after rupture, and peaks in 7–110 days and resolves in 14–21 days. Transcranial Doppler can be used to detect vasospasm.
- Delayed cerebral ischemia—This is defined as a clinical syndrome of focal neurological deficits occurring 4–14 days after rupture. Nimodipine prevents the risk of DCI. Dose is 60 mg orally every 4 hours for 21 days. If it occurs treatment is double H therapy—hypervolemia and hypertension. DCI in a major vessel like middle cerebral artery (MCA) territory can be treated with angioplasty and selective intraarterial vasodilator therapy.
- Obstructive hydrocephalus
- Rebleeding
- Seizures

Medical Complications

Medical complications are listed in **Table 4**.

PREVENTION

Lifestyle modification: Encourage lifestyle changes such as smoking cessation, blood pressure control, and stress reduction to reduce the risk of recurrent SAH.

TABLE 4: Medical complications of subarachnoid hemorrhage.

Cardiac	Troponin elevation, arrhythmias, left ventricular dysfunction
Pulmonary	Neurogenic pulmonary edema, ARDS
Infective	Fever, VAP
Endocrine	Hyperglycemia
Electrolyte-sodium imbalance	SAIDH, CSWS, DI
Neurologic	Seizures, hydrocephalus
	Deep vein thrombosis

(ARDS: acute respiratory distress syndrome; CSWS: cerebral salt wasting syndrome; DI: diabetes insipidus; SAIDH: syndrome of inappropriate antidiuretic hormone; VAP: ventilator-associated pneumonia)

SUMMARY

Subarachnoid hemorrhage represents a critical neurological emergency requiring prompt diagnosis and management. The Hunt and Hess and Fisher classifications provide essential frameworks for assessing the severity and guiding treatment strategies. Early intervention, meticulous monitoring, and comprehensive rehabilitation are paramount to improving outcomes and minimizing the long-term impact on patients' lives.

SUGGESTED READING

1. Connolly Jr ES, Rabinstein AA, Carhuapoma JR, Derdeyn CP, Dion J, Higashida RT, et al. Guidelines for the management of aneurysmal subarachnoid hemorrhage: a guideline for healthcare professionals from the American Heart Association/American Stroke Association. Stroke. 2012;43(6):1711-37.
2. Fisher CM, Kistler JP, Davis JM. Relation of cerebral vasospasm to subarachnoid hemorrhage visualized by computerized tomographic scanning. Neurosurgery. 1980;6(1):1-9.
3. Hunt WE, Hess RM. Surgical risk as related to time of intervention in the repair of intracranial aneurysms. J Neurosurg. 1968;28(1):14-20.
4. Molyneux A, Kerr R, Stratton I, Sandercock P, Clarke M, Shrimpton J, et al. International Subarachnoid Aneurysm Trial (ISAT) of neurosurgical clipping versus endovascular coiling in 2143 patients with ruptured intracranial aneurysms: a randomised trial. Lancet. 2002;360(9342):1267-74.

CHAPTER 26

Status Epilepticus

Vivek Jain

INTRODUCTION

Status epilepticus (SE) is a neurological emergency requiring immediate medical intervention to prevent significant morbidity and mortality.

DIAGNOSIS

The diagnosis of convulsive status is clinical and is confirmed by verifying the presence of either an unremitting generalized convulsive seizure lasting longer than 5 minutes or multiple bilateral convulsive seizures without an interictal return to the baseline level of consciousness.

Treatment of SE is time sensitive.

URGENT EVALUATION

Focused history from a family member or caregiver to determine the following information:

- Patient history of epilepsy
- Precipitating factors
- Current medications, including prior or current use of antiseizure medications
- For patients with prior SE, history of treatment response
- Other active medical diagnoses

Initial physical examination include:

- A focused general medical evaluation should assess respiratory and circulatory status.
    - Attention to airway, breathing, and circulation is urgent.
    - Look for signs of head trauma, sepsis, anisocoria, or meningitis.
- A rapid neurologic examination to determine the type of SE and its etiology.

CLASSIFICATION

The length of time that patients are in uncontrolled SE is important for three reasons:

1. Increased risk of cerebral damage

2. Increased risk of systemic damage
3. Seizures become more resistant to treatment

ETIOLOGY

Status epilepticus can have various underlying causes, and identifying the etiology is crucial for appropriate management.

- *Epilepsy-related:* The most common cause of SE is the exacerbation of preexisting epilepsy, especially when antiseizure medication compliance is poor. In patients with known epilepsy, SE often occurs due to medication noncompliance, abrupt medication withdrawal, or inadequate seizure control.
- Acute symptomatic infections
- *Metabolic derangements:* Metabolic disturbances, such as hypoglycemia, hyponatremia, hypernatremia, and hypocalcemia.
- Cerebrovascular events including cerebral venous sinus thrombosis
- *Toxic and drug-induced:* Common substances associated with SE include alcohol withdrawal, drug intoxication (e.g., cocaine, amphetamines), and overdose of certain medications (e.g., tricyclic antidepressants).
- Febrile seizures
- *Structural brain lesions:* Brain tumors, vascular malformations, and other structural brain lesions.
- Autoimmune and paraneoplastic
- Idiopathic or cryptogenic

Diagnostic modalities for SE will include electroencephalography (EEG) especially continuous EEG, interictal EEG, and video-EEG.

- *Blood tests:*
  - *Electrolyte levels:* Serum electrolyte levels (sodium, potassium, calcium, and magnesium)/*Glucose:* Rule out hypoglycemia induced seizures.
  - Toxicology screen-urine toxicology
- *Neuroimaging:* Computed tomography (CT) scan and magnetic resonance imaging (MRI).
- Lumbar puncture
- Cardiac evaluation to evaluate for arrhythmias or cardiac causes of syncope, which can sometimes mimic seizures.

MANAGEMENT

The management of a patient with SE is a medical emergency that requires immediate and aggressive intervention to terminate the seizure, stabilize the patient, identify and treat the underlying cause, and prevent complications. **Flowchart 1** detailing the stages and management of SE. The stages are divided into four steps: (1) Early SE (5–10 minutes), (2) established SE

Flowchart 1: Key steps in the management of status epilepticus (SE).

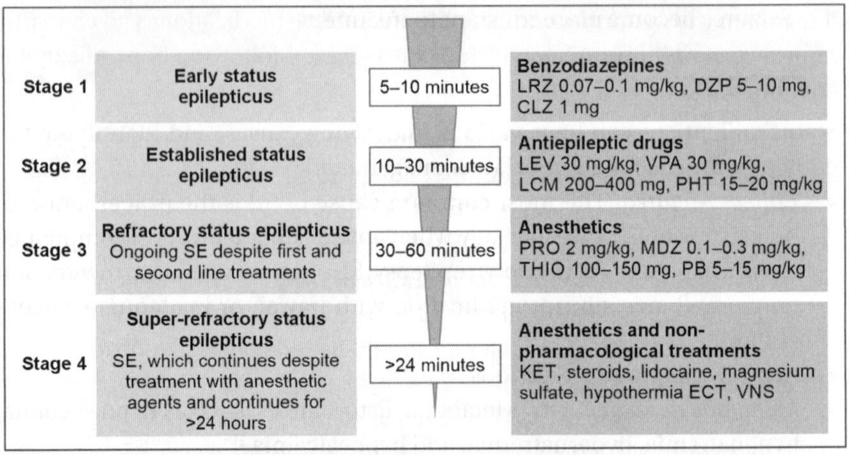

(CLZ: clozapine; DZP: diazepam; ECT: electroconvulsive therapy; KET: ketamine; LCM: lacosamide; LEV: levetiracetam; LRZ: lorazepam; MDZ: midazolam; PB: pentobarbital; PHT: phenytoin; PRO: propofol; THIO: thiopental; VNS: vagus nerve stimulation; VPA: valproic acid)

(10–30 minutes), (3) refractory SE (30–60 minutes), and (4) super-refractory SE (beyond 24 minutes). Each stage lists corresponding treatments, such as benzodiazepines for early SE and anesthetics for refractory SE.

Ensure Patient Safety and Immediate Assessment

Ensure a safe environment to prevent injury during convulsions. Assess the patient's vital signs and level of consciousness. Within 5 minutes of arrival in the emergency room (ER), airway should be secured, breathing and circulation optimized, and blood sugar checked. Thiamine 100 mg intravenous (IV) in all patients should be given. Physiological disturbances in the form of acidosis hypoxia and hypotension should be addressed.

Terminate Seizure Activity

- *First-line treatment*: Benzodiazepines
    - Lorazepam (preferred) 0.1 mg/kg IV (maximum 4 mg), if IV access is present.
    - Diazepam 0.15–0.2 mg/kg IV (maximum 10 mg) per rectum, if IV is not present.
    - Midazolam is preferred for intramuscular (IM), intranasal, or buccal administration. Dose—0.2 mg/kg (maximum 10 mg).
- If the seizure persists after the initial dose, repeat the benzodiazepine or use a different one.

Second-line Agents

Treatment with a nonbenzodiazepine antiseizure medication is given to prevent recurrence, even if convulsions have ceased following benzodiazepine treatment.

Second-line agents are levetiracetam, fosphenytoin, or valproate.

- *Levetiracetam:* Levetiracetam is given at a loading dose of 60 mg/kg (maximum 4,500 mg) infused over 15 minutes.
- *Fosphenytoin and phenytoin:* Fosphenytoin is started with a loading dose of 20 mg phenytoin equivalents (PE)/kg infused at 100–150 mg PE/min; phenytoin is started with a loading dose of 20 mg/kg and infused at 25–50 mg/min. The infusion rate should be reduced if significant adverse effects occur. An additional dose of fosphenytoin 5–10 mg PE/kg (or phenytoin 5–10 mg/kg) can be given 10 minutes after the loading infusion if seizures persist, up to a maximum cumulative dose of 30 mg/kg.
    - Phenytoin (but not fosphenytoin) is incompatible with any of the benzodiazepines and will precipitate if infused through the same IV line; the same applies to phenytoin and any fluid with glucose/dextrose. (See Fosphenytoin and phenytoin below)
- *Valproate:* Valproate is given with a loading dose of 40 mg/kg and infused at a rate of 10 mg/kg per minute in adults (maximum dose 3,000 mg); thus, the full dose can be given in 4 minutes, with no significant risk of acute adverse effects.

Fosphenytoin and phenytoin may require cardiac monitoring to prevent arrhythmias.

Anesthetic Agents (Refractory Status Epilepticus)

If seizures persist despite benzodiazepines and second-line agents, consider continuous IV infusion of anesthetic agents such as propofol, midazolam, or pentobarbital in an intensive care unit (ICU) setting.

Identify and Treat Underlying Cause

Simultaneously, investigate and treat the underlying cause of SE, such as infection, metabolic disturbance, or drug overdose, based on clinical and laboratory findings.

- *Monitor for complications:* Continuously monitor for complications, including respiratory depression, hypoxia, and organ dysfunction. Address complications such as rhabdomyolysis, hyperthermia, and electrolyte imbalances.
- *Evaluate for long-term management:* After stabilization, determine the need for long-term management, which may include optimizing antiseizure medication regimens or considering surgical interventions.

- *Neurology consultation:* Involve a neurologist for expert guidance in managing SE and determining long-term treatment plans.
- *Supportive care:* Provide supportive care, including nutrition, hydration, and rehabilitation, as needed.

SUMMARY

A multidisciplinary approach, incorporating neurologists, intensivists, and other healthcare professionals, is often necessary to optimize patient outcomes. Advances in diagnostic modalities and therapeutic strategies continue to improve our ability to manage SE effectively.

SUGGESTED READING

1. Brophy GM, Bell R, Claassen J, Alldredge B, Bleck TP, Glauser T, et al. Guidelines for the evaluation and management of status epilepticus. Neurocrit Care. 2012;17(1):3-23.
2. Lowenstein DH, Alldredge BK. Status epilepticus. N Engl J Med. 1998;339(14): 970-6.
3. Shorvon S, Ferlisi M. The treatment of super-refractory status epilepticus: A critical review of available therapies and a clinical treatment protocol. Brain. 2011;134(10):2802-18.
4. Trinka E, Cock H, Hesdorffer D, Rossetti AO, Scheffer IE, Shinnar S, et al. A definition and classification of status epilepticus–Report of the ILAE Task Force on Classification of Status Epilepticus. Epilepsia. 2015;56(10):1515-23.

CHAPTER 27

Delirium in ICU

Vivek Jain

INTRODUCTION

Delirium is a common and serious neurological complication observed in critically ill patients admitted to the intensive care unit (ICU). Delirium is characterized by acute disturbances in attention, awareness, and cognitive function, often accompanied by altered levels of consciousness. It can manifest as hypoactive (quiet and withdrawn), hyperactive (agitated and restless), or mixed (fluctuating between hypoactive and hyperactive) subtypes. Delirium in the ICU is a significant concern due to its association with increased morbidity, mortality, prolonged hospital stays, and long-term cognitive impairment.

PREVALENCE

Delirium affects a substantial proportion of ICU patients, with reported prevalence rates ranging from 20 to 80%, depending on the patient population and the tools used for assessment.

RISK FACTORS

Understanding the risk factors associated with ICU delirium is essential for identifying high-risk patients and implementing preventive measures. Risk factors include:

- *Advanced age:* Older adults are at higher risk due to age-related changes in brain function and comorbidities.
- *Severity of illness:* Patients with more severe physiological derangements are at increased risk.
- *Prolonged ICU stay:* Longer durations of ICU admission increase the likelihood of delirium.
- *Mechanical ventilation:* Patients requiring mechanical ventilation are particularly susceptible.
- *Sedative and analgesic medications:* The use of certain medications such as sedatives, opioids, and hypnotics in ICU care can contribute to delirium.
- *Infections:* Sepsis and other infections can trigger delirium.

- *Metabolic disturbances:* Electrolyte imbalances and organ dysfunction may precipitate delirium.
- *Preexisting cognitive impairment:* Patients with dementia or cognitive impairment are at higher risk.
- *Environmental factors:* Noise, light, and disrupted sleep patterns in the ICU can exacerbate delirium.

PATHOPHYSIOLOGY

Delirium in the ICU is a multifactorial syndrome with a complex pathophysiology involving several key mechanisms:

- *Neuroinflammation and oxidative stress:* Critical illness triggers neuroinflammation and oxidative stress, leading to blood-brain barrier disruption and microglial activation, contributing to cognitive dysfunction.
- *Neurotransmitter imbalance:* Alterations in cholinergic, dopaminergic, and serotonergic pathways are implicated in delirium. Reduced acetylcholine levels, dysregulated dopamine, and serotonin may play a role.
- *Brain network disruption:* Delirium may be linked to disturbances in large-scale brain networks, affecting attention, memory, and consciousness.
- *Neurocognitive vulnerability:* Individual factors such as preexisting cognitive impairment, genetics, and brain reserve capacity influence susceptibility to delirium.

The interplay of these mechanisms contributes to the development of delirium in the ICU and understanding them is vital for targeted interventions.

ASSESSMENT: SCALES AND TOOLS

Accurate assessment of delirium in the ICU is crucial for early detection and appropriate management. Several validated scales and tools have been developed to aid healthcare professionals in assessing delirium in critically ill patients. Here, we present some of the commonly used scales:

- *Confusion assessment method for the ICU (CAM-ICU):*
    - *Description:* The CAM-ICU is a widely used tool for delirium assessment in the ICU setting. It is based on the Diagnostic and Statistical Manual of Mental Disorders (DSM) criteria for delirium and assesses four features: acute onset or fluctuating course, inattention, disorganized thinking, and altered level of consciousness.
    - *Advantages:* It is easy to administer and has high interrater reliability. It can be used for mechanically ventilated patients.

- *Intensive care delirium screening checklist (ICDSC):*
  - *Description:* The ICDSC is another commonly used tool that assesses eight features of delirium, including altered consciousness, inattention, disorientation, hallucinations, psychomotor agitation or retardation, inappropriate speech or mood, sleep/wake cycle disturbances, and symptom fluctuation.
  - *Advantages:* It provides a comprehensive assessment of delirium symptoms and is easy to administer.

PREVENTION

Preventing delirium in the ICU is a crucial aspect of patient care, as it can significantly improve outcomes and reduce the burden on patients, their families, and healthcare systems. Various strategies have been identified to mitigate the risk of delirium in critically ill patients. Here are some evidence-based prevention strategies:

- *Early mobility and physical therapy:*
  - *Rationale:* Early mobility programs and physical therapy interventions in the ICU can prevent muscle atrophy, reduce immobilization, and promote cognitive function.
- *Sleep enhancement:*
  - *Rationale:* Promoting better sleep hygiene and reducing sleep disturbances in the ICU can help prevent delirium.
- *Medication management:*
  - *Rationale:* Minimizing the use of sedatives, benzodiazepines, and other psychoactive drugs, particularly in high-risk patients, can reduce the risk of delirium.
- *Delirium assessment and multicomponent interventions:*
  - *Rationale:* Regular delirium assessment using validated tools like the CAM-ICU, combined with multicomponent interventions that address modifiable risk factors, can significantly reduce the incidence and duration of delirium.
- *Adequate nutrition and hydration:*
  - *Rationale:* Malnutrition and dehydration can contribute to delirium. Ensuring patients receive adequate nutrition and fluids is essential for prevention.
- *Targeted geriatric care models:*
  - *Rationale:* Implementing targeted care models, such as the Hospital Elder Life Program (HELP), that focus on the specific needs of older adults in the ICU can be effective in delirium prevention.
- *Environmental modifications:*
  - *Rationale:* Creating a more patient-friendly environment in the ICU, including reducing noise and optimizing lighting, can promote sleep and reduce delirium risk.

TREATMENT

Managing delirium in the ICU is essential to improve patient outcomes and minimize distress for both patients and their families. The treatment of delirium involves addressing its underlying causes, providing supportive care, and minimizing its impact. Below are key components of delirium treatment:

- *Identification and management of underlying causes:*
  - *Rationale:* Identifying and addressing the underlying causes or contributing factors of delirium is crucial. These may include infections, medication side effects, metabolic disturbances, or organ dysfunction.
  - *Infections:* Prompt diagnosis and treatment of infections, such as pneumonia or urinary tract infections, are essential.
  - *Medication review:* Evaluate and adjust medications that may be contributing to delirium, such as sedatives, opioids, or anticholinergic drugs.
  - *Correction of metabolic imbalances:* Address electrolyte imbalances and manage organ dysfunction.
- *Symptom management:*
  - *Rationale:* Managing the symptoms of delirium, including agitation, hallucinations, and disorientation, is vital for patient comfort and safety.
  - *Pharmacological interventions:* In some cases, medications like antipsychotics (e.g., haloperidol or quetiapine) may be used to manage severe agitation or psychosis associated with delirium.
  - *Nonpharmacological approaches:* Nonpharmacological interventions, such as reorientation techniques, minimizing environmental stimuli, and maintaining a consistent daily routine, can help reduce distress and agitation.
- *Prevention of complications:*
  - *Rationale:* Delirium can lead to complications, such as pressure ulcers, falls, or self-extubation in mechanically ventilated patients. Preventing these complications is crucial.
  - *Fall prevention:* Implement fall precautions, such as bed alarms and bed rails, for patients at risk of falls.
  - *Skin integrity:* Ensure frequent repositioning and skin assessments to prevent pressure ulcers.
- *Multidisciplinary team collaboration:*
  - *Rationale:* Delirium management often requires input from various healthcare professionals, including physicians, nurses, pharmacists, and physical therapists.
  - *Collaborative care plans:* Develop and implement collaborative care plans that address the patient's specific needs and delirium risk factors.

- *Family and caregiver involvement:*
    - *Rationale:* Providing support and education to family members and caregivers is essential for managing delirium.
    - *Family education:* Educate family members about delirium, its causes, and the importance of maintaining a calm and supportive environment.
- *Reevaluation and monitoring:*
    - *Rationale:* Continuously monitor the patient's mental status and reevaluate the treatment plan as needed.
    - *Regular assessment:* Conduct regular delirium assessments using validated tools like the CAM-ICU to track changes in the patient's condition.
- *Addressing pain and discomfort:*
    - *Rationale:* Pain and discomfort can exacerbate delirium. Adequate pain management is essential.
    - *Pain assessment:* Continuously assess and manage pain using appropriate analgesics and nonpharmacological techniques.

SUMMARY

Delirium in the ICU is a common, serious, and often under-recognized condition associated with prolonged hospital stays, increased morbidity and mortality, and long-term cognitive decline. Early identification, prevention through minimizing sedation, ensuring adequate pain control, promoting sleep, and engaging patients in early mobility and cognitive activities are crucial. Multidisciplinary approaches and the use of tools like the CAM-ICU help in timely diagnosis and management, improving patient outcomes and overall ICU care quality.

SUGGESTED READING

1. Barr J, Fraser GL, Puntillo K, Ely EW, Gélinas C, Dasta JF, et al. Clinical practice guidelines for the management of pain, agitation, and delirium in adult patients in the intensive care unit. Crit Care Med. 2013;41(1):263-306.
2. Bergeron N, Dubois MJ, Dumont M, Dial S, Skrobik Y. Intensive Care Delirium Screening Checklist: evaluation of a new screening tool. Intensive Care Med. 2001;27(5):859-64.
3. Ely EW, Inouye SK, Bernard GR, Gordon S, Francis J, May L, et al. Delirium in mechanically ventilated patients: validity and reliability of the confusion assessment method for the intensive care unit (CAM-ICU). JAMA. 2001;286(21):2703-10.
4. Ely EW, Shintani A, Truman B, Speroff T, Gordon SM, Harrell FE Jr, et al. Delirium as a predictor of mortality in mechanically ventilated patients in the intensive care unit. JAMA. 2004;291(14):1753-62.
5. Girard TD, Pandharipande PP, Ely EW. Delirium in the intensive care unit. Crit Care. 2008;12(Suppl 3):S3.
6. Gélinas C, Fillion L, Puntillo KA, Viens C, Fortier M. Validation of the critical-care pain observation tool in adult patients. Am J Crit Care. 2009;18(2):136-43.

7. Hshieh TT, Yang T, Gartaganis SL, Yue J, Inouye SK. Hospital elder life program: systematic review and meta-analysis of effectiveness. Am J Geriatr Psychiatry. 2018;26(10):1015-33.
8. Inouye SK, Bogardus ST, Charpentier PA, Leo-Summers L, Acampora D, Holford TR, et al. A multicomponent intervention to prevent delirium in hospitalized older patients. New Engl J Med. 1999;340(9):669-76.
9. Kamdar BB, Needham DM, Collop NA, Sakamuri S, Colantuoni E, Neufeld KJ, et al. The effect of a quality improvement intervention on perceived sleep quality and cognition in a medical ICU. Crit Care Med. 2012;40(2):402-9.
10. Leslie DL, Inouye SK. The importance of delirium: economic and societal costs. J Am Geriatr Soc. 2011;59(Suppl 2):S241-3.
11. MacLullich AMJ, Ferguson KJ, Miller T, de Rooij SE, Cunningham C. Unravelling the pathophysiology of delirium: a focus on the role of aberrant stress responses. J Psychosom Res. 2008;65(3):229-38.
12. Meagher DJ, Leonard M, Donnelly S, Conroy M, Adamis D, Trzepacz PT, et al. A longitudinal study of motor subtypes in delirium: frequency and stability during episodes. J Psychosom Res. 2011;71(6):395-9.
13. Pandharipande P, Shintani A, Peterson J, Pun BT, Wilkinson GR, Dittus RS, et al. Lorazepam is an independent risk factor for transitioning to delirium in intensive care unit patients. Anesthesiology. 2006;104(1):21-6.
14. Salluh JI, Soares M, Teles JM, Ceraso D, Raimondi N, Nava VS, et al. Delirium Epidemiology in Critical Care Study Group. Delirium epidemiology in critical care (DECCA): an international study. Crit Care. 2015;19(1):1-8.
15. Schweickert WD, Pohlman MC, Pohlman AS, Nigos C, Pawlik AJ, Esbrook CL, et al. Early physical and occupational therapy in mechanically ventilated, critically ill patients: a randomised controlled trial. Lancet. 2009;373(9678):1874-82.
16. Shafi MM, Santarnecchi E, Fong TG, Jones RN, Marcantonio ER, Pascual-Leone A, et al. Advancing the neurophysiological understanding of delirium. J Ame Geriatr Soc. 2017;65(6):1114-8.
17. Siddiqi N, Harrison JK, Clegg A, Teale EA, Young J, Taylor J, et al. Interventions for preventing delirium in hospitalised non-ICU patients. Cochrane Database Syst Rev. 2016;3(3):CD005563.
18. van den Boogaard M, Pickkers P, van der Hoeven H, Roodbol G, van Achterberg T, Schoonhoven L. Implementation of a delirium assessment tool in the ICU can influence haloperidol use. Crit Care. 2012;16(3):R13.
19. van Gool WA, van de Beek D, Eikelenboom P. Systemic infection and delirium: when cytokines and acetylcholine collide. Lancet. 2010;9(9):934-44.

CHAPTER

28 Brain Death and Care of Brain Dead Donor

Vivek Jain

INTRODUCTION

Brain death is a complex clinical condition defined by the irreversible cessation of all cerebral and brainstem activities.

ETIOLOGY OF BRAIN DEATH

- Traumatic brain injury (TBI)
- Cerebrovascular events
- Anoxic brain injury
- Intracranial mass lesions
- Neurological diseases

CONFOUNDING FACTORS IN THE CLINICAL DIAGNOSIS OF BRAIN DEATH

- Hypothermia (core temperature <32°C)
- Sedative medications
- Neuromuscular blockade
- Metabolic disturbances
- High spinal cord injury
- Miscellaneous condition includes neurotoxic snake envenomation, brainstem encephalitis, Guillain–Barré syndrome, and encephalopathy.

DIAGNOSIS OF BRAIN DEATH

Flowchart 1 shows the steps to diagnose brain death in a comatose, ventilator-dependent patient. It covers the confirmation of irreversible brain damage, exclusion of reversible causes, and clinical examination of motor responses, brainstem reflexes, and apnea. If criteria are met, brain death is confirmed; otherwise, reassessment or treatment withdrawal is considered.

Prerequisites to Diagnosing Brain Death

There should be catastrophic brain injury. The patient's comatose condition and apnea must be due to irreversible brain damage of known etiology.

Flowchart 1: Diagnosis of brain death.

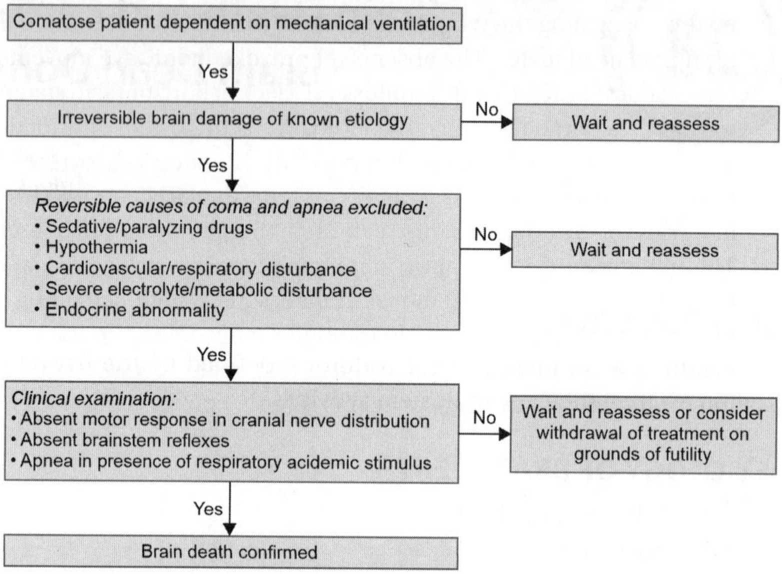

This process involves three critical components:

1. *Coma documentation:*
   a. Evaluation for the absence of motor response following the application of a standardized painful stimulus along a cranial nerve pathway (such as pressure on the supraorbital groove, temporomandibular joints, or trapezius squeeze).
   b. Caution should be exercised to avoid misinterpreting spontaneous or stimulus-induced motor movements resulting from local spinal reflexes.
2. *Documentation of the absence of brainstem reflexes:*
   a. Brainstem reflexes progressively cease in a cranial-to-caudal manner as brain death ensues, with reflexes in the medulla oblongata being the last to dissipate.
   b. The absence of the pupillary reflex is characterized by round or oval pupils, midposition dilatation (ranging from 4 to 9 mm), and no response to bright light. This evaluation targets cranial nerves II and III. Factors that can disrupt the pupillary reflex include conditions such as orbital trauma, head injuries, the presence of cataracts, as well as the influence of medications such as high doses of dopamine, glutethimide, scopolamine, atropine, bretylium, or monoamine oxidase inhibitors.
   c. The oculocephalic movements, also known as the "doll's eye reflex". The test involves rapidly turning the head horizontally and vertically while observing for any eye movements. In the presence of brainstem dysfunction, there should be no movement of the eyes toward the opposite side. This assesses cranial nerves III and IV.

d. The oculovestibular reflex, assessed through the cold calorie test, involves irrigating the tympanum with 50 mL of ice-cold water while tilting the head to 30°. The absence of provoked tonic eye movement toward the side of the cold stimulus and a lack of horizontal nystagmus toward the contralateral side are indicative of brainstem dysfunction. This evaluation targets cranial nerves VIII, III, and VI. Labyrinthine, injury tricyclic antidepressants (TCAs), particularly certain classes like tricyclic antidepressants, can alter the oculovestibular reflex. These medications have anticholinergic properties, which can affect the normal functioning of the central nervous system, including the pathways involved in the oculovestibular reflex. This alteration may lead to diminished or atypical reflex responses, complicating the interpretation of neurological exams that rely on this reflex, such as in the assessment of brain death or other conditions involving cranial nerve function.
e. The corneal reflex can be examined by instilling a few drops of sterile saline over the cornea. The absence of a response to this test indicates brainstem dysfunction and assesses cranial nerves V and VII.
f. Lastly, the cough reflex is best evaluated by passing a suction catheter through the endotracheal tube. Its absence suggests brainstem dysfunction and assesses cranial nerves IX and X.

3. *Documenting the apnea test:* Before conducting the apnea test, certain conditions must be satisfied, as outlined in references:
   a. The core temperature should be ≥36.5°C (or 97.7°F).
   b. The patient should be in a state of euvolemia or exhibit a positive fluid balance in the preceding 6 hours.
   c. Arterial PCO_2 levels should be within the normal range or ≥40 mm Hg.
   d. Adequate preoxygenation with 100% oxygen for 15 minutes is essential. The goal is to achieve an arterial PO_2 of ≥200 mm Hg for safe administration of the test.
   e. The apnea test is conducted only after confirming the absence of brainstem reflexes and aims to stimulate the respiratory center located in the medulla oblongata.
   f. Initially, the patient is preoxygenated with 100% oxygen for 15 minutes, and an arterial blood gas (ABG) analysis is obtained.
   g. Subsequently, the patient is disconnected from mechanical ventilation, and oxygenation is sustained through a tracheal catheter with oxygen flowing at a rate of 4–6 L/min. Alternatively, a T-piece system with oxygen flow at 12 L/min or continuous positive airway pressure (CPAP) at 10 cmH_2O with FiO_2 adjusted to maintain oxygen saturation above 95% may be used.
   h. The gradual increase in $PaCO_2$ is allowed (typically at a rate of 3 mm Hg/min). The threshold for maximal stimulation of the

respiratory center is considered to be a $PaCO_2$ of 60 mm Hg or a $PaCO_2$ of 20 mm Hg above the normal baseline value.

i. Within approximately 8–10 minutes of disconnecting from mechanical ventilation, another ABG is performed to document the rise in $PaCO_2$.

j. Standard visual observation for about 8–10 minutes is employed to detect respiratory movement. If, during this observation period, spontaneous respiration is not observed, and arterial PCO_2 reaches 60 mm Hg (or increases by 20 mm Hg from the baseline arterial PCO_2), the apnea test result is considered positive, supporting the clinical diagnosis of brainstem death.

k. The test should not be initiated or should be terminated if the patient experiences hemodynamic instability (systolic pressure ≤90 mm Hg, arrhythmia) or becomes hypoxemic (SpO_2 ≤85% for >30 seconds).

l. If the test yields inconclusive results but the patient remains hemodynamically stable during the procedure, it may be repeated for an extended duration (10–15 minutes) after adequate preoxygenation.

m. If, for any reason, the apnea test cannot be performed or must be terminated due to the aforementioned factors, consider conducting ancillary confirmatory tests to establish brain death. It should be noted that, in India, the "Transplantation of Human Organs Act" (THOA) does not mandate the use of ancillary confirmatory tests for diagnosing brainstem death.

Ancillary Tests

Ancillary test includes electroencephalography (EEG), cerebral angiography, transcranial Doppler, and radionuclide scan which are not mandatory as per THOA.

Ancillary tests may be warranted in the following situations:

- Patients with cranial or cervical injuries or those experiencing cardiovascular instability.
- Individuals with severe facial trauma, otorrhagia, or eye agenesis.
- When certain aspects of the clinical examination cannot be conducted, or when providing reassurance to both family members and medical personnel is deemed necessary.
- In cases where a panel of doctors faces uncertainty or disagreement regarding the diagnosis.

CERTIFICATION OF BRAINSTEM DEATH

Brain death assessments necessitate two separate evaluations conducted by distinct medical teams. Typically, the second evaluation is performed approximately 6 hours after the initial one, and it is this comprehensive process that confirms the diagnosis of brainstem death in adult patients.

Certifying brainstem death involves a panel consisting of four medical professionals:

1. The attending physician responsible for the patient's care.
2. The physician overseeing the hospital where the patient is being treated.
3. An independent specialist with an unspecified specialty, chosen from a list of approved names by the relevant authority (including physicians, surgeons, or intensivists).
4. A neurologist or neurosurgeon.

Criteria for excluding organ donation encompass:

- Infection with human immunodeficiency virus, human T-cell leukemia-lymphoma virus, systemic viral infections (such as measles, rabies, adenovirus, and parvovirus), and herpetic meningoencephalitis.
- Active malignant disease or a history of malignancy with a high risk of transmission, regardless of the apparent disease-free period (e.g., melanoma, choriocarcinoma).

MANAGEMENT OF POTENTIAL ORGAN DONOR

Maintaining physiological stability in brain dead patients is a critical aspect of their care. It involves several key components to ensure the preservation of organ function and optimize the suitability of organs for transplantation.

Hemodynamic Stability

Hemodynamic stability is paramount in brain dead patients. The absence of neurological control can lead to significant cardiovascular instability, which can have adverse effects on organ perfusion and viability. Measures to maintain hemodynamic stability include:

- Continuous monitoring of blood pressure, heart rate, and central venous pressure (CVP).
- Administration of vasopressors and inotropes to support blood pressure and cardiac output.
- Adequate volume resuscitation to optimize intravascular volume and tissue perfusion.
- Frequent assessments and adjustments to ensure adequate tissue perfusion.
- A simple rule 100 can be followed, which includes:
  - Systolic arterial pressure >100 mm Hg
  - Urine output >100 mL/h
  - PaO_2 >100 mm Hg
  - Hemoglobin concentration >100 g/L
  - Blood sugar 100 mg/dL.

Fluid and Electrolyte Balance

Proper fluid and electrolyte management is essential to prevent complications such as electrolyte imbalances, edema, and organ dysfunction. Key considerations include:

- Monitoring of fluid intake and output to maintain an euvolemic state.
- Electrolyte monitoring and correction of imbalances, particularly sodium and potassium.
- Prevention of fluid overload, which can lead to pulmonary edema and compromise oxygenation.

Hormone Replacement Therapy for Brain Dead Patients

Brain death is often associated with a state of panhypopituitarism, where the normal hormonal regulation by the pituitary gland ceases. This condition can lead to hemodynamic instability, making hormone replacement therapy an essential part of patient management.

Hormone replacement therapy serves several critical roles in brain dead patients:

- *Correcting hemodynamic instability:* One of the primary objectives is to correct hemodynamic instability, which can be refractory to standard treatments. Adequate hormone levels are essential for maintaining blood pressure and overall cardiovascular stability.
- *Improving organ procurement:* Proper hormone replacement has been shown to improve the condition of organs intended for transplantation, increasing the likelihood of successful organ procurement.
- *Enhancing graft function:* Hormone replacement therapy contributes to better graft function in transplant recipients.

Commonly Replaced Hormones

Several hormones are commonly replaced in brain dead patients:

- *Thyroid hormones:* Levothyroxine (T4) is initiated in hemodynamically unstable patients, particularly in potential cardiac donors with a left ventricular ejection fraction <45%. The recommended dosing is an initial 20 μg intravenous (IV) bolus followed by an infusion at 10 μg/h. T4 has demonstrated greater effectiveness than T3. If IV formulation is not available, one can also use thyroxine (T4) 300–400 μg through nasogastric route.
- *Triiodothyronine (T3):* T3, when used, is administered initially as a 4 μg IV bolus, followed by an infusion at 3 μg/h.
- *Corticosteroids:* Methylprednisolone is commonly used and can be administered in different dose regimens, such as 15 mg/kg IV OD, 100 mg IV OD, or a 250 mg IV bolus followed by an infusion of 100 mg/h. This treatment helps improve donor hemodynamics, organ procurement, graft function, and recipient survival.

- *Hydrocortisone:* In some cases, lower doses of hydrocortisone are employed, reducing the need for vasopressors. Recommended doses include a 50 mg IV bolus followed by a 10 mg/h infusion or 300 mg IV OD.
- *Insulin:* Brainstem death often leads to hyperglycemia, which can have adverse effects on organ function. Initiating insulin therapy aims to maintain blood glucose levels below 140 mg/dL. The standard starting rate is 1 unit/h IV infusion, with frequent monitoring and adjustment to achieve the target.
- *Vasopressin and desmopressin:* Vasopressin deficiency can contribute to persistent hypotension and diabetes insipidus. Replacement therapy involves vasopressin infusion or desmopressin (DDAVP) administration, with dosages adjusted based on clinical parameters.

Initiating hormone replacement: The timing of initiating hormone replacement therapy may vary among institutions. Some prefer to start components of the therapy soon after the first brain death declaration, while others begin all hormones simultaneously. The decision is often influenced by the patient's clinical status, including hemodynamic stability and the presence of diabetes insipidus.

Monitoring and Caution

- Careful monitoring of patients' blood sugar levels is essential when administering corticosteroids and insulin, as they can impact blood glucose levels.
- Regular assessment and adjustment of vasopressin and desmopressin doses are necessary, along with monitoring for potential side effects.

  Hormone replacement therapy plays a pivotal role in managing brain dead patients, aiming to correct hemodynamic instability, improve organ suitability for transplantation, and enhance graft outcomes. The specific hormone regimen and timing may vary, but close monitoring and tailored interventions are essential components of this therapy.

Oxygenation and Ventilation

In cases of brainstem death, neurogenic pulmonary edema and ischemia-reperfusion injury can give rise to a condition resembling acute respiratory distress syndrome (ARDS). This resultant hypoxia, when not appropriately addressed, can negatively impact organ procurement. Additionally, inadequate ventilatory management may contribute to lung injury.

Ensuring adequate oxygenation and ventilation is crucial to maintain oxygen delivery to vital organs and prevent hypoxia. Key strategies include:

- Mechanical ventilation with careful attention to lung protective strategies.
- Frequent ABG analysis to assess oxygenation and acid-base status.
- Optimization of oxygen delivery to maintain adequate oxygen saturation.

Management of Infections

- Comprehensive screening and assessment of donor infections before transplantation are imperative.
- In cases of donor bacteremia and sepsis, it is crucial to initiate appropriate antibiotic therapy at least 48 hours prior to organ procurement. Importantly, the presence of bacteremia or sepsis alone does not preclude organ donation, unless accompanied by shock, multiorgan failure, or an inadequate response to antibiotic treatment.

Metabolic Abnormalities

Brain dead patients may develop metabolic abnormalities that need to be addressed promptly. Some considerations include:

- Monitoring metabolic parameters such as glucose levels.
- Correcting metabolic acidosis, if present, with appropriate interventions.
- Addressing any hypernatremia or other electrolyte disturbances.

Nutrition

Nutrition should be continued as per standard ICU protocol. Potential donors who continue to get enteral nutrition may aid to improve organ function.

Aggressive Temperature Management

Temperature control is essential in brain dead patients to minimize the risk of organ dysfunction and enhance transplant outcomes. Measures include:

- Maintaining a core temperature of ≥35°C to prevent hypothermia.
- Utilizing temperature management devices to regulate body temperature.
- Monitoring and managing fever, if present, as it can exacerbate metabolic demands.

SUMMARY

The care of a brain dead patient is a crucial and sensitive aspect of health care, primarily focused on preserving the viability of organs for transplantation. Despite the absence of brain activity, the body's physiological functions, such as circulation and respiration, must be maintained through intensive medical support. This involves managing blood pressure, fluid balance, and oxygenation, as well as preventing infections and other complications. The care team, including doctors, nurses, and specialists, must work collaboratively to monitor the patient's condition closely and make timely interventions. Effective communication with the patient's family is also essential, providing them with clear information and support during this difficult time. The ultimate goal is to honor the donor's gift by ensuring that the organs remain suitable for transplantation, offering the chance of life to others.

SUGGESTED READING

1. Bernat JL. Chronic disorders of consciousness. Lancet. 2006;367(9528):2060.
2. Dhanwate AD. Brainstem death: a comprehensive review in Indian perspective. Indian J Crit Care Med. 2014;18(9):596-605.
3. Goila AK, Pawar M. The diagnosis of brain death. Indian J Crit Care Med. 2009;13(1):7-11.
4. Greer DM, Varelas PN. Assessment of brain death in adults. In: Greer DM, Varelas PN (Eds). Seminars in Neurology. New York: Thieme Medical Publishers; 2010. pp. 519-28.
5. McKeown DW, Bonser RS, Kellum JA. Management of the heartbeating brain-dead organ donor. Br J Anaesth. 2012;108(Suppl 1):i96-107.
6. Powner DJ, Darby JM, Kellum JA. Proposed treatment guidelines for donor care. Prog Transplant. 2004;14(1):16-26.
7. Saposnik G, Redelmeier D, Ruff CC, Tobler PN. Cognitive biases associated with medical decisions: a systematic review. BMC Med Informa Decis Mak. 2016;16(1):138.
8. Sethi NK, Sethi PK. Brainstem death: Implications in India. J Assoc Physicians India. 2003;51:910-1.
9. Singer P, Shapiro H, Cohen J. Brain death and organ damage: The modulating effects of nutrition. Transplantation. 2005;80(10):1363-8.
10. Vaghadia H. Atropine resistance in brain-dead organ donors. Anesthesiology. 1986;65(6):711-2.
11. Van der Jagt M, Lin MS, Briegel J. Optimizing apnea testing to determine brain death. Intensive Care Med. 2016;42(1):117-8.
12. Westphal GA, Garcia VD, Souza RL, Franke CA, Vieira KD, Birckholz VR, et al. Guidelines for the assessment and acceptance of potential brain-dead organ donors. Rev Bras Ter Intensiva. 2016;28(3):220-55.
13. Wijdicks EF. The diagnosis of brain death. N Engl J Med. 2001;344:1215-21.
14. Wood KE, Becker BN, McCartney JG, D'Alessandro AM, Coursin DB. Care of the potential organ donor. N Engl J Med. 2004;351(26):2730-9.

CHAPTER

29 Spinal Cord Injuries

Vivek Jain

DEFINITION

A spinal cord injury (SCI) is a traumatic or nontraumatic insult to the spinal cord resulting in a disruption of normal spinal cord function. This can lead to a range of motor, sensory, and autonomic impairments, depending on the location and severity of the injury. SCIs are often classified based on the level of injury (cervical, thoracic, lumbar, or sacral) and the extent of neurological compromise.

CAUSES

Spinal cord injuries can result from various traumatic and nontraumatic causes.

PATHOPHYSIOLOGY

The pathophysiology of SCI involves a complex series of events that occur following the initial trauma.

- *Primary injury:*
  - *Mechanical damage:* The initial trauma, often caused by compression, contusion, laceration, or distraction, leads to immediate physical damage to the spinal cord.
  - *Vascular changes:* Blood vessels may be disrupted, leading to hemorrhage and ischemia in the affected area.
- *Secondary injury:*
  - *Inflammatory response:* Within hours to days, an inflammatory cascade is triggered, involving immune cells and releasing proinflammatory molecules.
  - *Excitotoxicity:* Excessive release of neurotransmitters, especially glutamate, leads to excitotoxic damage to nearby cells.
  - *Oxidative stress:* Reactive oxygen species (ROS) contribute to cellular damage.
  - *Apoptosis:* Programmed cell death pathways are activated, leading to further loss of neural tissue.

- *Ischemia and edema:*
    - *Vascular changes:* Continued disruption of blood flow contributes to ischemia, exacerbating damage.
    - *Edema formation:* Swelling occurs, further compressing the spinal cord and impeding blood flow.
- *Blood-brain barrier disruption:*
    - *Breakdown of barrier:* The blood-brain barrier is compromised, allowing substances that would normally be restricted to enter the spinal cord tissue.
- *Axonal degeneration:*
    - *White matter damage:* Axons may undergo Wallerian degeneration, leading to the loss of communication between neurons.
- *Glial scar formation:*
    - *Astrogliosis:* Reactive astrocytes form a glial scar, which, while providing structural support, can hinder axonal regeneration.
- *Cyst formation:*
    - *Cavitation:* Fluid-filled cysts may form at the injury site, contributing to the physical disruption of spinal cord tissue.

CLINICAL FEATURES DEPENDING ON THE LEVEL OF TRANSACTION OF CORD

The clinical manifestations of SCI vary based on the specific level of cord injury. Here is an overview of the clinical features according to the level of transaction:

- *Cervical SCI (C1–C8):*
    - *Tetraplegia (Quadriplegia):* Paralysis or weakness in all four limbs.
    - *Impaired respiratory function:* Potential need for mechanical ventilation, especially with higher cervical injuries (C1–C4).
    - *Loss of sensation:* Variable loss of sensation below the level of injury.
    - *Altered bowel and bladder function:* Often requires assistive devices for toileting.
- *Thoracic SCI (T1–T12):*
    - *Paraplegia:* Paralysis or weakness in the lower limbs.
    - *Impaired trunk function:* Limited or no control over abdominal muscles.
    - *Altered sensation:* Loss of sensation below the level of injury.
    - *Potential for autonomic dysreflexia:* Especially with injuries above T6.
- *Lumbar and sacral SCI (L1–S5):*
    - *Variable motor impairment:* Depending on the specific level, there may be weakness or paralysis in the lower limbs.

- *Altered sensation:* Loss of sensation in the lower limbs or specific dermatomes.
- *Potential bowel and bladder dysfunction:* Depending on the level of injury.

DIAGNOSTIC INVESTIGATIONS

Accurate and timely diagnosis of SCI is crucial for appropriate management. Diagnostic investigations include clinical assessments and various imaging modalities. Here is an overview of diagnostic investigations:

- *Clinical assessment:*
  - *Neurological examination:* Assess motor and sensory function, reflexes, and the level of injury.
  - *Clinical history:* Gather information on the mechanism of injury, symptoms, and associated trauma.
- *Imaging studies:*
  - *X-rays:* Assess spinal alignment, fractures, or dislocations.
  - *Computed tomography (CT) scan:* Provide detailed images of bone structures and detect fractures.
  - *Magnetic resonance imaging (MRI):* Visualize soft tissues, ligaments, and the spinal cord for detailed assessment.
- *Electrophysiological studies:*
  - *Somatosensory evoked potentials (SSEPs):* Measure electrical signals along the spinal cord's sensory pathways.
  - *Motor evoked potentials (MEPs):* Evaluate motor pathway integrity.
- *Urodynamic studies:*
  - *Assessment of bladder function:* Important for identifying neurogenic bladder dysfunction.

TREATMENT

Medical management of SCI aims to stabilize the spine, prevent secondary damage, and manage complications.

- *Stabilization of the spine:*
  - *Immobilization:* Use of cervical collars, thoracolumbar orthoses, or spinal traction to prevent further movement and potential exacerbation of injury.
- *Pharmacological management:*
  - *Methylprednisolone:* Steroid therapy, although controversial, may be considered within the first 8 hours postinjury for selected cases.
- *Surgical interventions:*
  - *Decompression:* Timely decompression of the spinal cord by removing bone fragments, hematoma, or other compressive elements.

- *Spinal fusion:* Stabilization of the spine through fusion procedures, which may involve instrumentation.
- *Complication management:*
  - *Respiratory support:* Mechanical ventilation may be necessary for individuals with high cervical injuries.
  - *Autonomic dysreflexia control:* Management of elevated blood pressure and other symptoms.
- *Rehabilitation:*
  - *Physical therapy:* Focus on improving mobility, strength, and independence.
  - *Occupational therapy:* Assistive device training and activities of daily living.
  - *Psychological support:* Address emotional and psychological challenges.

SUMMARY

Ultimately, effective management of spinal cord injuries requires a multidisciplinary approach, timely intervention, and ongoing rehabilitation to optimize recovery and enhance the quality of life for affected individuals.

SUGGESTED READING

1. American Spinal Injury Association. (2019). International Standards for Neurological Classification of Spinal Cord Injury. [online] Available from: https://www.asia-spinalinjury.org/isncsci-2022-revision/ [Last assessed July, 2024].
2. Anderson KD, Targett PS, Nicholas JS, Brown AW. Spinal cord injury and the neurogenic bowel. In: Anderson KD, Targett PS, Nicholas JS, Brown AW (Eds). Seminars in Neurology. New York: Thieme Medical Publishers; 2004. pp. 405-17.
3. Bracken MB, Shepard MJ, Collins WF, Holford TR, Young W, Baskin DS, et al. A randomized, controlled trial of methylprednisolone or naloxone in the treatment of acute spinal-cord injury. New Engl J Med. 1990;322(20):1405-11.
4. Fehlings MG, Vaccaro A, Wilson JR, Singh A, Cadotte DW, Harrop JS, et al. Early versus delayed decompression for traumatic cervical spinal cord injury: results of the Surgical Timing in Acute Spinal Cord Injury Study (STASCIS). PloS one. 2012;7(2):e32037.
5. Fehlings MG, Wilson JR, Cho N. Methylprednisolone for the treatment of acute spinal cord injury: counterpoint. Neurosurgery. 2014:61(Suppl 1):36-42.
6. Furlan JC, Sakakibara BM, Miller WC, Krassioukov AV. Global incidence and prevalence of traumatic spinal cord injury. Can J Neurol Sci. 2013;40(4): 456-64.
7. Kirshblum SC, Burns SP, Biering-Sorensen F, Donovan W, Graves DE, Jha A, et al. International standards for neurological classification of spinal cord injury (revised 2011). J Spinal Cord Med. 2011;34(6):535-46.

8. National Institute of Neurological Disorders and Stroke. (2022). Spinal Cord Injury. [online] Available from: https://www.ninds.nih.gov/health-information/disorders/spinal-cord-injury [Last assessed July, 2024].
9. Pannek J, Göcking K. Current status of neurogenic lower urinary tract dysfunction after spinal cord injury. World J Urol. 2016;34(6):813-9.
10. Rowland JW, Hawryluk GW. Advances in spinal cord protection during surgery for spinal deformities. World Neurosurg. 2016;90:176-80.
11. Tator CH, Fehlings MG. Review of the secondary injury theory of acute spinal cord trauma with emphasis on vascular mechanisms. J Neurosurg. 1991; 75(1):15-26.
12. White AA, Panjabi MM. The problem of clinical instability in the human spine: a systematic approach. In: White AA, Panjabi MM (Eds). Clinical biomechanics of the spine, 2nd edition. Philadelphia, PA: Lippincott Williams & Wilkins; 1990. pp. 277-378.

CHAPTER 30

Intensive Care Unit-acquired Weakness

Kesari Masaipeta

INTRODUCTION

Intensive care unit-acquired weakness (ICU-AW) is a skeletal muscle dysfunction occurring in ICU patients commonly following systemic inflammatory response system (SIRS), sepsis, immobility, usage of neuromuscular blocking agents, glucocorticoid usage, hyperglycemia, vasoactive drugs usage, and bedridden status. Also associated with female gender, renal replacement therapies.

It may result in difficult weaning from ventilator, decreased reflexes, muscular atrophy, paresis, and even quadriplegia. It may develop as early as few hours after mechanical ventilation or on second day of ICU admission. It results in prolonged mechanical ventilation and extended hospitalization.

PATHOPHYSIOLOGY

Local immune activation due to cytokines accompanied by neurogenic and myogenic damage leads to ICU-AW. Though previously it was thought critical illness neuropathy (CIN) and critical illness polyneuropathy (CIP) as different entities, now the concept of critical illness polyneuromyopathy (CIPMN) explains the multifactorial pathophysiology of the disease. It occurs due to imbalance between protein synthesis and degradation. Muscle biopsy shows selective loss of thick filaments—loss of myosin and myoglobin related protein and necrosis. There is no demyelination. Neuromuscular junction (NMJ), motor neuron, and mitochondria play role in pathogenesis. Ubiquitin proteasome pathway calpain, caspase 3, and autophagy lysosome system are the possible mechanisms for muscle atrophy.

CLINICAL MANIFESTATIONS

Symmetrical limb weakness, proximal more than distal without sensory loss viz critical illness myopathy (CIM) and distal muscle weakness more than proximal with sensory loss viz CIP or a combination of both—CIPMN/critical illness neuromyopathy (CINM) can be the spectrum of the disease. Weakness occurs in generalized fashion, usually affecting limb and respiratory (diaphragmatic and extra diaphragmatic) muscles. Facial muscles are generally spared but may cause ophthalmoplegia. Brainstem reflexes are preserved. Diffuse encephalopathy may occur if central nervous system is involved.

DIAGNOSIS

It is a diagnosis of exclusion. Two tier muscle strength assessment is done—where both hand grip dynamometry (HGD) and Medical Research Council (MRC) sum score are used to identify ICU-AW.

If the patient is cooperative, then HGD is used. If HGD >11 kg in males and ≥7 kg in females, then ICU-AW is excluded. If HGD is less than cut off, then MRC sum scoring is done. Six muscle group testing is done (grades 0–5) viz—wrist flexion, forearm flexion, shoulder abduction, ankle dorsiflexion, knee extension, and hip flexion, a score ranging from 0 to 60. If it is <48, ICU-AW is likely.

In patients who are unable to do voluntary muscle examination, e.g., septic shock patients in deep sedation, then *peroneal nerve test (PENT)* can be done where reduction in compound muscle action potential may need further electrophysiological studies.

Neuromuscular ultrasound can identify muscle mass and architectural changes in limb by measuring muscle layer thickness and echo-intensity and cross sectional area, and also muscle necrosis, fascial inflammation, and fasciitis.

Ultrasound can also be used to measure the *diaphragmatic thickness fraction* (DTF), a predictor for ventricular failure.

Ergometers can be used to measure force by combining electrical and magnetic supramaximal stimulation to muscle or motor nerve.

In quadriplegic ICU-AW patients, sternal or nail bed pressure will lead to facial grimacing as facial muscles are unaffected.

Electrophysiological features in CIP may reveal axonal damage with reduced amplitude of compound muscle action potential (CMAP) and sensory nerve action potential (SNAP) with normal CMAP duration. Abnormal spontaneous potentials and polyphasic motor unit potentials are seen in electromyography (EMG).

The EMG of CIN shows reduced motor responses (amplitude <80% of normal) in at least two nerves without conduction block, preserved sensory response (amplitude >80% of normal), with increased CMAP duration. Myopathy pattern in needle EMG or muscle nonexcitability on direct muscle stimulation (DMS) can be seen.

Normal response to repetitive nerve stimulation (can be variable depending on stage of CIP) in both CIP and CIM, differentiated from long-term neuromuscular blocking agents where it gradually reduces **(Table 1)**.

Muscle biopsy reveals elevated creatinine kinase (CK) levels and myosin loss in CIM but is invasive and no longer advised.

TABLE 1: Diagnosis of critical illness myopathy (CIM) and critical illness polyneuropathy (CIP).

Investigation	*CIP*	*CIM*
Nerve conduction studies	Reduced motor and *reduced* sensory action potential amplitudes, normal conduction velocity	Reduced motor and *normal* sensory action potential amplitudes, normal conduction velocity
Electromyography	Spontaneous fibrillation potentials with *long* duration, *high* amplitude motor unit potentials	Spontaneous fibrillation potentials with *short* duration, low amplitude motor unit potentials

TABLE 2: Neuromuscular differential diagnosis of "Failure to Wean from Ventilator."

Motor neuron	• Amyotrophic lateral sclerosis • Poliomyelitis • Guillain–Barré syndrome • Critical illness polyneuropathy • Critical illness polyneuropathy/myopathy • Heavy metal toxicity • Vasculitis • Sarcoidosis • Mononeuritis multiplex
Neuromuscular junction	• Myasthenia gravis • Neuromuscular blockade • Lambert–Eaton myasthenic syndrome • Botulinum toxicity • Organophosphate toxicity • Tetrodotoxin toxicity
Muscle	• Rhabdomyolysis • Mitochondrial myopathy • Muscular dystrophy (e.g., myotonic dystrophy) • Critical illness myopathy • Acid maltase deficiency

DIFFERENTIAL DIAGNOSIS

Table 2 shows the neuromuscular differential diagnosis of "failure to wean from ventilator."

MANAGEMENT

- *Reduction of risk factors:*
  - Sepsis treatment
  - Curtailing use of neuromuscular agents
  - Hyperglycemia prevention—Intensive insulin therapy—RCT showing reduction in overall mortality.
  - Minimal usage of steroids—controversial

- Screening and early diagnosis
- Physiotherapy and training
- Early mobilization
- Therapies to prevent ICU-AW—nutritional interventions, supplement therapies, antioxidant therapies, electrolyte replacement as a part of ABCDEFG (awake and breathing coordination, choose light sedation, delirium management, early mobilization, feeding early and nutrition, and gain function and grow muscle)
- Use of testosterone derivatives, growth hormones, and immunoglobulins.
  - High doses of recombinant human growth hormone can improve nitrogen balance and peripheral muscle strength.
  - Intravenous immunoglobulins G (IVIG) useful when within first 3 days of gram-negative sepsis.
- Plasmapheresis
- Electrical muscle stimulation
- Conscious effort to wean mechanical ventilation
- Prevention of complications—bed sores, deep vein thrombosis

PROGNOSIS

Most of the patients with ICU-AW remain weak at the time of transfer out from ICU but gradually recover over time. Improvement in upper limbs generally precedes lower limbs. Follow-up studies reveal that about 28% of patients have sequela of weakness.

A clear understanding, early detection, and treatment of the disease will improve the prognosis.

SUMMARY

It is a diagnosis of exclusion. HGD and MRC sum score are used to identify ICU-AW. Electrophysiological studies help in diagnosis. Early diagnosis and application of preventive measures/reduction of risk factors are needed. Multidisciplinary approach is needed for proper management.

SUGGESTED READING

1. Appleton RT, Kinsella J, Quasim T. The incidence of intensive care unit-acquired weakness syndromes: A systematic review. J Intensive Care Soc. 2015;16(2):126-36.
2. Godoy D, Vaz de Mello L, Masotti L, Di Napoli M. Intensive Care Unit Acquired Weakness (ICU-AW): a brief and practical review. Reviews in Health Care. 2015;6(1):9-35.
3. Hermans G, Wilmer A, Meersseman W, Milants I, Wouters PJ, Bobbaers H, et al. Impact of intensive insulin therapy on neuromuscular complications and ventilator dependency in the medical intensive care unit. Am J Respir Crit Care Med. 2007;175(5):480-9.

4. Hermans G, Casaer MP, Clerckx B, Güiza F, Vanhullebusch T, Derde S, et al. Effect of tolerating macronutrient deficit on the development of intensive-care unit acquired weakness: a subanalysis of the EPaNIC trial. Lancet Respir Med. 2013;1(8):621-9.
5. Hermans G, De Jonghe B, Bruyninckx F, Van den Berghe G. Interventions for preventing critical illness polyneuropathy and critical illness myopathy. Cochrane Database Syst Rev. 2009;(1):CD006832.
6. Hermans G, van Mechelen H, Clerckx B, Vanhullebusch T, Mesotten D, Wilmer A, et al. Acute outcomes and 1-year mortality of intensive care unit-acquired weakness. A cohort study and propensity-matched analysis. Am J Respir Crit Care Med. 2014;190:410-20.
7. Kalamgi RC, Larsson L. Mechanical Signaling in the Pathophysiology of Critical Illness Myopathy. Front Physiol. 2016;7:23.
8. Kelmenson DA, Quan D, Moss M. What is the diagnostic accuracy of single nerve conduction studies and muscle ultrasound to identify critical illness polyneuromyopathy: a prospective cohort study. Crit Care. 2018;22(1): 342.
9. Lad H, Saumur TM, Herridge MS, Dos Santos CC, Mathur S, Batt J, et al. Intensive Care Unit-Acquired Weakness: Not Just Another Muscle Atrophying Condition. Int J Mol Sci. 2020;21(21):7840.
10. Latronico N, Bolton CF. Critical illness polyneuropathy and myopathy: a major cause of muscle weakness and paralysis. Lancet Neurol. 2011;10:931-41.
11. Latronico N, Nattino G, Guarneri B, Fagoni N, Amantini A, Bertolini G; et al. Validation of the peroneal nerve test to diagnose critical illness polyneuropathy and myopathy in the intensive care unit: the multicentre Italian CRIMYNE-2 diagnostic accuracy study. F1000Res. 2014;3:127.
12. Le Stang V, Latronico N, Dres M, Bertoni M. Critical illness-associated limb and diaphragmatic weakness. Curr Opin Crit Care. 2024;30(2):121-30.
13. Minnaard R, Drost MR, Wagenmakers AJ, van Kranenburg GP, Kuipers H, Hesselink MK. Skeletal muscle wasting and contractile performance in septic rats. Muscle Nerve. 2005;31(3):339-48.
14. Ozdemir M, Bomkamp MP, Hyatt HW, Smuder AJ, Powers SK. Intensive Care Unit Acquired Weakness is Associated with Rapid Changes to Skeletal Muscle Proteostasis. Cells. 2022;11(24):4005.
15. Patel BK, Pohlman AS, Hall JB, Kress JP. Impact of early mobilization on glyce-mic control and ICU-acquired weakness in critically ill patients who are mechanically ventilated. Chest. 2014;146(3):583-9.
16. Penuelas O, Muriel A, Frutos-Vivar F, Fan E, Raymondos K, Rios F, et al. Prediction and outcome of intensive care unit-acquired paresis. J Intensive Care Med. 2018;33:16-28.
17. Puthucheary ZA, Phadke R, Rawal J, McPhail MJ, Sidhu PS, Rowlerson A, et al. Qualitative Ultrasound in Acute Critical Illness Muscle Wasting. Crit Care Med. 2015;43(8):1603-11.
18. Shepherd S, Batra A, Lerner DP. Review of Critical Illness Myopathy and Neuropathy. Neurohospitalist. 2017;7(1):41-8.
19. Showalter CJ, Engel AG. Acute quadriplegic myopathy: analysis of myosin isoforms and evidence for calpain-mediated proteolysis. Muscle Nerve. 1997;20(3):316-22.

20. Silva AP, Maynard K, Cruz MR. Effects of motor physical therapy in critically ill patients: literature review. Rev Bras Ter Intensiva. 2010;22(1):85-91.
21. Stoian A, Bajko Z, Maier S, Cioflinc RA, Grigorescu BL, Moțățăianu A, et al. High-dose intravenous immunoglobulins as a therapeutic option in critical illness polyneuropathy accompanying SARS-CoV-2 infection: A case-based review of the literature (Review). Exp Ther Med. 2021;22(4):1182.
22. Supinski GS, Westgate P, Callahan LA. Correlation of maximal inspiratory pressure to transdiaphragmatic twitch pressure in intensive care unit patients. Crit Care. 2016;20:77.
23. Tiao G, Hobler S, Wang JJ, Meyer TA, Luchette FA, Fischer JE, et al. Sepsis is associated with increased mRNAs of the ubiquitin-proteasome proteolytic pathway in human skeletal muscle. J Clin Invest. 1997;99(2):163-8.
24. Vanhorebeek I, Gunst J, Derde S, Derese I, Boussemaere M, Güiza F, et al. Insufficient activation of autophagy allows cellular damage to accumulate in critically ill patients. J Clin Endocrinol Metab. 2011;96(4):E633-45.
25. Vanhorebeek I, Latronico N, Van den Berghe G. ICU-acquired weakness. Intensive Care Med. 2020;46(4):637-53.
26. Wang W, Xu C, Ma X, Zhang X, Xie P. Intensive Care Unit-Acquired Weakness: A Review of Recent Progress with a Look Toward the Future. Front Med (Lausanne). 2020;7:559789.
27. Wischmeyer PE, San-Millan I. Winning the war against ICU-acquired weakness: new innovations in nutrition and exercise physiology. Crit Care. 2015;19 Suppl 3 (Suppl 3):S6.
28. Yang T, Li Z, Jiang L, Wang Y, Xi X. Risk factors for intensive care unit-acquired weakness: A systematic review and meta-analysis. Acta Neurol Scand. 2018;138(2):104-14.
29. Yang T, Li Z, Jiang L, Xi X. Corticosteroid use and intensive care unit-acquired weakness: a systematic review and meta-analysis. Crit Care. 2018;22(1):187.
30. Zhou C, Wu L, Ni F, Ji W, Wu J, Zhang H. Critical illness polyneuropathy and my-opathy: a systematic review. Neural Regen Res. 2014;9(1):101-10.

SECTION

7

Endocrine Disorders

CHAPTER

31 Diabetes Mellitus and Acute Diabetic Emergencies

Jitendra Choudhary

INTRODUCTION

Diabetes mellitus (DM) is a chronic metabolic disease that affects millions of people worldwide. It is characterized by high blood glucose levels due to insufficient or ineffective insulin production or action. DM can lead to serious complications such as cardiovascular diseases, kidney failure, blindness, and lower limb amputation. The epidemiology of DM varies across regions and countries, depending on the prevalence of risk factors such as obesity, physical inactivity, and unhealthy diets. According to the World Health Organization, the number of people with DM rose from 108 million in 1980 to 422 million in 2014, and it is expected to increase further to 783 million by 2045. The majority of cases are type 2 DM, which is largely preventable by adopting a healthy lifestyle. In 2019, DM was the direct cause of 1.5 million deaths worldwide, and another 460,000 deaths were attributed to kidney disease due to diabetes. In addition, raised blood glucose was responsible for around 20% of cardiovascular deaths. In the United States, 37.3 million people have DM, of which 8.5 million are undiagnosed. Another 96 million adults have prediabetes, a condition that increases the risk of developing type 2 DM.

INSULIN AND TARGET ORGAN

Insulin is a hormone that regulates glucose metabolism in the body. It is produced by the beta cells of the pancreas and secreted into the bloodstream in response to high blood glucose levels. Insulin binds to insulin receptors on various target organs, such as the liver, muscle, and adipose tissue, and stimulates the uptake of glucose from the blood into the cells. Insulin also inhibits the breakdown of glycogen, fat, and protein, and promotes the synthesis of glycogen, fat, and protein. Insulin plays a key role in maintaining glucose homeostasis and preventing hyperglycemia or hypoglycemia.

PATHOPHYSIOLOGY AND CLASSIFICATION OF DIABETES MELLITUS

Diabetes mellitus is a chronic metabolic disorder characterized by hyperglycemia, or high blood glucose levels, resulting from defects in insulin secretion, insulin action, or both. Insulin is a hormone produced by the pancreatic beta cells that regulates glucose uptake and utilization by the body's cells. When insulin secretion or action is impaired, glucose accumulates in the blood, leading to various complications affecting the eyes, kidneys, nerves, heart, and blood vessels.

Diabetes mellitus can be classified into four main types: Type 1 diabetes, type 2 diabetes, gestational diabetes, and other specific types. Type 1 diabetes is caused by an autoimmune destruction of the pancreatic beta cells, resulting in absolute insulin deficiency. Type 2 diabetes is caused by a combination of insulin resistance and relative insulin deficiency. Gestational diabetes is a form of glucose intolerance that occurs during pregnancy and usually resolves after delivery. Other specific types of diabetes are caused by genetic defects, diseases of the pancreas, drug or chemical induced diabetes, or infections.

ACUTE HYPERGLYCEMIC EMERGENCIES

Diabetic ketoacidosis (DKA) and hyperglycemic hyperosmolar state (HHS) are decompensated acute hyperglycemic decompensated hyperglycemic state, which present as acute emergencies.

In DKA, insulin deficiency causes increased counter-regulatory hormone production leading to abnormal lipid and carbohydrate metabolism, this causes hyperglycemia and ketosis. In HHS, there is relative insulin deficiency, with insulin adequate enough to prevent lipolysis and ketogenesis. Diagnostic criteria for DKA and HHS are given in **Table 1**.

Pathophysiology

The DKA is state of insulin deficiency which leads to elevated counter-regulatory hormones (glucagon, growth hormone, and catecholamines). Liver, adipose tissues, and skeletal muscles are unable to utilize glucose in absence of insulin deficit; which induces gluconeogenesis and glycogenolysis. This worsens hyperglycemia.

TABLE 1: Diagnostic criteria for DKA and HHS.

Diagnostic criteria for DKA	*Diagnostic criteria for HHS*
Serum glucose >250 mg/dL	Plasma glucose >600 mg/dL
Serum pH <7.3	pH >7.3
Bicarbonate <18 mEq/L	Bicarbonate >18
Positive ketones and anion gap >10 mEq/L	• Small or negative ketones • Serum osmolality greater than 320 mOsm/kg

(DKA: diabetic ketoacidosis; HHS: hyperglycemic hyperosmolar state)

Insulin deficiency and increased counterregulatory hormones increase lipolysis and release of free fatty acids (FFAs) in circulation. Hepatic oxidation of FFAs will lead to formation of ketone bodies (acetoacetate and hydroxybutyrate). Ketone bodies are weak acid; which are well dissociated at physiological pH. This produces excessive hydrogen ions, resulting in depletion of buffering system and acidosis.

The HHS, like DKA, also have insulin deficiency and increase anti-insulin hormones. But unlike DKA, insulin is adequate enough to prevent lipolysis, ketogenesis, and acidemia.

Hyperglycemia and glycosuria lead to osmotic diuresis. Excessive diuresis causes net loss of electrolytes (potassium, chloride, sodium, and phosphate). Acidosis also causes extracellular shift of potassium and leads to net negative potassium balance. In HHS, because of lack of ketoacidosis, glycosuria develops slowly over period of days. This causes severe dehydration, hypovolemia, and decrease glomerular filtration rate. Thus, hyperglycemia and osmotic diuresis result in hyperosmolarity.

Precipitating Cause

Acute hyperglycemic emergencies require trigger. Most common trigger are either infection or omission of antidiabetic therapy **(Table 2)**.

Clinical Presentation

Patients with DKA and HHS may present with symptoms of hyperglycemia (polyuria and polydipsia) and symptoms of volume depletion (weakness, fatigue, anorexia, and somnolence). In DKA with ketoacidosis, patients will have symptoms of nausea, vomiting, and abdominal pain. Symptoms in case of DKA can develop quickly, sometimes within 24 hours; while in HHS,

TABLE 2: Precipitating factors for acute hyperglycemic emergencies.

Lack of insulin	• New diagnosis of diabetes • Poor treatment compliance • Dietary mismanagement
Physiological stress	• Infection • Systemic inflammatory response • Myocardial infarction • Surgery
Drugs which trigger	• Corticosteroids • Catecholamines • SGLT-2 inhibitors • Atypical antipsychotics • Checkpoint inhibitors (e.g., pembrolizumab, nivolumab) • TPN

(SGLT-2: sodium-glucose cotransporter-2; TPN: total parenteral nutrition)

symptoms will develop slowly over days or weeks. In DKA, mentation can be intact or altered if acidosis is severe. In HHS, mental status changes vary from somnolence to coma.

Patients with DKA and HHS present with clinical signs of volume depletion such as tachycardia, hypotension, dry mucous membranes, and reduced skin turgor. In DKA, patient may have Kussmaul breathing and fruity odor to breath because of acetone.

Diagnosis

The DKA diagnosis will be made when pH <7.3, bicarbonate <18 mEq/L, anion gap >10 mEq/L, and glucose level >250 mg/dL along with ketonemia. Detecting β-hydroxybutyrate level in blood is gold standard for detecting *presence and extent of ketoacidosis in DKA*. Normal level of beta hydroxybutarate is 0–0.6 mmol/L. Level of betahydroxybutarate >3 mmol/L is consistent with diagnosis of DKA. Urine nitroprusside test can be used to detect acetoacetate and acetone level, which is very sensitive for DKA but not very specific. β-hydroxybutyrate is converted to acetoacetate as DKA is treated; thus, nitroprusside test to detect ketones can cause false negative ketones at presentation and false positive ketone levels during recovery. Other causes of high anion gap metabolic acidosis with ketosis (starvation ketoacidosis, alcoholic ketoacidosis) needs to be looked for when investigating DKA.

Although most cases will have glucose >250 mg/dL, DKA can occur with lower or normal glucose levels, including pregnant cases owing to increased counterregulatory hormones, decrease oral intake and dehydration. Euglycemic DKA is commonly seen in type 2 diabetic patient on insulin and sodium-glucose cotransporter-2 (SGLT-2) inhibitors. Also, patient with hepatic insufficiency also may predispose patient for euglycemic DKA. Diagnosis of HHS is based on glucose level >600 mg/dL, serum osmolarity >320 mOsm/kg and minimal or absent ketosis.

When assessing for DKA and HHS, electrolyte including serum phosphorus, creatinine, complete blood count, hepatic enzymes, and serum ketones levels should be measured. A detail history should be taken to determine the precipitating cause. 25% of patients with DKA can have elevated amylase and lipase levels.

Management of Acute Hyperglycemic Emergencies

Treatment of DKA and HHS has three main pillars—fluid resuscitation, insulin, and electrolyte correction along with treatment of precipitating event.

Fluid Resuscitation

The DKA and HHS are disease state with volume loss, dehydration, and hyperosmolarity. Fluid replacement is necessary to restore intravascular volume, improve tissue and renal perfusion, and reduce plasma osmolarity.

All guidelines recommend fluid infusion at 15–20 mL/kg/h over first 2 hours, then subsequent fluid replacement rate as per state of hydration, serum electrolytes, and hemodynamic status. In HHS, fluid deficit is larger and patient may require fluid replacement as high as 500 mL/h to correct 50% of fluid deficit within first 12 hours.

Once euvolemic state is reached, patient still needs maintenance fluid ~150–200 mL/h. Patient at risk of developing volume overload, follows volume status with ultrasound and cautious fluid replacement, and appropriate monitoring. Dextrose is added to fluids once glucose level is around 200–250 mg/dL. Adding glucose allows fixed dose insulin infusion for correction of ketoacidosis.

Choice of resuscitation fluid: All guidelines recommend resuscitation with normal saline. Advantage of isotonic saline is cheap and widely available and may result in rapid resolution of ketoacidosis and lactic acidosis in DKA. But large volume of isotonic saline infusion will lead to large chloride load and will promote normal anion gap metabolic acidosis. Balance crystalloid is preferred fluid for replacement as this will avoid worsening acidosis. Most recent evidence comparing a "balanced" resuscitation crystalloid solution with saline has suggested that though the metabolic acidosis resolves faster with balance crystalloid, the duration of intensive care unit (ICU) stay is not affected. In patients who are hypernatremic or eunatremic, 0.45% normal saline solution can be used instead of normal saline.

Insulin

If you can do little about the insulin resistance of the stress-response state, at least you can supplement the missing insulin.

Primary problem in DKA and HHS is absolute or relative insulin deficiency, thus, supplementation of insulin is important to reverse pathological process. Once serum potassium level of >3.3 mEq/L is confirmed, insulin infusion is usually started at 0.1 U/kg/h. However, for patients with severe acidosis (e.g., bicarbonate <5 mEq/L) or marked insulin resistance (with high chronic insulin requirements), higher doses will often be needed (e.g., 0.2–0.3 U/kg/h).

The target of therapy is to achieve the following metabolic goals:

- Increase the HCO_3^- by 3 mmol/L every hour
- Decrease the blood sugar level (BSL) by 50–70 mg/dL every hour
- Decrease the blood ketone concentration by 0.5 mmol/L every hour
- Maintain normal electrolyte balance while doing so.

Insulin infusion should be uptitrated if metabolic goals are not met. Also, glucose infusion may be needed so that insulin infusion can be continued. Once the glucose falls to ~250 mg/dL (14 mmol/L) the insulin infusion rate is typically reduced considerably (to ~0.05 U/kg/h).

If patient is on long-acting insulin, it should be continued.

Resolution of ketoacidosis (anion gap <12 mEq/L), glucose <200 mg/dL, and pH >7.3 indicate resolution of DKA. Resolution of HHS is defined by normalization of effective serum osmolality to <310 mmol/kg and return to normal mental status. Once DKA and HHS is resolved, fixed dose insulin infusion is transitioned to subcutaneous regimen. Subcutaneous insulin must be overlapped with infusion for at least 2 hours to avoid recurrence.

Once daily insulin requirement are assessed, half of total dose is given as long-acting insulin and rest half is administered as short-acting insulin to prevent meal related hyperglycemia.

Electrolyte Correction

Insulin deficiency, acidosis, and hyperosmolarity cause extracellular shift of potassium. If potassium at time of presentation is low or normal, it indicates relative state of potassium deficit. Before starting insulin infusion, potassium level needs to be >3.3 mEq/L. If patient is hypokalemic, insulin infusion should be delayed and potassium correction started. During treatment of DKA and HHS with insulin and fluids, potassium level will fall rapidly, thus, aggressive potassium correction should be started once potassium level starts falling below 5 mEq/L. Around 20–40 mEq of KCl can be added in each 1 liter of fluid infused, to maintain potassium level between 4 and 5 mEq/L.

Like potassium, phosphate also moves out to extracellular space in acidosis. As correction of ketoacidosis starts with insulin infusion, phosphate will move to intracellular compartment. Thus, patient may develop hypophosphatemia. Phosphate levels need to be monitored and correction given if phosphate levels are <1.0 mg/dL.

Bicarbonate correction is not recommended for correction of acidosis in management of DKA. Evidence is lacking to support use of bicarbonate for treating DKA; in fact bicarbonate may be associated with worsening hypokalemia and increased risk of cerebral edema.

Bicarbonate may have some role for treatment of normal anion gap metabolic acidosis treatment, which develops because of resuscitation with normal saline or half-normal saline, and excretion of ketoacid in the urine.

Complications of Hyperglycemic Emergencies

Severe dyselectrolytemia, hyperosmolarity and extreme acid-base changes can lead to various complications. Most common complications are:

- Cardiac arrest due to bizarre electrolytes
- Brain injury or stroke (due to hypocapnic vasoconstriction)
- Cerebral edema
- Renal failure due to hypotension and possibly other reasons [e.g., whatever the precipitant for the DKA was, be it sepsis or acute myocardial infarction (MI)]
- Disseminated intravascular coagulation (DIC)

Renal dysfunction in DKA and HHS is mostly reversible with fluid resuscitation, and very few patients actually require renal replacement therapy for acute kidney injury.

Most common complications of management of DKA and HHS are hypoglycemia, hypokalemia, and hypophosphatemia. Regular and repeated monitoring for glucose and electrolytes and appropriate correction is necessary to prevent these complications.

Most dreaded complication of treatment of DKA and HHS is cerebral edema. Adults at risk for cerebral edema might include younger patients (almost all affected are <25 years old), marked baseline hyperosmolarity (e.g., calculated serum osmolarity >~330 mOsm) and lack of the normal, expected rise in sodium (Na) level during DKA treatment. The mortality rate is 20–50% and 15–35% of survivors are left with permanent neurologic sequelae. Probable mechanism for cerebral edema includes intracellular water shift when plasma osmolarity declines rapidly.

Measures to prevent cerebral edema development include avoiding reducing glucose too fast or too low. Also avoid reducing the glucose below <200 mg/dL. Avoid hypotonic fluid for resuscitation. Rate of correction of serum osmolarity should not be >3 mOsm/kg/h.

HYPOGLYCEMIA

Hypoglycemia represents a disturbance in carbohydrate metabolism which is defined as glucose level <40 mg/dL. Symptomatic hypoglycemia is considered when Whipple's triad (symptoms and signs of hypoglycemia, a low plasma glucose concentration, and resolution of symptoms or signs after the plasma glucose is corrected) is present. Hypoglycemia is more worrisome problem especially in critically ill, sedated, and ventilated patient.

Symptoms

Symptoms of hypoglycemia can be because of either sympathoadrenal or neuroglycopenic responses.

Sympathoadrenal Symptoms

Sympathoadrenal symptoms develop because of noradrenaline release leading to diaphoresis, tremulousness, and anxiety. Tachycardia, palpitations, increased blood pressure, and hunger as cholinergic stimulation.

Neuroglycopenic Symptoms

As glucose level drops, brain dysfunction becomes manifest in the form of confusion, visual changes (blurred vision, diplopia), slurred speech, dizziness, seizures, and eventually, lethargy, stupor, and coma.

Diagnosis

Point of care glucose monitoring is most important test in diagnosing hypoglycemia because of ease and speed of diagnosis. Glucose level between 40 and 70 mg/dL is defined as moderate hypoglycemia and level <40 mg/dL is classified as severe hypoglycemia. Fingerstick glucose monitoring may not be reliable in patients with poor peripheral perfusion, in that scenario, blood sample can be taken from arterial or venous catheters, or blood could be sent in laboratory for glucose measurement, which is gold standard for glucose monitoring.

Causes

Normal response to drop in blood glucose level is reduced insulin secretions causing decreased glucose uptake by skeletal muscles and adipose tissues along with reduced inhibition of glucagon. This causes increased glycogenolysis and glucogenesis. As glucose levels drop further, there is increase secretions of glucagon and epinephrine, and also elevated anti-insulin hormones (cortisol, growth hormone), leading to hepatic glucogenesis and gluconeogenesis, help in avoiding hypoglycemia. Epinephrine is a critical defense against hypoglycemia by mobilizing gluconeogenic substrates such as amino acids, lactate, and glycerol. When these mechanisms fail, hypoglycemia develops and neuroglycopenic symptoms will manifest. Important causes of hypoglycemia are mentioned in **Table 3.**

TABLE 3: Important causes of hypoglycemia.

Drugs	*Disease process*	*Consumption-utilization mismatch*
Insulin	Sepsis	Starvation
Diabetic medications	Hepatic failure	Exercise
Antibiotics (fluoroquinolones, sulfonamides, pentamidine, and artemisinin antimalarials)	Renal failure	Alcohol binge
Phenytoin, valproate	Adrenal insufficiency	Pregnancy
Haloperidol, fluoxetine, and lithium	Myxedema coma	
Nonselective beta-blockers (propranolol, nadolol), angiotensin-converting enzyme (ACE) inhibitors	Insulinoma	
Salicylate intoxication	Malignancies (e.g., mesenchymal tumors, hematologic malignancies)	
	Postgastric bypass	

Workup

Patients with Whipple's triad should only be evaluated for hypoglycemia. A thorough clinical history and laboratory data can give clues to the reason behind hypoglycemia.

When cause is not clear, evaluation during episode of hypoglycemia is necessary. This includes measurement of plasma glucose level, insulin level, C-peptide level, proinsulin, β-hydroxybutyrate, and oral hypoglycemic agent levels. When antibody induced hypoglycemia is suspected, insulin antibodies should be measured. Some patients may require 72 hours fast to induce spontaneous hypoglycemia to do workup. **Table 4** shows various diagnosis of cause of hypoglycemia based on various test results.

Patients with documented endogenous fasting or postprandial hyperglycemia, with a negative screen for oral hypoglycemic agents, and no circulating insulin antibodies insulinoma is suspected, and should undergo computed tomography (CT) or magnetic resonance imaging (MRI) scans or transabdominal ultrasonography to localize an insulinoma.

Treatment of Severe Hypoglycemia

Severe hypoglycemia with threatened brain injury will need urgent correction of blood glucose level. Traditional treatment is intravenous (IV) dextrose bolus. Commonly, D50W bolus is used to achieve safe blood glucose level, which is very easily available. D10W is another option (several 50 mL boluses) to increase glucose level. Advantages of D10W over D50W are less risk of overshoot hyperglycemia and less hypertonic toxicity (local skin irritation, thrombophlebitis, and tissue necrosis after skin extravasation). There are few small, randomized control trials which suggest that higher concentrations of dextrose-containing fluids do not expedite reversal of hypoglycemia as compared to lower concentrations, and that lower concentration formulations are more likely to achieve normal glycemic targets.

Once patient is awake, oral carbohydrate dense food is the most efficient way to correct hypoglycemia. Ice cream or chocolate are good choices (100 g of Dairy Milk bar = 534 kcal). In intubated patients, nasogastric feeding should be started.

In case of recurrent hypoglycemia and oral feeding is not tolerated, either D5W or D10W are safe for peripheral infusion. Rate of infusion depends on severity of hypoglycemia. In case of central access, infusion of D25W or D50W can also be considered. Frequent blood glucose monitoring is necessary to titrate dextrose infusion.

Octreotide as continuous infusion may be considered in patients with sulfonylurea intoxication. Steroids can be used for patients who are refractory to usual measures used to treat hypoglycemia, especially useful in adrenal insufficiency and large dose insulin overdose. Steroids counteract effects

TABLE 4: Diagnosis of cause of hypoglycemia.

Symptoms/ Signs	*Glucose (mg/dL)*	*Insulin (μU/mL)*	*C-peptide (nmol/L)*	*Proinsulin (pmol/L)*	*β-hydroxy-butyrate (mmol/L)*	*Glucose increase after glucagon (mg/dL)*	*Circulating oral hypoglycemic agent*	*Antibody to insulin*	*Diagnostic interpretation*
No	<55	<3	<0.2	<5	>2.7	<25	No	No	Normal
Yes	<55	>>3	<0.2	<5	5.2.7	>25	No	Negative (positive)	Exogenous insulin
Yes	<55	3	0.2	5	5.2.7	>25	No	Negative	Insulinoma, postgastric bypass hypoglycemia
Yes	<55	3	0.2	5	5.2.7	>25	Yes	Negative	Oral hypoglycemic agent
Yes	<55	3	>0.2	>5	5.2.7	>25	No	Positive	Insulin autoimmune
Yes	<55	<3	<0.2	<5	5.2.7	>25	No	Negative	IGF-mediated
Yes	<55	<3	<0.2	<5	>2.7	<25	No	Negative	Not insulin (or IGF)-mediated

(IGF: insulin-like growth factor)

of insulin. Steroid administration helps reduce dextrose requirement to manageable levels, thus helps in avoiding volume overload, electrolyte abnormalities. Short acting IV steroids act rapidly with effect lasting for 8–12 hours. Hydrocortisone with starting dose of 100 mg is reasonable and subsequent doses and interval titrated as per glucose trends.

Patients with no IV access, approach is to use 1 mg glucagon intramuscular (IM). Disadvantages of glucagon are: (1) Glucagon may not work, if liver glucagon stores are depleted; (2) Glucagon can cause nausea and vomiting, which limit oral feeding and can be dangerous in drowsy patients; (3) Glucagon takes 10–15 minutes to start acting, which is a long time in severely hypoglycemic patients.

GLYCEMIC CONTROL IN ICU

Acute hyperglycemia is adaptive response to stress. Both hyperglycemia and hypoglycemia are associated to poor outcome in critically-ill patients.

Stress hyperglycemia is transient hyperglycemia during acute illness—usually restricted to patients without prior evidence of diabetes with reversion to normal after discharge. Stress hyperglycemia results from increased hepatic glucose production and impaired glucose utilization in peripheral tissues. Excess counterregulatory hormones (glucagon, cortisol, catecholamines, and growth hormone) increase lipolysis and protein breakdown (proteolysis), and impair glucose utilization by peripheral tissues.

Hyperglycemia can increase blood glucose levels at the cellular level, resulting in mitochondrial injury by generating reactive oxygen species, and endothelial dysfunction by inhibiting nitric oxide production. It also increases levels of proinflammatory cytokines such as tumor necrosis factor (TNF)-α and interleukin (IL)-6, causing immune system dysfunction. Immune dysfunction increases plasminogen activator inhibitor-1 and fibrinogen, causing platelet aggregation and hypercoagulable state. These changes can eventually lead to increased risk of infection, impaired wound healing, multiple organ failure, prolonged hospital stay, and death.

Early observational studies of patients with MI, stroke, and critical illness revealed that acute hyperglycemia is associated with increased in-hospital mortality in patients with and without DM.

In 1995, DIGAMI (Diabetes Mellitus, Insulin Glucose Infusion in Acute Myocardial Infarction) study was published, which was study of diabetics with MI. This study found mortality benefits for tight blood glucose control group. This made clear that greater attention is needed to stress induced hyperglycemia.

In 2001, Van den Berge evaluated intensive insulin therapy (glucose target 80–110 mg/dL) versus conventional treatment (glucose target 180–200 mg/dL) in surgical ICU (Leuven trial). Intensive glucose control group was associated with a dramatic reduction in mortality, septicemia, length of stay in ICU, and number of transfusions required. However, not all was well. European trials of this protocol did not find the expected benefit, and in fact had to stop prematurely because too many patients were having hypoglycemic episodes. Reason probably why Leuven trial had such dramatic results as compared to following studies, could be because 87% of study patients were on total parenteral nutrition (TPN). Thus, control group (where sugar fluctuated) experienced all the mortality-increasing disadvantages of TPN-associated hyperglycemia, whereas the tightly controlled group was protected from them.

In 2009, Finfer published NICE-SUGAR (Normoglycemia in Intensive Care Evaluation–Survival Using Glucose Algorithm Regulation) trial, which was huge multicenter trial comparing effects of intensive glucose control (81–108 mg/dL) versus conventional glucose control (<180 mg/dL) in critically-ill patients. There was increased mortality (2.6%) in intensive control group. A post hoc analysis of NICE-SUGAR data published in 2012 concluded that there was direct correlation in hypoglycemia and death and episodes of hypoglycemia were 10 times higher in intensive glucose control group.

Despite strong evidence against tight glucose control, interest in intensive glucose control has not weaned. Recently, trials have tried using computerized algorithms and close loop automatic systems to control blood sugar level in tight control. None of these studies have shown long-term mortality benefits.

Current recommendation including from the Surviving Sepsis Campaign, the American Association of Clinical Endocrinologists, the Endocrine Society and American Diabetes Association, is to maintain glucose between 140 mg/dL and 180 mg/dL in ICU patients.

SUMMARY

Diabetic emergencies are very important endocrine complications seen in critically ill patient and if not dealt with immediately can cause significant morbidity and mortality in patients.

SUGGESTED READING

1. Alsahli M, Gerich JE. Hypoglycemia. Endocrinol Metab Clin North Am. 2013;42(4):657-76.
2. American Diabetes Association. Classification and diagnosis of diabetes. Sec. 2. In standards of medical care in diabetes-2016. Diabetes Care. 2016;39(suppl 1): S13-S22.
3. Bode BW, Braithwaite SS, Steed RD, Davidson PC. Intravenous insulin infusion therapy: indications, methods and transition to subcutaneous insulin therapy. Endocr Pract. 2004;10(suppl 2):71-80.

4. Chiasson JL, Aris-Jilwan N, Ekoé JM, et al. Diagnosis and treatment of diabetic ketoacidosis and the hyperglycemic hyperosmolar state. CMAJ. 2003;168(7): 859-66. Erratum in: CMAJ. 2003;168(10):1241.
5. Chua HR, Venkatesh B, Stachowski E, Schneider AG, Perkins K, Ladanyi S, et al. Plasma-Lyte 148 vs 0.9% saline for fluid resuscitation in diabetic ketoacidosis. J Crit Care. 2012;27(2):138-45.
6. Cornwell B, Knight B, Olivieri L, Willis GC. Current diagnosis and treatment of hyperglycemic emergencies. Emerg Med Clin North Am. 2014;32(2): 437-52.
7. Cryer PE, Axelrod L, Grossman AB, Heller SR, Montori VM, Seaquist ER, et al. Evaluation and management of adult hypoglycemic disorders: an endocrine society clinical practice guideline. J Clin Endocrinol Metab. 2009;94(3): 709-28.
8. Cryer PE, Davis SN, Shamoon H. Hypoglycemia in diabetes. Diabetes Care. 2003;26(6):1902-12.
9. Cryer PE. Glucose homeostasis and hypoglycemia. In: Melmed S, Polonsky KS, Larsen PR, Kronenberg HM (Eds). Williams Textbook of Endocrinology, 13th edition. Philadelphia: Elsevier; 2016. pp. 1503-33.
10. Cryer PE. Mechanisms of sympathoadrenal failure and hypoglycemia in diabetes. J Clin Invest. 2006;116(6):1470-3.
11. Evans L, Rhodes A, Alhazzani W, Antonelli M, Coopersmith CM, French C, et al. Surviving sepsis campaign: international guidelines for management of sepsis and septic shock 2021. Intensive Care Med. 2021;47(11):1181-247.
12. Falciglia M, Freyberg RW, Almenoff PL, D'Alessio DA, Render ML. Hyperglycemia-related mortality in critically ill patients varies with admission diagnosis. Crit Care Med. 2009;37(12):3001-9.
13. Farrokhi F, Smiley D, Umpierrez GE. Glycemic control in non-diabetic critically ill patients. Best Pract Res Clin Endocrinol Metab. 2011;25(5):813-24.
14. Goldenberg RM, Berard LD, Cheng AY, Gilbert JD, Verma S, Woo VC, et al. SGLT2 inhibitorassociated diabetic ketoacidosis: clinical review and recommendations for prevention and diagnosis. Clin Ther. 2016;38(12):2654-64.
15. Gouveia CF, Chowdhury TA. Managing hyperglycaemic emergencies: an illustrative case and review of recent British guidelines. Clin Med (Lond). 2013;13(2):160-2.
16. Hegazi MO, Mashankar A. Central pontine myelinolysis in the hyperosmolar hyperglycaemic state. Med Princ Pract. 2012;22(1):96-9.
17. Hsia DS, Tarai SG, Alimi A, Coss-Bu JA, Haymond MW. Fluid management in pediatric patients with DKA and rates of suspected clinical cerebral edema. Pediatr Diabetes. 2015;16(5):338-44.
18. Jaber S, Paugam C, Futier E, Lasocki S, Lescot T, Pottecher J, et al. Sodium bicarbonate therapy for patients with severe metabolic acidaemia in the intensive care unit (BICAR-ICU): a multicentre, open-label, randomised controlled, phase 3 trial. The Lancet. 2018;392(10141):31-40.
19. Kiefer M, Gene H, Alter H, Barger J. Dextrose 10% in the treatment of out-of-hospital hypoglycemia. Prehosp Disaster Med. 2014;29(2):190-4.
20. Kitabchi AE, Umpierrez GE, Fisher J, Murphy MB, Stentz FB. Thirty years of personal experience in hyperglycemic crises: diabetic ketoacidosis and hyperglycemic hyperosomar state. J Clin Endocrinol Metab. 2008;93(5):1541-52.

21. Kitabshi A, Umpierrez G, Miles JM, Fisher JN. Hyperglycemic crises in patients with diabetes. Diabetes Care. 2009;32(7):1335-43.
22. Leelarathna L, English SW, Thabit H, Caldwell K, Allen JM, Kumareswaran K, et al. Feasibility of fully automated closed-loop glucose control using continuous subcutaneous glucose measurements in critical illness: a randomized controlled trial. Crit Care. 2013;17(4):R159.
23. Mahmoodpoor A, Hamishehkar H, Beigmohammadi M, Sanaie S, Shadvar K, Soleimanpour H, et al. Predisposing factors for hypoglycemia and its relation with mortality in critically ill patients undergoing insulin therapy in an intensive care unit. Anesth Pain Med. 2016;6(1):e33849.
24. Maletkovic J, Drexler A. Diabetic ketoacidosis and hyperglycemic hyperosmolar state. Endocrinol Metab Clin North Am. 2013;42(4):677-95.
25. Maletkovic J, Drexler A. Diabetic ketoacidosis and hyperglycemic hyperosmolar state. Endocrinol Metab Clin North Am. 2013;42(4):677-95.
26. Malmberg K, Rydén L, Efendic S, Herlitz J, Nicol P, Waldenström A, et al. Randomized trial of insulin-glucose infusion followed by subcutaneous insulin treatment in diabetic patients with acute myocardial infarction (DIGAMI study): effects on mortality at 1 year. J Am Coll Cardiol. 1995;26(1):57-65.
27. Moghissi ES, Korytkowski MT, DiNardo M, Einhorn D, Hellman R, Hirsch IB, et al. American Association of Clinical Endocrinologists and American Diabetes Association consensus statement on inpatient glycemic control. Endocr Pract. 2009;15(4):1-17.
28. Moore C, Woollard M. Dextrose 10% or 50% in the treatment of hypoglycaemia out of hospital? A randomised controlled trial. Emerg Med J. 2005;22(7): 512-5.
29. NICE-SUGAR Study Investigators; Finfer S, Chittock DR, Su SY, Blair D, Foster D, Dhingra V, Bellomo R, et al. Intensive versus conventional glucose control in critically ill patients. N Engl J Med. 2009;360(13):1283-97.
30. Nyenwe EA, Kitabchi AE. Evidence based management of hyperglycemic emergencies in diabetes mellicus. Diabetes Res Clin Pract. 2011;94(3): 340-51.
31. Nyenwe EA, Kitabchi AE. The evolution of diabetic keroacidosis: an update of its etiology, pathogenesis and management. Metabolism. 2016;65(4):507-21.
32. Pasquel FJ, Umpierrez GE. Hyperosmolar hyperglycemic stare: a historic review of the clinical presentation, diagnosis and treatment. Diabetes Care. 2014;37(11):3124-31.
33. Preiser JC, Devos P, Ruiz-Santana S, Mélot C, Annane D, Groeneveld J, et al. A prospective randomised multi-centre controlled trial on tight glucose control by intensive insulin therapy in adult intensive care units: the Glucontrol study. Intensive Care Med. 2009;35(10):1738-48.
34. Rui L. Energy metabolism in the liver. Compr Physiol. 2014;4(1):177-97.
35. Saltiel AR, Kahn CR. Insulin signalling and the regulation of glucose and lipid metabolism. Nature. 2001;414(6865):799-806.
36. Scott AR; Joint British Diabetes Societies (JBDS) for Inpatient Care; JBDS hyperosmolar hyperglycaemic guidelines group. Management of hyperosmolar hyperglycemic state in adults with diabetes. Diabet Med. 2015;32(6): 714-24.

37. Taniguchi CM, Emanuelli B, Kahn CR. Critical nodes in signalling pathways: insights into insulin action. Nat Rev Mol Cell Biol. 2006;7(2):85-96.
38. Tariq K, Tariq S, Denny AM. Role of steroids in refractory hypoglycemia due to an overdose of 10,000 units of insulin glargine: a case report and literature review. AACE Clinical Case Rep. 2018;4(1):70-4.
39. Umpierrez G, Koryrkowski M. Diabetic emergencies-ketoacidosis, hyperglyaemic hyperosmolar state and hypoglycemia. Nat Rev Endocrinol. 2016;12(4):222-32.
40. Van den Berghe G, Wilmer A, Hermans G, Meersseman W, Wouters PJ, Milants I, et al. Intensive insulin therapy in the medical ICU. New Engl J Med. 2006;354(5):449-61.
41. van den Berghe G, Wouters P, Weekers F, Verwaest C, Bruyninckx F, Schetz M, et al. Intensive insulin therapy in critically ill patients. New Engl J Med. 2001;345(19):1359-67.
42. Yamada T, Shojima N, Noma H, Yamauchi T, Kadowaki T. Glycemic control, mortality, and hypoglycemia in critically ill patients: a systematic review and network meta-analysis of randomized controlled trials. Intensive Care Med. 2017;43(1):1-15.

CHAPTER

32 Adrenal Emergencies

Jitendra Choudhary

ADRENAL INSUFFICIENCY

Adrenal insufficiency is a state of cortisol deficiency and can be classified as primary, secondary, or tertiary adrenal deficiency depending on where the defect in production is. Primary adrenal insufficiency is a state of disorder due to partial or complete dysfunction of adrenal gland. Secondary adrenal insufficiency is a state of adrenal suppression in presence of normal adrenal glands. Secondary adrenal insufficiency could be because of drugs, critical illness, or hypothalamic-pituitary malfunction. Tertiary adrenal insufficiency is because of exogenous glucocorticoid treatment, causing suppression of hypothalamus. Tertiary adrenal insufficiency is the most common form of adrenal dysfunction.

PATHOPHYSIOLOGY

Adrenal steroid secretions are tightly regulated at multiple levels. Hypothalamic corticotropin releasing hormone (CRH) stimulates pituitary adrenocorticotropic hormone (ACTH) secretion, which stimulates cortisol production in the adrenal cortex. Cortisol shows negative feedback regulation of ACTH and CRH secretion. This regulation is adaptable and circadian, which causes secretory bursts every 60–90 minutes. Aldosterone secretion is regulated by renin-angiotensin system, but also exhibits circadian variation caused by hypothalamic-pituitary-adrenal axis. **Figures 1A and B** shows regulation of cortisol and aldosterone.

Primary adrenal insufficiency is caused because of direct effect on adrenal gland, cause could be vascular, autoimmune, or neoplastic cause. Secondary adrenal insufficiency is caused because of suppressed stimulus to otherwise normal adrenal gland. This is secondary to damaged pituitary or dysregulated pituitary because of drugs. Tertiary adrenal insufficiency is caused because of stopping corticosteroids or relative adrenal insufficiency of septic shock. Hypothalamic-pituitary-adrenal axis is intact in tertiary adrenal insufficicency.

CAUSES

Table 1 shows the causes of adrenal insufficiency.

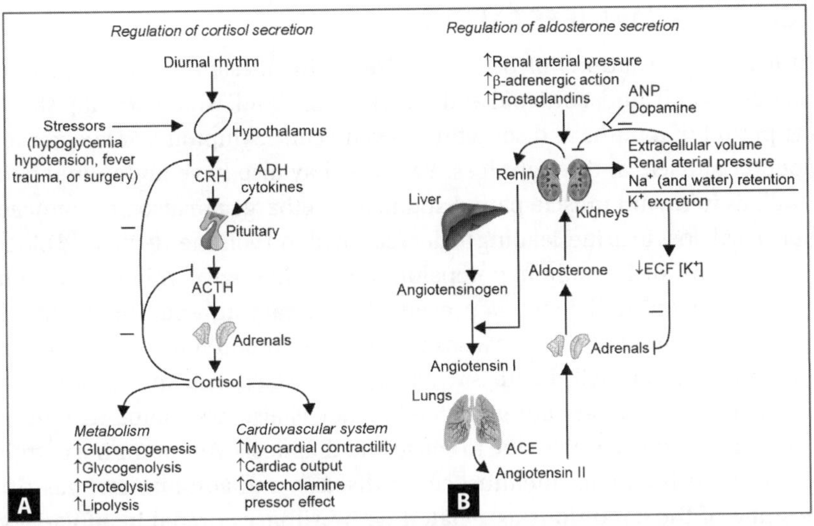

Figs. 1A and B: *Regulation of cortisol and aldosterone secretion:* (A) Regulation of cortisol; (B) Regulation of aldosterone. (ADH: antidiuretic hormone; ACTH: adrenocorticotropic hormone; ANP: atrial natriuretic peptide; CRH: corticotrophin-releasing hormone; ECF: extracellular fluid)

TABLE 1: Causes of adrenal insufficiency.

Autoimmune destruction: Addison's disease	*Congenital causes:* • Adrenal dysgenesis • Adrenoleukodystrophy • Impaired steroidogenesis • Empty sella syndrome	*Vascular etiologies:* • Infarction due to arterial embolism • Infarction due to AAA • Postpartum pituitary necrosis
Infection: • Sepsis • Tuberculosis • Histoplasmosis • Cytomegalovirus • Coccidioidomycosis • Meningococcal sepsis, purpura fulminans • Human immuno-deficiency virus (HIV)	*Neoplastic invasion:* • Renal cell carcinoma • Adrenal carcinoma • Breast carcinoma • Lung (NSCLC) • Malignant melanoma • Pituitary tumor	*Infiltrative systemic disease:* • Amyloid • Sarcoidosis • Hemochromatosis
Traumatic destruction	*Drugs:* • Corticosteroid withdrawal • Etomidate (causes primary adrenal insufficiency) • Azole antifungals—Fluconazole, ketoconazole • Rifampicin (increases steroid metabolism) • Phenytoin (increases steroid metabolism)	*Environmental factors:* Hypothermia

(AAA: abdominal aortic aneurysm; NSCLC: non-small cell lung cancer)

CLINICAL MANIFESTATIONS

Clinical manifestations of primary adrenal insufficiency are because of absence of both glucocorticoid and mineralocorticoid, which develop slowly over period of months and sometimes even years. Symptoms are decreased appetite, nausea, and weight loss. Patients may also have abdominal pain as well as joint and muscle pain. Fatigue and lethargy are also pronounced. There is salt loss in urine, leading to decreased blood volume, decreased blood pressure, and orthostatic hypotension. Severe hypoglycemia can present if glucocorticoid deficiency is present. In primary adrenal insufficiency, high concentration of ACTH causes increased skin and mucous membrane pigmentation, especially in areas which are exposed to sun and friction.

Patient with primary adrenal insufficiency is also associated with other conditions which may give clue to cause and diagnosis. Autoimmune thyroid disease, type 1 diabetes mellitus, celiac disease, and autoimmune gastritis are some of the conditions associated with primary adrenal insufficiency. The presence of hypoparathyroidism or *Candida* infections should prompt investigation for autoimmune polyendocrine syndrome type 1.

Presentation may be milder in secondary adrenal insufficiency as mineralocorticoid production is intact and adrenal insufficiency is partial. Predominant symptoms may be because of associated hormone deficiencies.

Adrenal crisis (AC) is a life-threatening exacerbation of adrenal insufficiency when an increased demand fails to increase hormone production. This is life-threatening emergency, which require immediate treatment. Presentation of AC are profound fatigue, malaise, headache, and muscle pain. Also, will have nausea, vomiting and abdominal pain, cramps, and dehydration leading to hypotension and shock. Increased confusion, loss of consciousness, and coma is also common during AC. Metabolic abnormalities manifest are hyponatremia, hyperkalemia, and hypoglycemia. Increase serum creatinine and sometimes mild hypercalcemia can present because of prerenal failure.

Adrenal crisis occurs in patients with primary or secondary adrenal insufficiency because of triggering event. The main triggers for AC include interruption of glucocorticoid intake, infections, surgery, gastroenteritis, and stress (physical or emotional).

DIAGNOSIS

To diagnose adrenal insufficiency, clinician must suspect about possibility of adrenal insufficiency based on metabolic and clinical clues. Unexplained hyponatremia or hypoglycemia should warrant evaluation of adrenal function. Important clues which should arouse suspicion of underlying adrenal Insufficiency are hyponatremia, hyperkalemia, nonanion gap metabolic acidosis, hypotension out of proportion to severity of illness, and refractory hypoglycemia despite glucose repletion.

Assess for serum cortisol level to diagnose adrenal insufficiency. A random cortisol level of >20 μg/dL excludes adrenal insufficiency. If cortisol level is <5–7 μg/dL in presence of physiologic stress, it strongly suggests adrenal insufficiency. Cortisol level <20 μg/dL warrants ACTH stimulation test. Intravenous (IV) ACTH 250 μg is given, and cortisol levels are checked at baseline and at 60 minutes after ACTH administration. If cortisol level does not rise above >20–25 μg/dL, this confirms the diagnosis of adrenal insufficiency. A normal response to ACTH stimulation test rules out primary adrenal insufficiency. Abnormal response to ACTH stimulation test establishes diagnosis of adrenal insufficiency. The cause of adrenal insufficiency is then investigated with a morning ACTH level measurement. ACTH levels will be elevated in case of primary adrenal insufficiency, while it will be normal or reduced in secondary insufficiency.

Secondary adrenocortical insufficiency (caused by pituitary dysfunction) can be distinguished from primary adrenal insufficiency by normal or low plasma ACTH level after rapid ACTH, absence of hyperpigmentation, no significant impairment of aldosterone secretion (because aldosterone secretion is under control of the renin-angiotensin system) and additional evidence of hypopituitarism (e.g., hypogonadism, hypothyroidism).

Once diagnosis of adrenal insufficiency is made, it is mandatory to determine cause of insufficiency. For primary adrenal insufficiency, autoantibody assays can be advised to diagnose autoimmune adrenal destruction. Also, computed tomography (CT) imaging is useful to diagnose infections, tumors, and bleeding in adrenal gland.

In cases of secondary adrenal insufficiency, the status of other pituitary hormones must be assessed together with magnetic resonance imaging (MRI) of the pituitary region, to detect the presence of a tumor or other infiltrative processes.

Drug-induced adrenal insufficiency is not immediately apparent. A detailed history must be taken including use of dermal, inhaled, and injected steroids. Also, opiates are second most common drugs to cause adrenal insufficiency.

TREATMENT

Management of Adrenal Crisis

Adrenal crisis is acute emergency characterized by circulatory collapse, hypoglycemia, dehydration, nausea, vomiting, and electrolyte disturbance. Important components of management of AC include treating an underlying etiology, stress dose steroids, IV fluid resuscitation, and glucose and electrolyte correction.

Treatment of patient with possible AC should not be delayed for diagnosis and investigations. Immediate IV steroid administration should be followed by blood testing for serum sodium, potassium, creatinine, urea, glucose, cortisol, ACTH, and other biochemistry for precipitating causes (for bacterial or viral infections).

In patient with known adrenal insufficiency 100 mg hydrocortisone should be given followed by 50 mg IV hydrocortisone IV q6h as a maintenance dose for next 24–48 hours until the patient can take oral medication. For patient with suspected adrenal insufficiency, dexamethasone 4–6 mg should be preferred, as dexamethasone does not interfere with measurement of cortisol levels (unlike most other steroids).

Along with steroid therapy, volume resuscitation with rapid infusion of IV fluids is equally important. Volume resuscitation should be based on hemodynamic assessment. IV glucose should be used to treat hypoglycemia. Also, vasopressors should be considered early in resuscitation and should be weaned as per hemodynamic.

Adrenal crisis patients will improve rapidly with steroids and volume resuscitation. Failure to improve with these should prompt to search and treat underlying secondary stressors.

Maintenance Therapy

Glucocorticoid Replacement

Daily requirement in nonstressed individual can be met with hydrocortisone dose of 15–20 mg given in 2–3 divided doses. Further dose should be adjusted by monitoring clinical symptoms and monitoring serum ACTH levels.

Mineralocorticoid Replacement

Usual starting dose of mineralocorticoid replacement is fludrocortisone 50–100 μg orally, and adjusted based on electrolytes (i.e., serum potassium and sodium), salt cravings, postural hypotension, or other symptoms of mineralocorticoid deficiency.

Treatment for Illness or Stress

For minor febrile illness, glucocorticoid doses should be increased to 2–3 times of daily requirement for few days of illness. There is no need for adjusting mineralocorticoid doses.

For moderate illness, hydrocortisone 50 mg bid PO or IV is given and rapidly tapered to maintenance doses as patient recovers.

For severe illness, hydrocortisone 100 mg IV q8h should be the starting dose and tapered to maintenance level gradually as per course of illness.

For moderately stressful procedures such as endoscopy, or arteriography, give a single 100 mg IV dose of hydrocortisone just before the procedure. For major surgery, stress dose steroids should be given just before induction and continued for first 24 hours after surgery, and then tapered rapidly to maintenance level.

SUMMARY

Adrenal insufficiency often present with nonspecific signs and symptoms, but unexplained hypotension, hypoglycemia, hyponatremia, and hyperkalemia should arouse suspicion and warrant workup for adrenal insufficiency. Along with steroid replacement, finding stressor which precipitated adrenal insufficiency and treating it is also equally important. AC should be considered in any patient who appears to be septic but does not have an obvious source of infection. This is a classic sepsis-mimic.

SUGGESTED READING

1. Allolio B. Extensive expertise in endocrinology. Adrenal crisis. Eur J Endocrinol. 2015;172(3):R115-24.
2. Amrein K, Martucci G, Hahner S. Understanding adrenal crisis. Intensive Care Med. 2018;44(5):652-5.
3. Bancos I, Hahner S, Tomlinson J, Arlt W. Diagnosis and management of adrenal insufficiency. Lancet Diabetes Endocrinol. 2015;3(3):216-26.
4. Bornstein SR, Allolio B, Arlt W, Barthel A, Don-Wauchope A, Hammer GD, et al. Diagnosis and treatment of primary adrenal insufficiency: An Endocrine Society Clinical Practice Guideline. J Clin Endocrinol Metab. 2016;101(2):364-89.
5. Chakera AJ, Vaidya B. Addison disease in adults: diagnosis and management. Am J Med. 2010;123(5):409-13.
6. Chan S, Debono M. Replication of cortisol circadian rhythm: new advances in hydrocortisone replacement therapy. Ther Adv Endocrinol Metab. 2010;1(3):129-38.
7. Charmandari E, Nicolaides NC, Chrousos GP. Adrenal insufficiency. Lancet. 2014;383(9935):2152-67.
8. Dorin RI, Qualls CR, Crapo LM. Diagnosis of adrenal insufficiency. Ann Intern Med. 2003;139(3):194-204.
9. Gjerstad JK, Lightman SL, Spiga F. Role of glucocorticoid negative feedback in the regulation of HPA axis pulsatility. Stress. 2018;21(5):403-16.
10. Lightman SL, Conway-Campbell BL. The crucial role of pulsatile activity of the HPA axis for continuous dynamic equilibration. Nat Rev Neurosci. 2010;11(10):710-18.
11. Marik PE. Mechanisms and clinical consequences of critical illness associated adrenal insufficiency. Curr Opin Crit Care. 2007;13(4):363-9.
12. Michels A, Michels N. Addison disease: early detection and treatment principles. Am Fam Physician. 2014;89(7):563-8.
13. Oelkers W. Adrenal insufficiency. N Engl J Med. 1996;335(16):1206-12.
14. Sun ZH, Nomura K, Toraya S, Ujihara M, Horiba N, Suda T, et al. Clinical significance of adrenal computed tomography in Addison's disease. Endocrinol Jpn. 1992;39(6):563-9.

CHAPTER 33

Thyroid Emergencies

Jitendra Choudhary

INTRODUCTION

Thyroid dysfunction is very common in critically-ill patient, but they are rarely primary cause of admission in intensive care unit (ICU). Emergencies related to thyroid gland requiring ICU admission are either because of overt dysfunction or marked enlargement of the gland that jeopardize the life of patients.

THYROID EMERGENCIES

Severe thyroid disorder can be because of either excess or deficiency of thyroid hormone. Both thyrotoxicosis and hypothyroidism have effect on cardiovascular, digestive system and also basal metabolism, muscles, and skin.

Hypothyroidism in ICU

"Subclinical hypothyroidism" was defined as a condition characterized by normal thyroid hormone levels and high serum thyroid-stimulating hormone (TSH) concentrations. "Overt hypothyroidism" was defined as a condition with serum TSH concentrations exceeding the normal range associated to low serum free thyroid hormone level.

Hypothyroid (myxedema) coma is endocrine emergency because of severe untreated hypothyroid state, which warrants ICU admission and management. It is state characterized by decreased level of consciousness, altered thermoregulation, and cardiovascular collapse.

Precipitating Factor

In known hypothyroid patients, myxedema coma is initiated by various precipitating factors. Most common precipitating factors are low temperature, systemic infections, cerebrovascular events, congestive cardiac failure, and drugs such as anesthetics, neuroleptics, amiodarone, lithium, phenytoin, and opiates.

Clinical Features

Main presenting features of myxedema coma are hypothermia and decreased sensorium. Patient may be bradycardic also. There is reduced hypoxic respiratory drive leading to CO_2 retention and narcosis, causing progressive somnolence and drowsiness. There is respiratory muscle weakness also causing inadequate ventilation. Severe hypothyroidism causing ascites, pleural effusion, and pericardial effusion also contribute to ineffective ventilation.

Hypothermia is noted in majority patients and temperature could be as low as 80°F.

There is also impaired cardiac function because of decreased cardiac contractility, reduced stroke volume, and cardiac output. Cardiac contractility can be further impaired by pericardial effusion and reduced intravascular volume. Rewarming can cause vasodilatation and subsequent hypotension because of impaired cardiac function, and body is not able to compensate for effects of vasodilatation.

Neuropsychiatric effects of myxedema coma range from increased somnolence to unresponsiveness and seizures or delirium. Patients typically have short-term memory loss, cerebellar signs, and overall slow verbal response.

Patient can also have constipation, paralytic ileus, and bladder atony with large residual urine retention. There is also total body fluid retention with hyponatremia, caused because of impaired water diuresis. Hypoglycemia is common and may be associated with underlying adrenal insufficiency.

Diagnosis

Diagnosis of hypothyroid coma depends on history of previous thyroid diseases, low serum free T4 and free T3 levels, along with high serum TSH concentration, along with progressive lethargy, and particular signs and symptoms. The presence of severe, nonthyroidal illness may reduce the degree of TSH elevation expected for particular patients. In addition, if a patient has myxedema coma related to central hypothyroidism, the TSH level may be low or normal.

Along with free T3, free T4, and TSH levels, blood gas analysis to detect hypoxia, hypercapnia, and respiratory acidosis should be done. Also, biochemistry panel to detect hyponatremia and hypoglycemia.

Electrocardiography done usually to demonstrate sinus bradycardia, Q–T prolongation, and low voltage QRS complex (because of pericardial effusion). Echocardiogram to disclose cardiomegaly, measure cardiac output, and assess pericardial effusion, and also to rule out impending cardiac tamponade. Neuroimaging will be normal in cases of primary hypothyroidism. In patients with secondary hypothyroidism, neuroimaging is done to detect pituitary macroadenoma or an empty sella.

Treatment

Important pillars of myxedema coma treatment are replacement of thyroid hormone, treatment of predisposing condition, and supportive care.

Hormone Replacement

Intravenous correction is preferred in acute ill patient. Starting regimen recommended is high-dose intravenous (IV) T4 300–400 μg/daily. Rapid correction of hypothyroidism may not be tolerated by all patients, and sudden cardiac death has been reported with rapid correction.

Other regimens which can be used are liothyronine 10–20 μg IV as bolus initially, followed by 10 μg every 4 hours for the first 24 hours, and every 6 hours for days 2–3, and then to start oral administration if feasible. Otherwise T3 plus T4 regimen can be used. In this regimen, initial dose of 250 μg of IV T4 administered, followed by 100 μg 24 hours later, and 50 μg every day either oral or IV. Simultaneously with T4 bolus, 10 μg T3 as IV bolus followed by 10 μg IV every 8–12 hours until patient is conscious and can take oral maintenance T4.

Because of rare occurrence of myxedema coma, there are studies lacking comparison of various regimens for thyroid hormone replacement.

Other Supportive Measures

Along with thyroid hormone replacement, hydrocortisone 100 mg 6 hourly should be given to patients with myxedema coma, as hypothyroidism can be associated with autoimmune adrenal insufficiency. Also, in cases of central hypothyroidism, there will be associated adrenocorticotropic hormone (ACTH) and subsequent adrenal insufficiency.

Fluid and electrolyte imbalance needs to be corrected along with hormone replacement. Most common abnormality is hyponatremia, and it could also cause mental status changes and seizures. Severe symptomatic hyponatremia will need correction of hypertonic saline to gradually raise sodium levels to >120 mEq/L. Care must be taken to avoid fluid overload and rapid correction of hyponatremia. Asymptomatic mild hyponatremia (>120 mEq/L) usually resolves with thyroid hormone replacement therapy only. Hypoglycemia needs to be detected and corrected urgently with IV glucose.

Hypothermia needs to be corrected gradually with passive warming. Active warming measures are not recommended as it can cause vasodilatation and shock.

Hypoventilation and CO_2 narcosis can be present and will warrant endotracheal intubation and mechanical ventilation. Also, these patients require frequent blood gas analysis to guide further therapy.

Cardiac arrhythmias, acute myocardial infarction, acute pulmonary edema, and cardiac shock are common complications in patient with myxedema coma and may cause death also. Reduced stroke volume and decreased cardiac contractility could be because of reduced cardiac contractility or cardiac tamponade. Prolong Q-T interval can lead to ventricular tachycardia, and these patients needs to be monitored closely.

IV diuretics should be part of treatment of myxedema coma, especially when suspecting acute pulmonary edema. In patient with myxedema coma, acute coronary events are not uncommon and can be precipitated by high doses of thyroxine needed to treat myxedema coma in patient with underlying myocardial ischemia. As myxedema coma patients have impaired mentation, clinical alert regarding ischemic events may not be present, and thus, cardiac enzymes should be routinely measured in absence of typical electrocardiographic features of myocardial infarction also.

Myxedema patients have high risk of bleeding because of acquired von Willebrand syndrome and reduction in coagulation factors V, VII, VIII, IX, and X. This risk is reversible with hormone replacement therapy.

Thyroid Storm

Thyroid storm is an acute life-threatening clinical situation of hyperthyroidism, which requires immediate intensive care monitoring and management. Hyperthyroidism can become thyroid storm when manifestations become life-threatening, which happens in patients with clinically overt hyperthyroidism.

Thyroid storm is defined as life-threatening exacerbation of hyperthyroid state with one or more organ dysfunction. Thyroid storm is a rare event and mostly affect hyperthyroid patients who are either inadequately treated or stopped treatment. Prevalence of thyroid storm can be 1% in patients with hyperthyroidism. Prognosis of untreated thyroid storm is unfavorable and can cause mortality as high as 10%, if urgent treatment initiated.

Precipitating Factors

Patient with hyperthyroidism will have history of partially treated hyperthyroidism or will have other manifestations of orbitopathy of Grave's disease. On this background, decompensation and precipitation of thyroid storm can happen because of secondary conditions such as surgery, stroke, diabetic ketoacidosis, infections, withdrawal of antithyroid medications, pregnancy, or radioiodine therapy. Also, use of iodinated contrast can precipitate thyroid storm.

Pathogenesis

It is difficult to predict which patient will decompensate, as levels of hormone remains same in patients with hyperthyroidism and thyroid storm. Mechanism with why thyroid storm occurs is uncertain. Several hypotheses are proposed for thyroid storm:

- Because of medical condition or acidosis, thyroid binding to carrier proteins become affected and leads to more free T3 and free T4 levels.
- There is effect at level of thyroid hormone receptor site at target tissues; leading to exaggerated response to adrenergic stimuli.

Signs and Symptoms

Thyroid storm is extreme spectrum of thyrotoxicosis, where one or more organ dysfunction happens. Thus, signs and symptoms can be varied. Cardiac symptoms are often predominant, and patient can present with tachyarrhythmias (atrial fibrillation, ventricular fibrillation), systolic hypertension with wide pulse pressure, systolic failure, and may be high output states with distributive heart failure states. Neurological manifestations include acute confusional state with delirium and psychosis.

Hyperthermia with temperature reaching 104–105°F is a very common finding in thyroid storm. Diarrhea, nausea, and abdominal pain are common gastrointestinal findings. Jaundice and hepatic failure can also be present. Other findings like weight loss, tremors, and restlessness are features which may suggest diagnosis of thyroid storm. These patients may have large goiter or have scar with history of partial thyroidectomy.

Diagnosis

Diagnosis of thyroid storm based on history of thyroid disease and eventual triggering factors; typical signs and symptoms and serum FT4 and FT3 concentrations exceeding the normal reference range and undetectable (<0.1 mIU/L) TSH levels. Diagnosis must be made on basis of clinical findings and waiting for results of test should not cause delay in initiation of effective urgent treatment.

Burch and Wartofsky introduced a score system to identify thyroid storm, which was based on following parameters: Temperature (ranging from 37.2 to >40°C); central nervous system effects (from mild agitation to coma, passing through the psychotic state); gastro-intestinal-hepatic dysfunction (including diarrhea, nausea/vomiting, abdominal pain, and unexplained jaundice); heartrate (ranging 90–140 bpm); atrial fibrillation; heart failure (low score pedal edema—high score pulmonary edema); and negative or positive precipitant history. A score of 45 or more is highly suggestive of thyroid storm; a score of 25–44 supports the diagnosis; a score below 25 makes thyroid storm unlikely.

As thyroid storm always occurs with stressor on background of partially treated or untreated thyrotoxicosis, immediate investigation to find out precipitating factors such as infections or other causes should be done. ECG and cardiac enzymes should be done to rule out acute coronary syndrome. Also, pregnancy should be excluded in women of childbearing age group.

Treatment

Once thyroid storm is identified, priority is resuscitation of patient, and these patients require urgent care. Main pillars of treatment are general supportive care and resuscitation and thyroid specific treatment. Thyroid specific treatment includes therapy to control the thyroid gland and therapy to block the effects of thyroid hormone on peripheral tissues. Along with these, equally important is detection and treatment of precipitating cause.

Initial Resuscitation and Supportive Care

Supportive care should include cooling measures, IV fluid for volume resuscitation, electrolyte replacement and nutritional support.

Temperature which can rise to as high as 104°F, needs urgent interventions with antipyretics and external cooling measures. Salicylates should be avoided as antipyretics, as they bind with thyroid binding proteins.

Tachyarrhythmias are other dreaded complication requiring urgent care. If tachyarrhythmias are associated with hemodynamic instability, it should be managed with urgent cardioversion. Antiarrhythmics should be the treatment if patients are hemodynamically stable. Along with antiarrhythmics, electrolyte correction is equally important.

In thyroid storm, patient may have increased metabolic and oxygen demands, and may need ventilatory support either with noninvasive or intubation and invasive ventilation.

Severe agitation and psychosis may interfere in assessment and appropriate treatment of patients. Sedatives such as benzodiazepines or haloperidol may be given to control agitation state.

Nutrition support is important and should include vitamin replacement. Thyroid storm patients need close monitoring of glucose levels, as there will be liver glycogen store depletion. Corticosteroids are routinely needed to be given to tackle underlying adrenal insufficiency.

Thyroid Specific Treatment

Goals of thyroid specific treatment are preventing synthesis and release of thyroid hormone, and also to decrease peripheral action of thyroid hormone. Therapy can be summarized as 5 B's—block synthesis, block release, block conversion, block peripheral effects, and block enterohepatic circulation.

Block thyroid hormone synthesis: Thiouracils (propylthiouracil) and imidazoles (methimazole or carbimazole) are two classes of drug, which prevent thyroid hormone synthesis by inhibiting thyroperoxidase, the enzyme responsible for oxidizing the iodide anion. Propylthiouracil also have some effect of preventing peripheral conversion of T4 to T3. Carbimazole has a longer half-life than propylthiouracil.

In nonthyroid storm patients' imidazole is a drug of choice. Studies comparing efficacy of methimazole versus propylthiouracil, showed better efficacy of low dose methimazole and thus propylthiouracil cannot be recommended as initial treatment because of poor efficacy and side-effects profile.

However, in thyroid storm patients, propylthiouracil should be the drug of choice as it has rapid onset of action and also prevents peripheral conversion, if T4 to T3, leading to rapid decrease in T3 levels.

Block release of thyroid hormone: Inorganic iodine (potassium iodide, ipodate sodium) blocks release of T4 and T3 from thyroid gland. Also, large doses of iodine inhibit organification of iodine (Wolff–Chaikoff effect). But iodine transport system gets used to higher concentration of iodine and will restart synthesis of thyroid hormone, thus, iodide therapy is best combined with methimazole, to block synthesis of thyroid hormone.

Lithium has demonstrated control of thyrotoxicosis in nonstorming patients having contraindication for propylthiouracil and carbimezole. Use of lithium in thyroid storm is limited, as more effective and less toxic agents exist. But lithium can be used in patient's intolerant of potassium iodide.

Blocks peripheral T4 to T3 conversion: Many drugs can stop peripheral conversion of T4 hormone to active T3 hormone. Drugs which can be used are propylthiouracil, corticosteroids, propranolol, and iodide contrast—ipodate sodium.

Blockade of the peripheral effects of thyroid hormone: To block adrenergic effects of thyroid hormone, β-blockers should be initiated immediately, as most immediate consequences of thyroid storm are cardiovascular. Propranolol is a β-blocker of choice, as it has effect on peripheral conversion of T4 to T3, but all β-blockers are equally effective in improving signs and symptoms of thyrotoxicosis. In thyroid storm, oral propranolol in dose of 60–120 mg 6 hourly is the starting dose. In severe cases, titrated doses of IV propranolol or rapid acting agents such as esmolol can be initiated.

Blockade of enterohepatic recirculation of thyroxine: Normally, T3 is metabolized in conjugation with glucuronide and sulfate, and then excreted in bile. Free thyroid hormone excreted in bile is reabsorbed in intestine and thus intestine becomes a large reservoir of thyroid hormone. Cholestyramine is bile sequestrant which blocks reabsorption of free thyroid hormone excreted in bile and thus reduces circulating free T3 and T4 levels.

Extracorporeal Therapies

Plasmapheresis can be used to remove circulating thyroid hormone, especially in refractory cases to medical therapies or severe thyroid storm with multiorgan system failure. Each session of plasmapheresis removes about 20% of T4 pool and even less of T4 pool, thus plasmapheresis needs to be repeated several times.

Charcoal hemoperfusion is another effective therapy which has shown clearance rate for T3 and was even higher than with plasmapheresis.

Thyroidectomy

Thyroidectomy is occasionally only option available in management of thyroid storm which is refractory to medical therapy. Thyroidectomy may be associated with exacerbation of thyroid storm, if preoperative thyroid hormone levels are very high.

SUMMARY

Thyroid emergencies are uncommon problems in ICU patients, but early identification and immediate treatment of both thyroid storm and myxedema coma may be lifesaving.

SUGGESTED READING

1. Binimelis J, Bassas L, Marruecos L, Rodriguez J, Domingo ML, Madoz P, et al. Massive thyroxine intoxication: evaluation of plasma extraction. Intensive Care Med. 1987;13(1):33-8.
2. Bogazzi F, Bartalena L, Campomori A, Brogioni S, Traino C, De Martino F, et al. Treatment with lithium prevents serum thyroid hormone increase after thionamide withdrawal and radioiodine therapy in patients with Graves' disease. J Clin Endocrinol Metab. 2002;87(10):4490-5.
3. Burch HB, Wartofsky L. Life-threatening thyrotoxicosis. Thyroid storm. Endocrinol Metab Clin North Am. 1993;22(2):263-77.
4. Burger AG, Philippe J. Thyroid emergencies. Baillieres Clin Endocrinol Metab. 1992;6(1):77-93.
5. Chabot J. Myxedematous coma and terminal forms of untreated myxedema. Cah Coll Med Hop Paris. 1964;258:215-20.
6. Cooper DS, Saxe VC, Meskell M, Maloof F, Ridgway EC. Acute effects of propylthiouracil (PTU) on thyroidal iodide organification and peripheral iodothyronine deiodination: correlation with serum PTU levels measured by radioimmunoassay. J Clin Endocrinol Metab. 1982;54(1):101-7.
7. Dillmann WH. Thyroid storm. Curr Ther Endocrinol Metab. 1997;6:81-5.
8. Herrmann J, Rudorff KH, Gockenjan G, Konigshausen T, Grabensee B, Kruskemper HL, et al. Charcoal haemoperfusion in thyroid storm. The Lancet. 1977;1(8005):248.
9. Holvey DN, Goodner CJ, Nikoloff JT, Dowling JT. Treatment of myxedema coma with intravenous thyroxine. Arch Intern Med. 1964;113:139-46.
10. Klubo-Gwiezdzinska J, Wartofsky L. Myxedema coma. In: Wass JAH, Stewart PM (Eds). Oxford Textbook of Endocrinology and Diabetes, 2nd edition. Oxford: Oxford University Press; 2011. pp. 537-43.
11. Klubo-Gwiezdzinska J, Wartofsky L. Thyroid emergencies. Med Clin North Am. 2012;96(2):385-403.
12. Kreisner E, Lutzky M, Gross JL. Charcoal hemoperfusion in the treatment of levothyroxine intoxication. Thyroid. 2010;20(2):209-12.
13. Lanska D, Harsch HH. Hypothermic coma associated with thioradizine in a myxedematous patient. J Clin Psychiatry. 1984;45(4):188-9.

14. Lechner MG, Angell TE. Severe Thyrotoxicosis and Thyroid Storm. In: Garg RK, Hennessey JV, Malabanan AO, Garber JR (Eds). Handbook of Inpatient Endocrinology, 1st edition. Switzerland AG: Springer Cham; 2020. pp. 33-42.
15. Manfredi E, vanZaane B, Gerdes VE, Brandjes DP, Squizzato A. Hypothyroidism and acquired vonWillebrand's syndrome: a systematic review. Haemophilia. 2008;14(3):423-33.
16. Moore AP, Macfarlane IA, Blumhardt LD. Neuroleptic malignant syndrome and hypothyroidism. J Neurol Neurosurg Psychiatry. 1990;53(6):517-8.
17. Nakamura H, Noh JY, Itoh K, Fukata S, Miyauchi A, Hamada N, et al. Comparison of methimazole and propylthiouracil in patients with hyperthyroidism caused by Graves' disease. J Clin Endocrinol Metab. 2007;92(6):2157-62.
18. Nayak B, Burman K. Thyrotoxicosis and thyroid storm. Endocrinol Metab Clin North Am. 2006;35(4):663-86.
19. Ng YW, Tiu SC, Choi KL, Chan FK, Choi CH, Kong PS, et al. Use of lithium in the treatment of thyrotoxicosis. Hong Kong Med J. 2006;12(4):254-9.
20. Pasleau R, Lederer J. The myxedematous coma. Ann Endocrinol (Paris). 1964;25:103-6.
21. Ringel MD. Management of hypothyroidism and hyperthyroidism in the intensive care unit. Crit Care Clin. 2001;17(1):59-74.
22. Roti E, Robuschi G, Gardini E, Montermini M, Salvi M, Manfredi A, et al. Comparison of methimazole, methimazole and sodium ipodate, and methimazole and saturated solution of potassium iodide in the early treatment of hyperthyroid Graves'disease. Clin Endocrinol. 1988;28(3):305-14.
23. Sarlis NJ, Gourgiotis L. Thyroid emergencies. Rev Endocr Metab Disord. 2003;4(2):129-36.
24. Shaheen M. Severe congestive heart failure patient on amiodarone presenting with myxedemic coma: a case report. Indian Heart J. 2009;61(4):392-3.
25. Solomon BL, Wartofsky L, Burman KD. Adjunctive cholestyramine therapy for thyrotoxicosis. Clin Endocrinol. 1993;38(1):39-43.
26. Tsatsoulis A, Johnson EO, Kalogera CH, Seferiadis K, Tsolas O. The effect of thyrotoxicosis on adrenocortical reserve. Eur J Endocrinol. 2000;142(3):231-5.
27. Turhan NO, Kockar MC, Inegöl I. Myxematous coma in a laboring woman suggested a pre-eclamptic coma: a case report. Acta Obstet Gynecol Scand. 2004;83(11):1089-91.
28. Wartofsky L. Myxedema coma. In: Braverman LE, Utiger RD (Eds). The Thyroid: A Fundamental and Clinical Text, 7th edition. Philadelphia: Lippincott-Raven; 1995. p. 871.
29. Weber C, Scholz GH, Lamesch P, Paschke R. Thyroidectomy in iodine induced thyrotoxic storm. Exp Clin Endocrinol Diabetes. 1998;107(7):468-72.
30. Zwillich CW, Pierson DJ, Hofeldt FD, Lufkin EG, Weil JV. Ventilatory control in myxedema and hypothyroidism. New Engl J Med. 1975;292(13):662.

SECTION 8

Oncological Emergencies

CHAPTER

34

Metabolic Oncological Emergencies

Pragnasree Ravulapalli

INTRODUCTION

Oncological emergencies are life-threatening conditions that can arise in cancer patients due to the disease itself or as a result of treatment. These emergencies are categorized into metabolic, hematologic, structural, and treatment-related emergencies. Here are the main oncological emergencies:

- *Metabolic emergencies:*
    - *Tumor lysis syndrome (TLS):* Caused by the rapid breakdown of tumor cells, leading to elevated levels of potassium, phosphate, and uric acid, which can cause renal failure, arrhythmias, and metabolic imbalances.
    - *Hypercalcemia of malignancy:* Elevated calcium levels due to cancer (commonly breast, lung, or multiple myeloma), which can cause confusion, dehydration, kidney failure, and cardiac arrhythmias.
    - *Syndrome of inappropriate antidiuretic hormone secretion (SIADH):* Syndrome of inappropriate antidiuretic hormone secretion, often seen in small cell lung cancer, leading to low sodium levels, confusion, seizures, and coma.
- *Hematologic emergencies:*
    - *Febrile neutropenia:* A fever in a patient with low neutrophil counts, often due to chemotherapy, which increases the risk of severe infections.
    - *Disseminated intravascular coagulation (DIC):* Widespread clotting throughout the body, leading to both clot formation and bleeding, often seen in leukemia, pancreatic cancer, or metastatic cancers.
    - *Hyperviscosity syndrome:* Seen in multiple myeloma or Waldenström's macroglobulinemia, where increased blood thickness can cause visual disturbances, headache, stroke, or heart failure.
- *Structural emergencies:*
    - *Spinal cord compression:* Caused by tumor invasion or metastasis to the vertebrae, leading to back pain, sensory and motor deficits, and potential paralysis if untreated.

    - *Superior vena cava (SVC) syndrome:* Compression or obstruction of the SVC, often due to lung cancer or lymphoma, leading to facial swelling, shortness of breath, and venous congestion.
    - *Increased intracranial pressure:* Due to brain metastases or primary brain tumors, which can cause headache, vomiting, vision changes, and altered mental status.
    - *Malignant pleural effusion:* Accumulation of fluid around the lungs, causing shortness of breath, chest pain, and hypoxia.
    - *Malignant pericardial effusion:* Fluid accumulation around the heart, leading to cardiac tamponade, with symptoms of hypotension, tachycardia, and shortness of breath.
    - *Airway obstruction:* Often due to head and neck cancers, lung tumors, or metastases compressing the trachea, causing respiratory distress or stridor.
- *Treatment-related emergencies:*
    - *Anaphylaxis from chemotherapy:* Severe allergic reaction to chemotherapy or biologic agents, leading to airway constriction, shock, and death if not treated immediately.
    - *Extravasation of chemotherapy agents:* Leakage of vesicant chemotherapy into surrounding tissues, causing severe tissue damage.
    - *Cytokine release syndrome (CRS):* Seen with immunotherapies like CAR-T cell therapy, leading to systemic inflammatory responses such as fever, hypotension, and multi-organ dysfunction.
    - *Radiation-induced emergencies:* Including radiation pneumonitis, pericarditis, or bowel perforation from excessive exposure to radiation therapy.

These oncological emergencies require prompt diagnosis and treatment to prevent serious complications or death.

HYPERCALCEMIA OF MALIGNANCY

Hypercalcemia, although can be associated with any malignancy but is most commonly associated with breast cancer, lung cancer, non-Hodgkin's lymphoma, and multiple myeloma. The incidence is noted to be around 10–30%. Hypercalcemia with levels >13 mg/dL at the time of presentation should raise suspicion of malignancy and needs to be ruled out.

Classification

Based on the levels of serum calcium, hypercalcemia is classified as mild 10–12 mg/dL, moderate 12–14 mg/dL, or severe >14 mg/dL. Ionized calcium levels should be measured. Corrected calcium level for serum albumin is calculated using the following formula: Serum calcium + 0.8 × (4 – patient's albumin level); 4.0 is the normal albumin level in g/dL.

Pathophysiology

The pathophysiology of hypercalcemia of malignancy is explained mainly through three mechanisms:

1. Excessive secretion of parathyroid hormone-related protein (PTHrP).
2. Bony metastases with the release of osteoclast activating factors.
3. The production of 1,25-dihydroxy vitamin D (calcitriol).

The PTHrP increases bone resorption, increased phosphate excretion from the proximal tubules, and calcium reabsorption from the distal tubules in the kidney. Lab findings include elevated PTHrP, low to normal parathyroid hormone (PTH), and normal 1,25-dihydroxy vitamin D levels. Bony metastases causing the release of osteoclast activating factors are commonly seen in patients with multiple myeloma and solid organ tumors, which metastasize to bones, such as breast cancer. Lab findings include skeletal metastasis with low to low-normal PTH, PTHrP, and 1,25-dihydroxy vitamin D levels. Granulomatous diseases such as sarcoidosis and tuberculosis as well as most Hodgkin and non-Hodgkin lymphomas cause hypercalcemia by increasing 1,25-dihydroxy vitamin D production. These patients respond well to steroids.

Clinical Manifestations

Hypercalcemia has nonspecific presentation and physical examination findings. Symptoms are often vague with most common presentation being anorexia, nausea, vomiting, and constipation but can present as malaise, polyuria, polydipsia, lethargy, confusion, cognitive disturbance, and even coma. These symptoms indicate a volume depleted state secondary to osmotic diuresis from hypercalcemia. Cardiac manifestations are usually rhythm disturbances with short QTc intervals. Gastrointestinal (GI) involvement presents as pancreatitis and peptic ulcer disease.

Hypercalcemia can result in nephrogenic diabetes insipidus and renal insufficiency to distal renal tubular acidosis secondary to nephrolithiasis. Musculoskeletal symptoms can manifest as muscle weakness and bone pain.

Investigations

A detailed medication history including calcium supplements, multivitamins and prescription drugs, family history, dietary history, and medical history suggestive of prior granulomatous disease along with baseline investigations can help identify the cause of hypercalcemia.

Baseline investigations should include PTH levels, 25 hydroxy vitamin D levels, 24-hour urinary calcium levels along with free and ionized calcium levels. If vitamin D levels are within the normal range serum electrophoresis, urine electrophoresis with immunofixation, and serum-free light chains can help rule out multiple myeloma.

Treatment

The goal of initial emergent treatment is to restore the intravascular volume and increase urinary calcium excretion. This is achieved by aggressive hydration with intravenous (IV) fluids, usually normal saline at the rate of 200–300 L/h and target a urine output of >100 mL/h. In patients with heart failure or renal failure intravenous fluid (IVF) needs to be used with caution.

In addition to IV hydration, loop diuretics, calcitonin, bisphosphonates, and denosumab play a significant role in treatment of hypercalcemia.

Loop diuretics, after adequate resuscitation help promote urinary calcium excretion by inhibiting calcium reabsorption at the loop of Henle.

Calcitonin is rapid acting within 4–6 hours and effects lasting for 2 days. It helps prevent bone resorption and increase urinary calcium excretion. Dose is 4 IU/kg.

Bisphosphonates have a delayed onset of action at 2–3 days with effects lasting for 3–4 weeks. Recommended dosing includes Zoledronic acid 4 mg IV over 15–30 minutes or pamidronate 60–90 mg IV over 2 hours once a month. Major side effects include osteonecrosis of the jaw and nephrotoxicity.

In patients with renal failure or nonresponse to bisphosphonates, *denosumab*-receptor activator of nuclear factor-kappa-B ligand (RANKL) inhibitor is preferred.

Glucocorticoids inhibit the conversion of 25-hydroxyvitamin D to calcitriol, decreasing gut absorption and renal reabsorption of calcium. A dose of IV hydrocortisone 200–300 mg/day is useful in patients with granulomatous diseases.

In patients dependent on hemodialysis or hypercalcemia secondary to parathyroid cancer calcimimetic agents, such as cinacalcet are preferred.

When all medical therapies fail, or in patients with fluid restriction such as heart failure patients hemodialysis is the treatment modality of choice.

The serum phosphorus levels need to be monitored and repleted along with other medical therapies as hypophosphatemia makes management difficult.

TUMOR LYSIS SYNDROME

Tumor lysis syndrome is one of the most common oncologic emergency which can be life-threatening. It can occur as a result of initiation of chemotherapy or even spontaneously. The rapid destruction of tumor cells causes an abrupt release of intracellular ions, nucleic acids, proteins

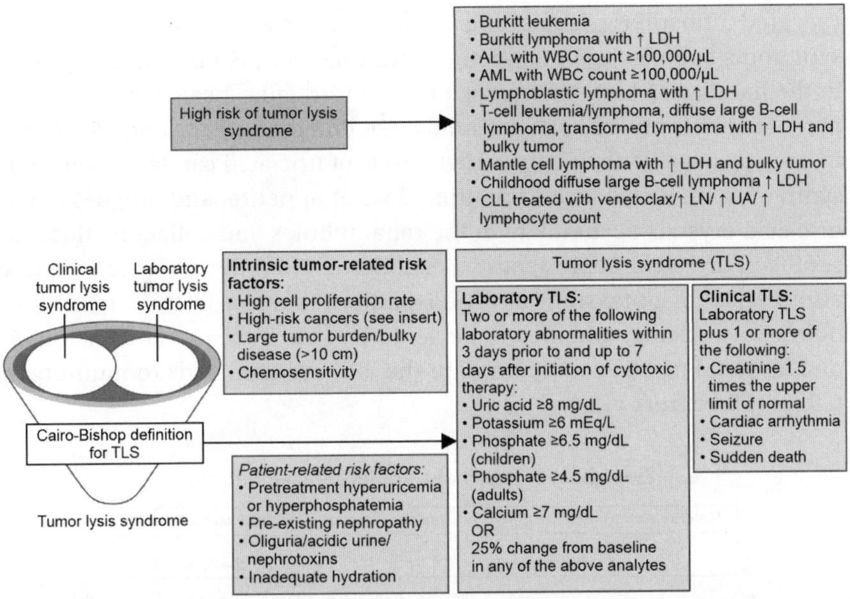

Fig. 1: Risk factors and diagnosis of "tumor lysis syndrome". (ALL: acute lymphoblastic leukemia; AML: acute myeloid leukemia; CLL: chronic lymphocytic leukemia; LDH: lactate dehydrogenase; LN: lymph node; UA: uric acid; WBC: white blood cell)
Source: Adapted from Puri I, Sharma D, Gunturu KS, Ahmed AA. Diagnosis and management of tumor lysis syndrome. J Community Hosp Intern Med Perspect. 2020;10(3):269-72.

and their metabolites into the extracellular space causing hyperkalemia, hyperphosphatemia, hypocalcemia, and hyperuricemia. These biochemical derangements can cause renal dysfunction, cardiac arrhythmias, central nervous system (CNS) toxicity, and sometimes even death **(Fig. 1)**.

Tumor lysis syndrome can occur within a few hours or even before chemotherapy but is most commonly seen 12–72 hours after initiation of treatment.

Diagnosis and Risk Factors

Cairo and Bishop classified TLS according to clinical and laboratory features.

Pathophysiology and Clinical Features

When cancer cells break down, they release potassium, phosphorus, and nucleic acids, which are then converted into hypoxanthine, followed by xanthine, and ultimately uric acid. Hyperkalemia can result in symptoms such as fatigue, nausea, vomiting, diarrhea, muscle weakness, tingling sensations, and ECG changes including elevated tented T waves, a widened QRS complex, and potentially life-threatening ventricular arrhythmias.

Elevated phosphate levels and subsequent low calcium can lead to symptoms such as loss of appetite, vomiting, confusion, muscle spasms in the hands and feet, tetany, seizures, and irregular heartbeats. Calcium pyrophosphate crystals can accumulate in different organs and play a role in causing acute kidney injury. High levels of uric acid can lead to general symptoms such as nausea, vomiting, loss of appetite, and fatigue. When uric acid crystals accumulate in the renal tubules and collecting ducts, it results in uric acid nephropathy. Renal dysfunction decreases the urinary elimination of potassium and phosphate, resulting in fluid retention, pulmonary edema, and metabolic acidosis. This increases the likelihood of additional urate accumulation in the kidneys and leads to multiorgan failure **(Flowchart 1)**.

Flowchart 1: Treatment stratification algorithm.

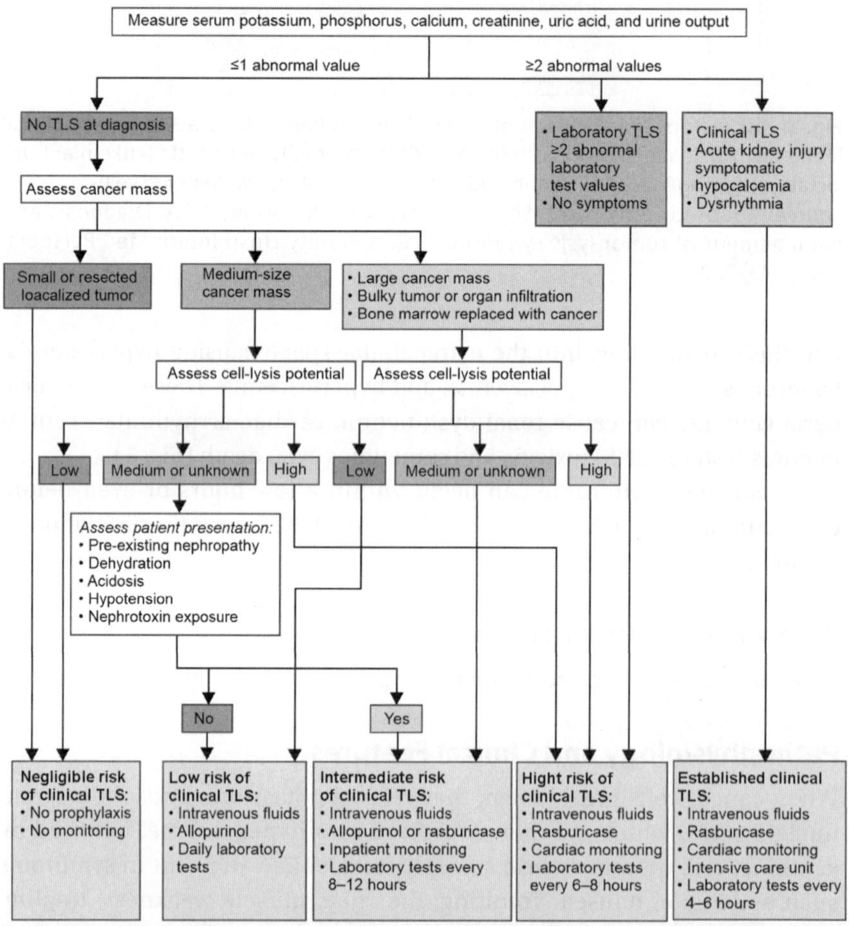

Source: Adapted from Howard SC, Jones DP, Pui CH. The tumor lysis syndrome. N Engl J Med. 2011;364(19):1844-54.

Risk Assessment

Flowchart 1 shows the algorithm of treatment stratification.

Management

The primary preventive strategies for patients at risk of TLS include monitoring, maintaining hydration, and administering hypouricemic therapy. Patients without existing clinical TLS can be classified into low, intermediate, and high-risk groups.

Preventive strategies for high-risk patients: Monitor urine output, fluid balance, and electrolytes. Perform biochemistry tests every 6 hours at first, then reduce frequency based on the patient's clinical response. Ensure proper hydration through intravenous fluids (typically $3L/m^2$/day, avoiding potassium) and target a urine output of 100 mL/h. Loop diuretics may be appropriate for patients with reduced urine output. Consider deferring chemotherapy for 24–48 hours to ensure proper hydration and urine output, based on the clinical urgency. On the other hand, a prephase treatment with reduced intensity, such as initial steroid treatment alone for individuals with acute lymphoblastic leukemia (ALL) should be considered.

Rasburicase (0.2 mg/kg in 50 mL of normal saline administered over 30 minutes) may be given for a duration of up to 7 days. This recombinant urate oxidase facilitates the conversion of uric acid into allantoin, a compound that is water soluble and excreted efficiently by the kidneys. Uric acid levels may decrease within 4 hours, enhance kidney function, and subsequently lower phosphate levels. No adjustment of the dose is necessary for those with kidney or liver impairment. Possible side effects include a rash and urticariia caused by an allergic reaction. Methemoglobinemia, glucose-6-phosphate dehydrogenase (G6PD) deficiency, or any conditions that may lead to hemolytic anemia are the contraindications for the use of rasburicase.

Allopurinol may be administered either orally or intravenously following the completion of rasburicase treatment. Allopurinol prevents the conversion of xanthines into uric acid. As this would diminish the effectiveness of rasburicase, they should not be administered simultaneously.

Prevention for moderate-risk patients: This should involve adequate hydration with intravenous fluids. It is advisable to monitor urine output in hospital inpatients alongside biochemical assessments, initially every 12 hours. Allopurinol should be initiated 1–2 days prior to treatment and continued for 3–7 days afterward. It can be administered either orally or intravenously at a dosage of 300 mg/m^2/day, with a maximum limit of 600 mg/day, divided into one to three doses. Dose adjustments are necessary for individuals with renal or hepatic impairment.

Low-risk patients can be monitored on outpatient basis by achieving hydration orally.

Urinary alkalization (e.g., with sodium bicarbonate) has been utilized to enhance uric acid excretion, but it reduces the solubility of calcium phosphate and lacks supporting evidence for its effectiveness. It is no longer advised and should be avoided in cases of established TLS, if rasburicase has been administered or if phosphate levels are high.

Established Tumor Lysis Syndrome

- *Renal management:* The treatment of TLS follows the basic principles as its prevention and rasburicase is advised. Electrolyte levels should be checked every 4–6 hours initially, along with ongoing cardiac monitoring. Fluid balance should be adjusted to achieve a urine output exceeding 100 mL/h. If hydration is adequate, a loop diuretic may be considered.

  The criteria for initiating renal replacement therapy are akin to other types of acute kidney injury, although the threshold for intervention is lower. Indications include early-stage renal failure, persistent electrolyte imbalances, fluid overload that does not respond to diuretics, and symptoms resulting from uremia, such as pericarditis or encephalopathy. Continuous venovenous methods (such as hemofiltration, hemodiafiltration, and hemodialysis) utilize filters with larger pore sizes, which may enable quicker phosphate removal in comparison to conventional dialysis.
- *Electrolyte imbalances:* Hyperkalemia necessitates ongoing cardiac monitoring. A rapid decrease in potassium (when levels exceed 6.5 or with associated ECG changes) can be achieved by administering 50 mL of a 50% dextrose solution containing 20 units of human "Actrapid" insulin over the course of 1 hour. Calcium gluconate (10 mL of 10% solution over 2–3 minutes) can be administered in cases of cardiac arrhythmias to help to stabilize the heart muscle; however, this effect is transient, and dialysis may be required.

  Hypocalcemia and hyperphosphatemia: Asymptomatic hypocalcemia does not need treatment (as treatment may lead to the formation of calcium phosphate). In symptomatic patients, short-term management can be achieved by infusing 10 mL of 10% calcium gluconate over 10 minutes. Cardiac monitoring is required throughout the infusion, and dialysis should be considered.

  The best approach to managing asymptomatic hyperphosphatemia initially involves providing optimal renal support. Phosphate binders like aluminum hydroxide (administered orally at 50–100 mg/kg/day for a maximum of 1–2 days) or sevelamer (2.4–4.8 g/day) can be considered, but may not be well-tolerated. In cases of severe hyperphosphatemia, dialysis is necessary.

SYNDROME OF INAPPROPRIATE ANTIDIURETIC HORMONE SECRETION

It is a significant metabolic oncological emergency. It occurs when excess antidiuretic hormone (ADH) is secreted, leading to water retention and dilutional "hyponatremia" (low sodium levels). This condition is commonly associated with certain cancers, particularly "small cell lung cancer", but can also be triggered by other malignancies like head and neck cancers, or as a side effect of chemotherapy.

Pathophysiology

In SIADH, the excessive ADH secretion causes the kidneys to retain water, diluting the sodium in the bloodstream and resulting in "hyponatremia". This water retention does not lead to edema but causes intracellular swelling, particularly affecting the brain.

Symptoms

- *Early:* Nausea, headache, fatigue.
- *Severe:* Confusion, seizures, coma, and potentially death due to cerebral edema from the hyponatremia.

Management

Treatment includes "fluid restriction", salt supplementation, and in severe cases, medications like "demeclocycline" or "vasopressin receptor antagonists". Rapid correction of sodium must be avoided to prevent osmotic demyelination syndrome.

SUMMARY

Oncologic metabolic abnormalities are life-threatening conditions that arise due to cancer or its treatment. Key metabolic emergencies include "TLS", "hypercalcemia of malignancy", and "SIADH".

- "Hypercalcemia of malignancy" results from increased calcium levels, commonly in cancers like breast or lung cancer, causing symptoms like confusion, dehydration, and arrhythmias.
- "TLS" occurs when cancer cells break down rapidly, releasing large amounts of potassium, phosphate, and uric acid into the bloodstream, leading to kidney failure, arrhythmias, and metabolic imbalances.
- "SIADH" leads to hyponatremia, or low sodium levels, seen in cancers like small cell lung cancer, causing confusion, seizures, or coma.

Early recognition and treatment of these metabolic disturbances, including hydration, medications, and electrolyte management, are crucial to prevent severe complications and improve patient outcomes.

SUGGESTED READING

1. Cairo MS, Bishop M. Tumour lysis syndrome: new therapeutic strategies and classification. Br J Haematol. 2004;127(1):3-11.
2. Cairo MS, Coiffier B, Reiter A, Younes A. Recommendations for the evaluation of risk and prophylaxis of tumour lysis syndrome (TLS) in adults and children with malignant diseases: an expert TLS panel consensus. Br J Haematol. 2010;149:578-86.
3. Howard SC, Jones DP, Pui CH. The tumor lysis syndrome. N Engl J Med. 2011;364(19):1844-54.
4. Klemencic S, Perkins J. Diagnosis and management of oncologic emergencies. West J Emerg Med. 2019;20(2):316-22.
5. Puri I, Sharma D, Gunturu KS, Ahmed AA. Diagnosis and management of tumor lysis syndrome. J Community Hosp Intern Med Perspect. 2020;10(3):269-72.
6. Vakiti A, Anastasopoulou C, Mewawalla P. Malignancy-related hypercalcemia. In: StatPearls [Internet]. Treasure Island (FL): StatPearls Publishing; 2023.

SECTION

9 Infectious Disorders

CHAPTER

35

Fever in ICU

Neha Patel

INTRODUCTION

The fever in the intensive care unit (ICU) could be a continued manifestation of the disease/disorder that prompted the ICU admission or other unique etiologies in the ICU which could result from interventions or therapies provided during ICU care or due to systemic inflammatory response syndrome (SIRS), septic, metabolic, or neuroendocrine response.

The infectious diseases society of America has defined fever as single oral temperature >37.8°C (~100°F), repeated temperature of >37.2°C (~99°F; oral) or >37.5°C (~99.5°F; rectal).

Immunocompromised or neutropenic patients do not mount an appropriate febrile response. Also, the clinical, laboratory, and radiological manifestations of inflammation/infection would be scanty or absent in these patients in the initial stages. In patients with neutropenia due to chemotherapy fever is defined as single oral temperature ≥38.3°C (101°F) or >38.0°C (~100.4°F) sustained over at least 1 hour.

Not all patients with infection manifest fever as in patients who are on extracorporeal membrane oxygenation (ECMO).

Not all febrile episodes will need investigations such as fever post-operative procedure is common because of SIRS. SIRS is an exaggerated defense response of the body to a noxious stress (surgery, infection, trauma, acute inflammation, ischemia, or reperfusion, etc.) to localize and then eliminate the endogenous or exogenous source of the insult.

Fever has been associated with an increased length of stay and cost of care. Fever may also result in poor outcomes in patients with pancreatitis, traumatic head injury, or subarachnoid hemorrhage.

ETIOLOGY

Common infectious causes in ICU are ventilator-associated pneumonia (VAP), catheter-related bloodstream infections, surgical site infections, urinary tract infections related to catheters, and bacteremias of various origins.

Central Nervous System

Infectious: Meningitis, encephalitis, brain abscess

Noninfectious: Cerebral infarction, cerebral hemorrhage, subarachnoid hemorrhage

Respiratory

Infectious: VAP, sinusitis

Noninfectious: Acute respiratory distress syndrome (ARDS), atelectasis, pulmonary embolism, chemical pneumonitis

Abdominal

Infectious: Nosocomial diarrhea

Noninfectious: Acalculous cholecystitis, ischemic bowel, gastrointestinal bleeding, acute pancreatitis

Cardiovascular

Infectious: Infective endocarditis, catheter-related bloodstream infection

Noninfectious: Myocardial infarction, deep vein thrombosis, pericarditis, thrombophlebitis

Renal

Pyelonephritis

Skin and Soft Tissue, Bone, and Joints

Infectious: Septic arthritis, osteomyelitis, cellulitis, abscess

Noninfectious: Decubitus ulcers, gout

Autoimmune

Systemic lupus erythematosus (SLE)

Endocrine

Noninfectious: Adrenal insufficiency, thyroid storm, pheochromocytoma

Miscellaneous

Infectious: Bacteremias of multifocal origin

Noninfectious: Drug fever, drug/alcohol withdrawal, postoperative fever, fat embolism, reaction to the contrast agent, transfusion reaction, malignancy, Stevens–Johnson syndrome.

Fever etiology unique or exclusive to the ICU setting include:
- Ventilator-associated pneumonia
- Central line-associated bloodstream infection (CLABSI)
- Catheter-associated urinary tract infection (CAUTI)
- *Clostridium difficile* colitis
- Pressure ulcer
- Surgical wound-related infection

CLINICAL EVALUATION

- A detailed history and a thorough physical examination.
- To check whether infectious and noninfectious cause of the fever.
- Need to examine vascular access sites, urinary catheters, drain sites, and surgical incision sites.
- Heart sounds to rule out a clue for infective endocarditis.
- Tracheal secretions for color, odor, purulence, and quantity.
- The skin and soft tissue evaluation for cellulitis, furunculosis, and paronychia.
- Skin findings such as ulcers, nodules, vesicles, pilonidal sinus, and lesions such as erythema multiforme and ecthyma gangrenosum might be the subtle sign of infectious etiology and need to look for in neutropenic or immunosuppressed patients specifically. Perianal infections are often missed in neutropenic patients.
- The subtle or silent sources of infection such as sinusitis, decubitus ulcers, dental or tonsillar infections, perineal wounds, and abscesses, all of which need a high degree of clinical suspicion.
- Drug history should be reviewed, and drug fever is a diagnosis of exclusion.

INVESTIGATIONS

Biochemistry and Microbiology

- *Lactate:* High lactate levels are usually seen in sepsis. This is due to the increased lactate production due to anaerobic metabolism and reduced clearance.
- Complete blood count and kidney and liver function tests
- Serum amylase and lipase
- Central venous line cultures (sampling at two lumens) and peripherally drawn cultures (fever without obvious source and who have a central venous catheter; and simultaneous collection from central catheter and peripheral to allow calculation of differential time to positivity).
- Blood cultures (when performing blood cultures in adults), at least two sets of blood cultures, ideally 60 mL of blood total, one after the other, from different anatomical sites.

- Urine cultures [patients with pyuria and whom urinary tract infection (UTI) is suspected, to replace the urinary catheter and obtaining urine cultures from the newly placed catheter].
- Severe acute respiratory syndrome coronavirus-2 (SARS COVID 2) polymerase chain reaction (PCR) (for critically-ill patient with new onset of fever), based on level of community transmission.
- Biomarkers such as C-reactive protein (CRP) and procalcitonin (PCT) with rapid turnover time can be used as adjuncts in the early diagnosis of sepsis while awaiting microbiological cultures results. When these biomarkers are used in conjunction with clinical assessment they may guide antimicrobial therapy.
  - *PCT:* A precursor hormone of calcitonin produced by the parafollicular cells of the thyroid gland and neuroendocrine cells of the lung and the intestine that is thought to discriminate the systemic response due to bacterial causes from viral and noninfectious etiologies, but recent studies show PCT may be elevated during severe viral infections.
  - *CRP:* An acute-phase protein synthesized in the liver which rises in response to inflammation/infection. CRP has cell-membrane-binding capability which occurs following attachment to the phosphocholine in exposed cell membranes during cell injury, and phosphocholine in polysaccharides from cell envelopes of bacterial pathogens present in infections. In deciding whether to use CRP or PCT, the literature does not strongly favor one over the other. PCT and CRP provide supportive and complementary information to clinical assessment.

RADIOLOGY

- Chest radiograph
- Ultrasound (in any patients with either abdominal symptoms or suspicion of an abdominal source or recent abdominal surgery)
- Computed tomography (CT) (in patients who have recently undergone thoracic, abdominal, or pelvic surgery if an etiology is not readily identified).

SUMMARY

Fever in patients admitted to ICU can have different clinical syndrome and accordingly different etiologies. It can be either infectious or non-infectious. When we discuss about new onset fever in ICU that will have unique causes which includes VAP, CLABSI, CAUTI, *C. difficile* infection, etc. In that case pathogens causing the illness can be multi-drug resistant and can be different on different floors, in different ICU of the same hospital. As we know in India carbapenem resistant organisms and colistin breakthrough pathogens are predominant pathogens for nosocomial infections which are also associated with high mortality and morbidity due to limited treatment options. It is crucial to identify cause of fever with appropriate scientific approach depending upon the clinical syndrome for better outcome.

SUGGESTED READING

1. Achaiah NC, Bhutta BS, AK AK. Fever in the Intensive Care Patient. [Updated 2023 Aug 17]. In: StatPearls [Internet]. Treasure Island (FL): StatPearls Publishing; Jan 2024. Available from: https://www.ncbi.nlm.nih.gov/books/NBK570583/
2. O'Grady NP, Alexander E, Alhazzani W, Alshamsi F, Cuellar-Rodriguez J, Jefferson BK. Society of Critical Care Medicine and the Infectious Diseases Society of America Guidelines for Evaluating New Fever in Adult Patients in the ICU. Crit Care Med. 2023;51(11):1570-86.

CHAPTER

36 Syndromic Approach to Antibiotic Use

Neha Patel

PNEUMONIA

COMMUNITY-ACQUIRED PNEUMONIA

Streptococcus pneumoniae is still the single most common pathogen in all age groups except newborns and accounts for two-thirds of bacteremia cases in adults and most frequent cause of lethal community-acquired pneumonia (CAP). *Mycoplasma pneumoniae, Legionella* spp., *Chlamydia pneumoniae, Haemophilus influenzae, Moraxella catarrhalis*, respiratory viruses, and presently coronavirus disease 2019 (COVID)/H1N1 influenza A form the other common spectrum as causative organisms for CAP. Other organisms such as *Mycobacterium tuberculosis*, influenza, histoplasma, etc., are pathogenic but noncolonizers. Aspiration from colonized upper airway is the most common route of acquisition of CAP. Other modes are inhalation, hematogenous spread, and direct inoculation from infected sites **(Table 1)**.

TABLE 1: Organisms specific to clinical settings.

Factors	*Possible etiological agents*
Alcoholism	*Pneumococcus, Klebsiella* spp., anaerobes, and tuberculosis
Chronic obstructive pulmonary disease and/or smoking	*Haemophilus influenzae, Moraxella catarrhalis, Pneumococcus*
Structural lung disease (e.g., bronchiectasis)	*Pseudomonas aeruginosa, Burkholderia cepacia, Staphylococcus aureus*
Decreased consciousness	Oral anaerobes, gram-negative enteric bacteria
Splenectomy	Encapsulated organisms (*Streptococcus Pneumoniae, H. influenzae*)
Acquired immunodeficiency syndrome (AIDS)	*Pneumocystis jiovecii, S. pneumoniae*
Travel to Southwest United States	Coccidioidomycosis

TREATMENT IN INTENSIVE CARE UNIT

- *Without antipseudomonal cover:* Intravenous (IV) second or third generation cephalosporin with or without macrolide or a fluroquinolone.
- *With antipseudomonal cover: Antipseudomonal* β-lactam such as ceftazidime (CAZ) or cefepime or β-lactam plus β-lactam inhibitor and plus to cover atypical with a macrolide or fluroquinolone.

Duration of treatment depends on severity of illness, associated comorbid conditions, and is usually 7–10 days for *streptococcal* pneumonia and 10–14 days for atypical organisms. Duration of treatment does not depend on the radiological improvement as it may take anywhere from 2 to 6 weeks for improvement, radiologically. Switching from IV to oral will depend upon leukocyte count, hemodynamics, and at least 24 hours of being afebrile. Failure to respond may be due to inadequate coverage, unusual pathogens, complications of pneumonia, and could be a noninfectious illness.

ASPIRATION PNEUMONIA

"Aspiration pneumonia" is acute lung infection that occurs after aspiration of oropharyngeal/nasopharyngeal secretions or upper gastrointestinal (GI) contents in large volumes. The aspirated contents are not acidic enough to induce chemical pneumonitis and capable of inducing lung infections due to their large volume and significant bacterial load followed by bacterial replication, consequence of host response, resultant inflammation, and tissue damage.

It is important to know the etiology of aspiration pneumonia which will be different in patients coming from community and patients who are hospitalized for longer period or have history of prior hospitalization. CAP resulting from less virulent organisms from oral cavity or nasopharynx such as *S. pneumoniae, H. influenzae,* and *Staphylococcus aureus,* whereas hospital-acquired pneumonias (HAPs) are resulting from more virulent organisms like predominantly gram-negative organisms most likely multidrug-resistant (MDR) organisms such as *Klebsiella, Acinetobacter, Pseudomonas* and rarely *Escherichia coli,* and all other above mentioned organisms causing CAP. Bacteria may colonize in oral cavity and nasopharynx of hospitalized patients. Gram-negative MDR organisms such as *Klebsiella, Acinetobacter,* and *Pseudomonas* are emerging in hospitalized patients which are otherwise not seen in healthy individuals coming from community without any history of previous hospitalization. Hospital-acquired organisms will be variable according to the different countries, different hospitals, and in the same hospital those will be different in different intensive care units (ICUs) and different wards.

In aspiration pneumonia, treatment of the causative factor is also important. In cases of aspiration pneumonia due to poor gag reflex, altered sensorium to put nasogastric or nasojejunal feeding tube, to keep the patient nil by mouth (NBM) for time being and feed via Ryle's tube (RT) feeding tube and to feed the patient in propped up position. To reverse the primary cause of aspiration pneumonia such as septic encephalopathy, intoxication, motility disorders, etc., and operative management for surgical causes such as head and neck trauma; removal of mass lesion, etc.

Coverage for anaerobes may be considered when lung abscess or empyema is suspected and it is reasonable when anaerobic infection is suspected on clinical grounds, e.g., a subacute to chronic clinical course, presence of periodontal disease, foul smelling sputum, high quality sputum Gram stain that shows numerous polys and mixed or oral-type flora.

Community-acquired aspiration pneumonia treatment would be IV/oral amoxicillin clavulanic acid or IV ceftriaxone + metronidazole.

NOSOCOMIAL PNEUMONIA

- *Hospital-acquired pneumonia:* Pneumonia not associated with mechanical ventilation not incubating at the time of hospital admission and occurring 48 hours or more after admission.
- *Ventilator-associated pneumonia (VAP):* Pneumonia that develops ≥48 hours of mechanical ventilation.

ETIOLOGIES

Early-onset: <5 days in the hospital, no risk factors for MDR; apart from organisms causing CAP as discussed earlier—*S. pneumoniae, H. influenzae,* enteric gram-negative bacilli, *M. catarrhalis, and S. aureus.*

Late-onset: ≥5 days in the hospital, risk factors for MDR organisms present; apart from organisms causing CAP as discussed earlier—gram-negative bacteria (GNB) and often MDR (common in India). *K. pneumoniae, Acinetobacter baumannii, Pseudomonas aeruginosa, Enterobacter* spp. *and E. coli* in patients who have aspiration. *S. aureus* [often methicillin-resistant *Staphylococcus aureus* (MRSA)]—not very common in India.

Possible role of viruses: One study showed that in nonventilated HAP, polymerase chain reaction (PCR) was positive for respiratory viruses in 22.4% and in VAP 22.5% had respiratory viruses [respiratory syncytial virus (RSV), influenza, or parainfluenza).

TREATMENT

- *Low risk of MDR pathogens:* IV cefepime/piperacillin-tazobactam/meropenem.
- *More severe disease and where MDR risk factors suspected:* IV polymyxin-based therapy alone or in combination, till results awaited.
- *If MDR-GNB suspected:* Drug that should be active against the ICU flora such as for MDR *Klebsiella* spp.—ceftazidime-avibactam + aztreonam (ATM), for *E. coli*—fosfomycin, for *Pseudomonas* spp.—carbapenems, etc.

- If VAP develops after prolonged ICU stay and if the patient has been exposed to polymyxin-based therapy, then consider colistin breakthrough pathogens such as *Elizabethkingia meningoseptica, Serratia marcescens, Stenotrophomonas maltophilia,* or *rarely Burkholderia cepacia.* In such cases, consider adding trimethoprim-sulfamethoxazole (TMP-SMX) or minocycline based therapy.

For relatively susceptible pathogens, treat for 7 days. For suspected GNB multidrug-resistant organism (MDRO) such as *Pseudomonas* spp., *Acinetobacter, Stenotrophomonas; S. aureus* (MRSA)—duration is 10–14 days.

CENTRAL LINE-ASSOCIATED BLOODSTREAM INFECTION

A central line-associated bloodstream infection (CLABSI) occurs when bacteria or other organisms enter from central line into bloodstream. These infections are serious but can often be treated successfully.

ETIOLOGY

In Indian ICU settings, the order of selected organisms causing CLABSI are as follows. Gram-negatives (*Klebsiella, Enterobacter, Pseudomonas, E. coli, Acinetobacter*) according to local flora of respective ICUs followed by gram-positive organisms (coagulase-negative staphylococci, enterococci, and rarely MRSA) followed by *Candida* species, and others like Colistin breakthrough pathogens (*Elizabethkingia; Stenotrophomonas,* etc.).

RISK FACTORS

Host factors that increase the risk of CLABSI are chronic illnesses such as hemodialysis, malignancy, GI disorders, organ transplant, diabetes mellitus, malnutrition, and total parenteral nutrition. Other risks such as extremes of age, loss of skin integrity (burns), and prolonged hospitalization.

Femoral central venous catheters are associated with the highest risk, followed by internal jugular and subclavian catheters causing CLABSI. The catheter type, insertion conditions, catheter care, and operator skill also influence the risk of CLABSI.

Candida is associated with risk factors—Femoral catheterization, total parenteral nutrition (TPN), prolonged administration of broad-spectrum antibiotics, GI surgery, burns, hematologic malignancy, or solid organ or hematopoietic stem-cell transplantation. Certain organisms such as staphylococci, *Pseudomonas,* and *Candida* produce extracellular polysaccharide-biofilm, which increased virulence, adherence to catheter surface, and resistance to antimicrobial therapy.

Indications for removal of hemodialysis access causing CLABSI include the following:

- Persistent symptoms >36 hours or severe sepsis, hemodynamic instability (shock).
- Blood cultures that remain positive >72 hours of appropriate antimicrobial therapy.
- Difficult to clear organisms such as *S. aureus, Pseudomonas,* or fungi.
- Recurrence of uncomplicated CLABSI by nonvirulent organism, when salvaged catheter for difficult access.

If unexplained fever or sepsis persisted in a patient with a short-term central venous or arterial catheter and paired peripheral venipuncture, and catheter blood cultures are sterile, in that case, the catheter should be removed, and the tip should be sent for culture.

All nontunneled catheters causing CLABSI should be removed promptly when clinical suspicion is high. Only for long-term catheters, salvage—systemic therapy coupled with antimicrobial lock can be attempted in limited instances.

TREATMENT

The local prevalence and antimicrobial susceptibility patterns should be considered.

The antibiotic choice for gram-negative coverage should be based on local flora and susceptibility patterns. If the risk of *Pseudomonas* is low, then a third-generation cephalosporin such as ceftriaxone followed by β-lactam/β-lactamase inhibitors (BL/BLIs) combinations are appropriate for extended-spectrum β-lactamases (ESBL) organisms. In patients with a critical illness or high risk for resistant organisms will require empirical combination therapy—carbapenems followed by polymyxins and other novel antimicrobial molecules according to the identification of the organism (it is discussed in detail in later part of the chapter in approach to MDROs).

Parenteral antistaphylococcal penicillin or cephalosporins such as nafcillin or cefazolin in case of coagulase-negative staphylococci (CoNS) or methicillin-sensitive *Staphylococcus aureus* (MSSA). For MRSA vancomycin; If MRSA isolates, exhibit a minimum inhibitory concentration (MIC) of >2 mg/mL for vancomycin or, in the case of vancomycin-resistant *Enterococcus* (VRE), daptomycin is the drug of choice.

For Candidemia empirical IV fluconazole followed by echinocandins (micafungin, caspofungin, and anidulafungin) if azole resistance is suspected as in cases of using prior azole or prevalent nonalbicans *Candida* such as *Candida glabrata* or *Candida krusei.* Antifungal therapy must be considered when there are risk factors for Candidemia as mentioned before.

UROSEPSIS

PYELONEPHRITIS

Patient will have fever, costovertebral tenderness, dysuria, etc. Complicated pyelonephritis will have risk factors such as presence of obstruction, underlying renal disease, male sex, immunosuppression, stone disease, and anatomic or functional urinary tract abnormality.

ETIOLOGY

- Enterobacterales (*E. coli, Klebsiella, Proteus,* etc.)
- Enterococci (elderly patients)
- *Pseudomonas aeruginosa*/other MDROs (patients with prior antibiotics, manipulation of urinary tract)

EVALUATION

- To obtain urine and blood culture prior to therapy.
- To obtain imaging [ultrasonography (USG) or computed tomography (CT)] in critically-ill patients to rule out obstructive uropathy, new renal failure, etc.

TREAMENT

Empirical Treatment

- Low risk for resistant bacteria
  - Ciprofloxacin, levofloxacin for 5–7 days
  - Ceftriaxone for 10 days
  - Transition to oral therapy—fluoroquinolones (FQs)
  - Treatment duration of 5–7 days
- High risk for resistant bacteria (i.e., prior highly-resistant bacteria in urine, recent inpatient healthcare facility stay, obstructive uropathy, recent fluoroquinolone, or β-lactam exposure)
  - Piperacillin-tazobactam, ceftazidime-avibactam, ertapenem
  - Meropenem (critically-ill patient, prior history of *Pseudomonas* infection)
  - Transitioning to oral therapy—TMP-SMX (total 10–14 days), cefixime/amoxicillin and clavulanate (Amox clav) (success rates may be lower with oral β-lactam therapy. Duration is a total of 14 days).
  - Treatment duration of 10–14 days.
    - *Febrile urinary tract infection (UTI) in men:* 14 days treatment is superior than 7 days.
    - In cases of bacteremia 7 days of antibiotic therapy may be as effective as 14 days.

In men to evaluate for benign prostatic hyperplasia (BPH), other causes of obstruction and chronic prostatitis if recurrent UTIs with same organisms.

When considering culture directed therapy: Enterococci are intrinsically resistant to cephalosporins and ertapenem; *Pseudomonas* is intrinsically resistant to Ertapenem.

In cases of MDRO organism causing urosepsis options are polymyxin based regime and other drugs—discussed in detail in approach to MDROs.

ACUTE PROSTATITIS

Acute prostatitis typically presents with fever, chills, malaise, myalgia, dysuria, pelvic/perineal pain, and cloudy urine.

Complications include bacteremia, epididymitis, prostatic abscess, extension, or metastasis to other locations (e.g., joints), and conversion to chronic prostatitis.

ETIOLOGY

- *Age <35 years: Neisseria gonorrhoeae, Chlamydia trachomatis*
- *Age ≥35 years:* Enterobacteriaceae, coliforms, *Enterococcus* spp.

TREATMENT

- *Uncomplicated, with risk of sexually transmitted disease (STD) (age <35 years):* Ceftriaxone or cefixime one dose and then doxycycline for 10 days.
- *Uncomplicated with low risk of STD:* Levofloxacin/ciprofloxacin/TMP-SMX for minimum 10–14 days. In chronic cases duration is for 6 weeks.
- *Chlamydial prostatitis:* Azithromycin for 4 weeks.
- *Resistant Enterobacteriaceae:* Ertapenem/meropenem and for MDRO polymyxin based regime or fosfomycin or ceftazidime + ATM for MDRO *Klebsiella* (for 2–4 weeks).
- *Resistant Pseudomonas:* Imipenem/meropenem for 4 weeks (for MDRO polymyxin based regime).
- FQs and not recommended for gonococcal infections because of significant rates of resistance.
- Antimicrobials with ability to penetrate the prostate, such as FQs in nongonococcal cases or TMP/SMX which has high degree of lipid solubility, low degree of ionization, high dissociation constant, low protein binding, and small molecular size.
- In acquired immunodeficiency syndrome (AIDS) patients think of *Cryptococcus neoformans.*
- Treat as an acute urinary infection for 14 days (may need 4–6 weeks of therapy).

MDROs—APPROACH TO MULTIDRUG-RESISTANT ORGANISMS

Carbapenem-resistant organisms (CRO) comprise carbapenem-resistant Enterobacteriaceae (CRE) and other carbapenem-resistant pathogens such as *Pseudomonas, Acinetobacter*, and colistin breakthrough pathogens such as *S. maltophilia* and *Elizabethkingia meningoseptica*. Therefore, CRO is different from CRE **(Table 2)**.

Enterobacteriaceae are common pathogens causing severe infections which include bloodstream infections (BSIs), CAP, HAP, VAP, UTIs, and intra-abdominal infections (IAIs).

POLYMYXINS

Polymyxin B and polymyxin E (colistin) are polymyxin class parenteral antibiotics, active against CRE, and among CRO *Pseudomonas* and *Acinetobacter*. Colistin has been studied more than polymyxin B and seems to be the preferred choice as colistin was available much before polymyxin B in the Indian market. Colistin and polymyxin B are like peas in a pod, or chalk and cheese? They both have indistinguishable microbiological activity in vitro but polymyxin B is administered as active form whereas colistin is inactive prodrug which gets converted in vivo. Apart from indications for a urosepsis, polymyxin B is preferred over colistin due to faster attainment of target serum levels, relatively less nephrotoxic, much lesser interpatient variability, and no dosage adjustment needed for mild-to-moderate increase in the serum creatinine. As far as efficacy is concerned both are fairly similar. It has a close to near complete sensitivity to the CRE organisms.

Empiric Combination Therapy in Suspected CRE *Klebsiella/E. Coli*

- Polymyxin B or E ± CAZ/avibactam (AVI) ± ATM [depends on oxacillinases β-lactamases (OXA-48) or OXA-48 + New Delhi metallo-β-lactamase (NDM)].
- Polymyxin B or E ± high dose of meropenem.

TABLE 2: According to the genotypic resistance of carbapenem-resistant Enterobacteriaceae (CRE) (phenotypic resistance testing is needed).

Organism	*CRE*		
Genotypic resistance	*NDM*	*OXA-48*	*NDM + OXA-48*
Antibiotics	Polymyxin-based therapy	Ceftazidime/avibactam (CAZ/AVI)	CAZ/AVI + aztreonam (ATM)/polymyxin-based therapy

(NDM: New Delhi metallo-β-lactamase; OXA-48: oxacillinases β-lactamases)

- CAZ/AVI ± High dose tigecycline.
- CAZ/AVI ± fosfomycin.
- Polymyxin B or E ± tigecycline/fosfomycin.

In urosepsis polymyxin B should not be used as it has no penetration in urinary system. Polymyxin E is the recommended drug for UTI but as it is nephrotoxic it will require creatinine monitoring, it causes hypokalemia, hence will require serum potassium monitoring.

CARBAPENEMS

Some CPE are even susceptible to carbapenems and this is observed in OXA-48-producing Enterobacteriaceae. Carbapenems work in CRE infections, particularly when used with lower MICs either in higher doses, in combination with other active anti-CRE agents. The strategy of high-dose (2 g q8h) carbapenem with prolonged infusion (over 3 hours) was also found to be associated with better outcomes in carbapenem-producing *K. pneumoniae* infections.

CEFTAZIDIME/AVIBACTAM (CAZ/AVI)

Ceftazidime/avibactam is a novel β-lactam/β-lactamase inhibitor combination approved for the treatment of complicated intra-abdominal infections cIAIs, complicated urinary tract infections (cUTIs), HAP, and VAP. Unlike most β-lactamase inhibitors, AVI is not a β-lactam. AVI is a new synthetic non-β-lactam (diazabicyclooctane)/β-lactamase inhibitor that inhibits a wide range of β-lactamases but does not cover all CRE isolates. The addition of AVI restores CAZ activity against various Enterobacteriaceae and *P. aeruginosa*, therefore expanding the activity spectrum of CAZ to MDR gram-negative bacteria. Nowadays, the emergence of CAZ/AVI-resistant strains has been reported. It has a major role to play against *Klebsiella* producing OXA-48 which is an excellent colistin sparer. Studies have shown equal efficacy of CAZ AVI versus colistin rather lesser morbidity and mortality considering the safety profile of CAZ. Most important to check the phenotypic sensitivity of CAZ. It does not act against metallo-β-lactamase (MBL).

CEFTAZIDIME/AVIBACTAM + AZTREONAM (CAZ + ATM)

The monobactam antibiotic ATM is stable against MBLs but is hydrolyzed by many other β-lactamases (ESBL, AmpC, and cephalosporinases) frequently coproduced by the MBL producing strains. Actually, it is ATM + AVI, rather than CAZ + AVI. We have to use CAZ in view of AVI is not available alone or ATM + AVI not available as one drug. It has good activity against NDM + OXA-48 producing *Klebsiella* but does not hold true for *E. coli* due to penicillin-binding protein (PBP)-3. It is most important to check for phenotypic sensitivity of this molecule. The combination of CAZ/AVI and ATM has been proposed as a potential therapeutic strategy against infections caused by MBL-producing bacteria.

HIGH-DOSE TIGECYCLINE

It is non-nephrotoxic compared to other potentially active antimicrobial agents for CRE, such as polymyxins and aminoglycosides. A high-dose tigecycline regimen consists of a 200 mg loading and a maintenance dose of 100 mg q12h, while a standard-dose tigecycline regimen consists of a loading dose of 100 mg and a maintenance dose of 50 mg q12h. High-dose tigecycline can be considered for bacteremia. Tigecycline is not good in bacteremia but very good for GI tract as it has very good tissue penetration. Tigecycline will require liver function monitoring.

FOSFOMYCIN

Fosfomycin is a phosphoenolpyruvate analog. It has bactericidal activity; it will inhibit one of the first steps in peptidoglycan synthesis. It is active against a wide range of gram-negative organisms, in particular *E. coli*. It has been used as an oral formulation for the treatment of uncomplicated UTIs for many years. Fosfomycin is active against the majority of CRE organisms and carbapenem-resistant *Pseudomonas* but not those of *Acinetobacter* or *Stenotrophomonas*. Monitoring of serum potassium and sodium is important as fosfomycin's side effects are hypernatremia and hypokalemia. In cases of fluid overload fosfomycin cannot be used as it causes fluid retention. Fosfomycin has good penetration in urinary, bone and joint, and central nervous system, hence can be considered in urosepsis, bone and joint infections, and central nervous system (CNS) infections.

CARBAPENEMASE-RESISTANT *PSEUDOMONAS*

Pseudomonas is one of the organism which has variable susceptibility due to multiple mechanisms of resistance, hence we have to follow according to the sensitivity. Options are as follows:

- Polymyxin-based therapy ± meropenem/doripenem (1 g q8h).
- If not detected with NDM then ceftolozane/tazobactam may work.
- ATM/aminoglycoside if susceptible is a very good option.

CARBAPENEMASE-RESISTANT *ACINETOBACTER*

- Polymyxin-based therapy ± tigecycline/minocycline (depending on susceptibility).
- Polymyxin-based therapy ± meropenem/imipenem.
- Polymyxin-based therapy ± sulbactam (dose is 6–8 g of sulbactam).

- In cases of pan-resistant *Acinetobacter* triple drug therapy is used—polymyxin-based therapy + ampicillin – sulbactam + carbapenems.

COLISTIN BREAKTHROUGH AND CARBAPENEM-RESISTANT PATHOGENS

- *Elizabethkingia meningoseptica:* Minocyclin or TMP-SMX. Glycopeptide such as vancomycin, linezolid drugs for gram-positive have activity against *Elizabethkingia.*
- *Stenotrophomonas maltophilia:* Options are minocycline, TMP-SMX, tigecycline, cefiderocol, ceftazidime-avibactam + ATM.

NOVEL ANTIMICROBIAL MOLECULES

Meropenem/Vaborbactam

The combination is approved for the treatment of complicated UTIs caused by *E. coli, K. pneumoniae, E. cloacae,* and other susceptible organisms. It does not increase the activity of meropenem against *A. baumannii, P. aeruginosa, or S. maltophilia.* Vaborbactam protects meropenem from degradation by extended-spectrum β-lactamases and serine carbapenemases (except class D OXA-enzymes).

Imipenem/Cilastatin/Relebactam

The food and drug administration (FDA) has approved imipenem/cilastatin/relebactam for three indications:

- HAP or VAP caused by *Acinetobacter calcoaceticus-baumannii, Enterobacter* cloacae, *E. coli, H. influenzae, Klebsiella* spp., *P. aeruginosa,* and *S. marcescens.*
- cUTI caused by *E. cloacae, E. coli, Klebsiella* spp., and *P. aeruginosa.*
- cIAI caused by *Bacteroides* spp., *Citrobacter freundii, E. cloacae, E. coli, Fusobacterium nucleatum, Klebsiella* spp., *Parabacteroides distasonis, P. aeruginosa.*

Cefepime Zidebactam

The combination theoretically works against class A, C, and D β-lactamase. Enterobacteriaceae with additional in vitro restored function to some group B β-lactamase Enterobacteriaceae, drug-resistant *Pseudomonas,* and drug-resistant *Acinetobacter.*

Plazomicin

It was approved in June 2018 by the FDA for the treatment of adults with cUTI. It has broad-spectrum activity against gram-positive cocci and gram-negative bacilli, including ESBL producers and CRE. It will not act against NDM.

Eravacycline

It has broad-spectrum antimicrobial activity against gram-positive, gram-negative, and anaerobic bacteria, except *Pseudomonas.* That was approved by the FDA in August 2018 for the treatment of cIAIs. Of note, eravacycline is not indicated for the treatment of cUTI as clinical trials have not demonstrated the efficacy for a clinical cure and microbiological success for UTI. Eravacycline has been shown to have effective in vitro against MDR pathogens with two-fold higher activity than tigecycline against CRE. It will not work against NDM.

Cefiderocol

Cefiderocol, a novel siderophore cephalosporin which has potent in vitro and in vivo activity against a variety of gram-negative bacteria, including CRE. It will work in NDM but no clinical experience in India. FDA has approved it for the treatment of UTI caused by *E. coli, Klebsiella, Proteus mirabilis, Pseudomonas,* and *E. cloacae* complex. Hospital-acquired and VAP caused by *Acinetobacter, E. coli, E. cloacae* complex, *Klebsiella, Pseudomonas,* and *Serratia.* It is not active against gram-positive and anaerobic bacteria.

Ceftolozane-Tazobactam

The combination of ceftolozane with tazobactam further improves its antipseudomonal activity and also imparts activity against strains producing ESBLs (but not any carbapenemases). It is not active against CRO *Acinetobacter,* or *Stenotrophomonas.*

Aztreonam/Avibactam

Aztreonam is an old β-lactam antibiotic, which is not hydrolyzed by MBLs. However, since many MBL producing organism strains coproduce enzymes (e.g., AmpC, ESBL) that can hydrolyze ATM, hence β-lactamase inhibitor such as AVI could be given as combination drug and the combination of ATM/AVI works against MBL producing CRE and *Pseudomonas.*

SUMMARY

Patients getting admitted in the ICU can present with different clinical syndromes such as pneumonia, urosepsis, abdominal infections, etc. Some patients get admitted with other conditions like neurological or surgical problems, etc. and can have longer ICU stay hence can developed multidrug-resistant organism infections. It is very important to know the clinical syndrome while treating and to differentiate whether the infection is community acquired or hospital acquired. Approach to start empirical antibiotics will depend on many factors like community/hospital acquired infection; site of the infection, pharmacokinetics and dynamics of the antimicrobials, etc. Community-acquired infection we would think of less resistant organisms and can spare higher class of antibiotics like carbapenems and polymyxins. Here we have mainly focused on important clinical syndromes such as pneumonia, urosepsis, line related infections and MDRO infections in various conditions due to various reasons and brief on future antimicrobials for difficult to treat gram negative infections.

SUGGESTED READING

1. Bennett JE, Dolin R, Blaser MJ. Mandell, Douglas, and Bennett's principles and practice of infectious diseases E-book, 9th edition. Amsterdam: Elsevier Health Sciences; 2019.
2. Doi Y. Treatment options for carbapenem-resistant gram-negative bacterial infections. Clin Infect Dis. 2019;69(Suppl_7):S565-75.
3. Ekren PK, Ranzani OT, Ceccato A, Li Bassi G, Muñoz Conejero E, Ferrer M, et al. Evaluation of the 2016 Infectious Diseases Society of America/American Thoracic Society guideline criteria for risk of multidrug-resistant pathogens in patients with hospital-acquired and ventilator-associated pneumonia in the ICU. Am J Respir Crit Care Med. 2018;197(6):826-30.
4. Enne VI, Personne Y, Grgic L, Gant V, Zumla A. Aetiology of hospital-acquired pneumonia and trends in antimicrobial resistance. Current opinion in pulmonary medicine. 2014;20(3):252-8.
5. Gupta K, Hooton TM, Naber KG, Wullt B, Colgan R, Miller LG, et al. Infectious Diseases Society of America; European Society for Microbiology and Infectious Diseases. International clinical practice guidelines for the treatment of acute uncomplicated cystitis and pyelonephritis in women: A 2010 update by the Infectious Diseases Society of America and the European Society for Microbiology and Infectious Diseases. Clin Infect Dis. 2011;52(5):e103-20.
6. Haddadin Y, Annamaraju P, Regunath H. Central Line–Associated Bloodstream Infections. Treasure Island (FL): StatPearls Publishing; 2024.
7. Hooton TM. Clinical practice. Uncomplicated urinary tract infection. N Engl J Med. 2012;366(11):1028-37.
8. Kalil AC, Metersky ML, Klompas M, Muscedere J, Sweeney DA, Palmer LB, et al. Management of adults with hospital-acquired and ventilator-associated pneumonia: 2016 clinical practice guidelines by the Infectious Diseases Society of America and the American Thoracic Society. Clin Infect Dis. 2016;63(5):e61-111.
9. Lipsky BA, Byren I, Hoey CT. Treatment of bacterial prostatitis. Clin Infect Dis. 2010;50(12):1641-52.
10. Nagvekar V, Shah A, Unadkat VP, Chavan A, Kohli R, Hodgar S, et al. Clinical Outcome of Patients on Ceftazidime–Avibactam and Combination Therapy in Carbapenem-resistant Enterobacteriaceae. Indian J Crit Care Med. 2021;25(7):780.
11. Rees J, Abrahams M, Doble A, Cooper A; Prostatitis Expert Reference Group (PERG). Diagnosis and treatment of chronic bacterial prostatitis and chronic prostatitis/chronic pelvic pain syndrome: a consensus guideline. BJU Int. 2015;116(4):509-25.
12. Sandford JP. Guide to antimicrobial therapy: 1994. Dallas: Antimicrobial therapy; 1994.
13. Sheu CC, Chang YT, Lin SY, Chen YH, Hsueh PR. Infections caused by carbapenem-resistant Enterobacteriaceae: an update on therapeutic options. Front Microbiol. 2019;10:80.
14. Soman R, Veeraraghavan B, Hegde A, Jiandani P, Mehta Y, Nagavekar V, et al. Indian consensus on the management of CRE infection in critically ill patients (ICONIC)—India. Expert Rev Anti Infect Ther. 2019;17(8):647-60.

SECTION

10 Nutrition

CHAPTER

37

Nutrition Practice for a Low Resource Unit

Eileen Canday, Vedika Premani

INTRODUCTION

Nutritional support is one of the essential components of a critical care setting. Its aim is to attenuate the detrimental effects of critical illness on the nutritional status. It favorably influences outcomes and prevent or reverse malnutrition. The general goals of nutritional care in all patients, including those with respiratory disorders and critical illness, are to provide adequate nutrition to support metabolic demands, to preserve lean body mass, and to prevent muscle wasting.

NUTRITION CARE PROCESS IN A CRITICAL CARE UNIT

The nutrition care process is composed of the following: Nutrition assessment and reassessment, nutrition diagnosis, nutrition intervention, nutrition monitoring and evaluation.

Nutrition Assessment

In order to have a uniform and accurate nutrition assessment, the dietician uses validated tools such as nutrition risk score (NRS, 2002) and subjective global assessment (SGA). These tools include various parameters such as the following:

- *Medical history:* Age, comorbidities, and loss of physical function.
- *Nutrition history:* Weight loss, reduced food intake, loss of appetite, and food allergies.
- *Physical examination:* Height, weight, body mass index (BMI), edema, and body composition.
- *Severity of disease:* Critically-ill patients are severely ill by definition.

A unit that does not have a qualified dietician, the nurse or the doctor may perform the nutrition screening, which will give an understanding of the nutritional status of the patient. This screening includes parameters such as weight loss, appetite loss, height, and weight.

When the patient cannot consume orally due to swallowing difficulty, unconsciousness, or loss of appetite; then enteral nutrition (EN) support is considered to be started within 48 hours of admission if hemodynamically stable. The decision to initiate parenteral nutrition (PN) is influenced by the patient's nutritional risk, clinical diagnosis and condition, gastrointestinal tract function, and duration of anticipated need.

Nutrition Intervention

The dietician usually calculates *energy targets* for the day by multiplying 24–30 kcal by the current body weight as per American College of Chest Physicians (ACCP) recommendations; similarly, *protein target* for the day by multiplying 1.0–2 g by the current body weight.

In a set up that has an in-house kitchen, blenderized feeds can by prepared, for set up which do not have a kitchen, a family member can prepare the feeds at home **(Table 1)**.

The foods that can be included in pureed forms, such as:

- *Carbohydrate rich foods:* Rice, ground chapatti, sprouted ragi atta
- *Protein rich foods:* Sattu powder, dal, roasted soya atta
- *Fats:* Peanut powder, sesame seed powder, sunflower, mustard oil, or locally available seeds
- *Micronutrients:* Fruits and vegetables such as papaya, guava, chickoo, carrots, beans, spinach, potato.

Feed Preparation Instructions for 100 mL of Feed

Ragi flour feed: Roast 1 tablespoon (tbsp) ragi/soya flour, slowly add 100 mL of whole milk and stir continuously for 3 minutes, cool and use for tube feeds.

TABLE 1: Sample low resource kitchen feeds.

Standard tube feeds	
Volume	***Feed components***
150	Milk or its substitutes + water + 1 tablespoon (tbsp) sesame seeds
150	One-third cup cooked rice puree + one-third cup moong dal puree + 1 tbsp roasted sesame seeds
150	Peanut powder feed with milk or one scrambled egg blended with 70 mL milk
150	One-third cup cooked rice + one-third cup curd + 2 tbsp oil + 1 g salt
150	2 tbsp powdered chapatti + one-third cup moong dal + 1 tbsp oil + 1 g salt
150	50 g of vegetable puree (carrots, beans, spinach, and potato) + 1 tbsp oil +1 g salt
150	Ragi or soya flour feed with 50 g fruit pulp (papaya, chickoo)
150	One-third cup cooked rice puree + one-third cup moong dal + 2 tbsp oil + 1 g salt
150	Soya flour feed
150	Milk or 2 tbsp sattu powder + water

Peanut powder feed: Blend 1 tbsp of roasted peanut powder + 2 tbsp milk powder with 100 mL of whole milk.

Tube Feed Instructions

Tube hygiene: Enteral feeding is an ideal environment for bacterial growth. Thus, hygiene is crucial to avoid contamination to the food and infection which could lead to diarrhea.

Thorough hand wash is necessary before contacting the tube, liquid food, or medication. It is also important to clean the skin around the nose with an aseptic cloth before and after each feed.

- All feeds should be strained before administration.
- Make use of measuring glass and spoons for accuracy.
- Always use boiled water for the preparation of the feeds and for flushing the tube.
- Feeds should be administered at room temperature, i.e., neither hot nor cold.
- Refrigerated feeds should be thawed and reheated before administration.
- All feed should be administered at 45° (propped up position).
- Flushing the tube with water after every feed is must.
- Wash the syringe with lukewarm water before and after administration of the feed.

Specific Feeds and Formulations

For patients who can afford to purchase ready to make formulations, dieticians can choose from the following based on the condition.

Specific feeds and formulations can be planned based on nutrition assessment and needs, physical assessment, gastrointestinal (GI) function considerations, overall medical condition including clinical history and metabolic abnormalities, and goals/outcomes for the patient.

- *Polymeric formulas:* Intact nutrients (e.g., whey protein).
- *Semielemental formula*: Partially hydrolyzed; used for individuals with dysfunction in the GI tract preventing standard enteral formulas to be digested or tolerated (e.g., whey peptides).
- *Elemental formula:* Fully hydrolyzed; used only for individuals who cannot tolerate semielemental formula [e.g., branched chain amino acids (BCAA)].
- *Disease-specific enteral formula:* Specialty formulas are available for medical conditions including diabetes, chronic obstructive pulmonary disease (COPD), acute respiratory distress syndrome (ARDS), wound healing, chronic kidney disease (on and off dialysis), liver failure, and compromised immune system. These products have varying differences in macronutrient and micronutrient content based on specific disease states (e.g., very high protein for wound healing).

- *Pharmacologic needs* such as immune modulation are covered in specialty EN products containing arginine, glutamine, dietary nucleotides, and ω-3 fatty acids.

Fluid and Electrolytes

Daily input and output of fluid should be closely monitored. Sodium and potassium should be prescribed depending on various factors such as their serum electrolyte levels, fluid retention, and renal function. If potassium is low, feeds like coconut water, fruit juices, and soups can be planned. If sodium is low then additional amount of salt can be added in the feeds, whereas if sodium is high then fluid restriction can be considered if coordination with the intensivists.

Nutrition Monitoring

Feeds need to be monitored daily by the healthcare personnel to check for diarrhea or constipation.

When a patient has persistent diarrhea, soluble fibers can be considered. This includes guar gum, wheat dextrin, inulin, or fructooligosaccharides, which do not gelatinize when dissolved and do not block the feeding tube.

When patient is having constipation, insoluble fiber rich sources such as psyllium husk should be considered. However, it is important to note that higher amount of water is required for its dissolution and should be administered immediately since it gelatinizes rapidly.

When diarrhea persists or if a patient has not been fed for >10 days, then trophic feeds can also be considered to prevent refeeding syndrome. Trophic feeding is a small volume of balanced EN insufficient for the patient's nutritional needs but producing some positive GI or systemic benefit.

Refeeding syndrome is a potentially fatal condition, caused by rapid initiation of feeding after a period of undernutrition. It is characterized by hypophosphatemia, associated with fluid and electrolyte shifts and metabolic and clinical complications. Awareness of refeeding syndrome and identification of patients at risk is crucial as the condition is preventable and the metabolic complications are avoidable. Patients at high risk include chronically undernourished patients and those who have had little or no energy intake for >10 days. Feeding should be started at a low level of energy replacement with a caloric intake restriction of 1,000 kcals in 48 hours (i.e., at 500 kcal per day) can be recommended. Once feeding is initiated, vitamin supplementation should also be started and continued for at least 10 days. As common risk factors fail to identify refeeding syndrome patients, regular phosphate and other electrolyte monitoring can be recommended at least once daily, in particular during the first 72 hours after the initiation of nutritional support.

SUMMARY

All the critically-ill patients should undergo nutrition assessment at the time of admission.

Observation of signs of malnutrition (e.g., cachexia, edema, muscle atrophy, BMI <20 kg/m^2) is critical. The EN should be started early, preferably within first 24–48 hours.

In case the nutrition requirement is not met adequately with EN even after 7 days of intensive care unit (ICU) admission, then usage of PN may be considered.

Nutritional support should be considered as of therapeutic benefits and not just supportive or adjunctive. Electrolytes should be strictly monitored in the patient on nutrition therapy.

Tube feeding to be considered if even 50–60% of nutrition targets are not met adequately within 72 hours of oral nutrition support.

SUGGESTED READING

1. Hill A, Elke G, Weimann A. Nutrition in the intensive care unit-A narrative review. Nutrients. 2021;13(8):2851.
2. Kolaček S. Enteral nutrition. World Rev Nutr Diet. 2013;108:86-90.
3. Lambell KJ, Tatucu-Babet OA, Chapple LA, Gantner D, Ridley EJ. Nutrition therapy in critical illness: a review of the literature for clinicians. Crit Care. 2020;24(1):35.
4. Lee JW. Fluid and electrolyte disturbances in critically ill patients. Electrolyte Blood Press. 2010;8(2):72-81.
5. Mehanna HM, Moledina J, Travis J. Refeeding syndrome: what it is, and how to prevent and treat it. BMJ. 2008;336(7659):1495-8.
6. Preiser JC, Arabi YM, Berger MM, Casaer M, McClave S, Montejo-González JC, et al. A guide to enteral nutrition in intensive care units: 10 expert tips for the daily practice. Crit Care. 2021;25(1):424.
7. Ridley EJ, Peake SL. Intermittent enteral nutrition as a sole intervention has no impact on muscle wasting in critical illness. Chest. 2020;158(1):183-94.
8. Singer P, Blaser AR, Berger MM, Alhazzani W, Calder PC, Casaer MP, et al. ESPEN guideline on clinical nutrition in the intensive care unit. Clinical Nutrition. 2019;38:48-79.

Index

Page numbers followed by *b* refer to box, *f* refer to figure, *fc* refer to flowchart, and *t* refer to table.

B

D

N

Q

R

T